# A SHARP BRAIN FOR LIFE

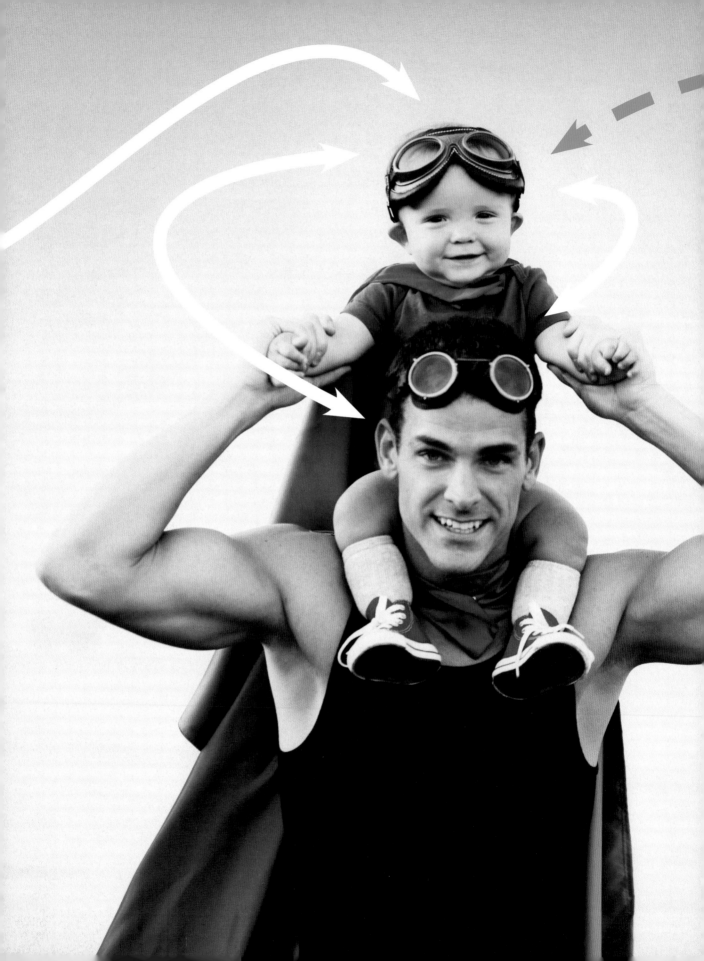

# A SHARP BRAIN FOR LIFE

## Proven ways to maintain your mind & memories

Published by The Reader's Digest Association, Inc.
London • New York • Sydney • Montreal

# CONTENTS

## Consultants

**Professor Robert Logie** PhD FRSE FBPsS FRSA
*Centre for Cognitive Ageing and Cognitive Epidemiology,*
*University of Edinburgh*

**Sheena Meredith** MB BS MPhil

**Fiona Hunter** BSc Nutrition Dip Dietetics

## Part 4 · Your brain fitness programme

## Part 5 · Resources

### Note to readers
While the creators of this work have made every
effort to be as accurate and up to date as possible, medical and
pharmacological knowledge is constantly changing. Readers are
recommended to consult a qualified medical specialist for individual advice.
The writers, researchers, editors and publishers of this work cannot be held
liable for any errors and omissions, or actions that may be taken as a
consequence of information contained within this work.

# Yes, you can CHANGE YOUR BRAIN

**Congratulations! This is an extraordinary time to be alive.** Modern medicine has developed cures and treatments for many of the health conditions that once felled us in our prime, giving us the most valuable gift of all: more years.

Wonderful indeed – but what kind of gift is extra longevity if our minds wear out before our bodies do? After all, the brain contains everything that makes us 'us': not only every talent and skill but also the records of all our experiences, our hopes and dreams, the jokes and friendships and births and achievements that give our lives purpose and meaning.

It's no wonder, then, that with every little 'brain hiccup' – forgetting a name, losing our car or house keys (again), a sudden losing streak in our regular bridge or whist game – we see our very lives slipping away. In fact, many people fear losing their memories more than they fear death itself.

The good news is that although the brain does shrink a little with age, its remaining capacity is still pretty large. This book was put together in consultation with some of the world's pre-eminent neurologists and psychologists, using hundreds of medical journal articles, and the message is positive.

It turns out that even with age most brains still retain the capability to learn and can continue to add new stores of information. Plus, a wealth of techniques have been discovered that can help you to make the maximum use of your mental abilities – you can effectively train your brain and improve the efficiency of your memory, whatever your age.

## AGE AND EXPERIENCE

Another piece of good news: the common saying 'You can't teach an old dog new tricks' isn't true. Although ageing may have some effect on memory and learning capacity, the experience and knowledge store that age brings can compensate for much of this.

What's more, taking heed of the information in this book, including the memory-improvement techniques, can help to preserve your mental functions into old age. And any slips can often be countered quite easily, for example, using aids such as diaries, Post-it notes or electronic reminders.

### EXPANDING OUR INTERESTS

As we age and our mental filing cabinets become packed full with the record of lives well-lived, the brain makes more complex associations between ideas and puts new learning in the context of a vast reservoir of experience. What this means is that it becomes easier to take in new information about topics of which we have some knowledge or experience. So someone who takes up stamp collecting as a hobby will gain more and more knowledge about stamp collecting and will find it easier to add to that knowledge.

The same is true of any area of interest, whether it is a hobby or a profession – football, rock music, playing bridge, choral singing, politics, birdwatching, medicine, psychology, astrophysics or television soap operas. And as well as helping to maintain your mental abilities, pursuing a serious new interest will make life more stimulating.

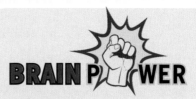

### BRAIN POWER

There are more potential connections between the cells in a single brain than atoms in the entire universe. The brain has about 100 billion neurons (nerve cells), and each neuron has up to 1,000 'docking points' where it can connect with others. If all of these potential connections were made, there would be 100 thousand billion information-exchanging links. In practice, of course, only a tiny fraction of these connections are ever established.

## TWO BREAKTHROUGHS THAT CHANGED THINGS

The brain, once a mysterious 'black box' that scientists couldn't decode, is finally revealing some of its biggest secrets, and the news offers huge promise to anyone who's ever wondered, 'Am I losing it?' High on the list are two major findings:

### WE DO GROW NEW BRAIN CELLS

Who doesn't remember knocking back a drink in their youth and joking to a friend, 'Well, there goes another thousand brain cells'? Many of us still believe that we start life with billions of brain cells, then slowly lose them with time (and alcohol). That we'll have fewer brain cells by our twenties and thirties, and by middle age, well, heaven help us. But, in fact, in a remarkable discovery, scientists have learned that the brain generates new cells every day, in a process called neurogenesis.

*Continued on page 12*

# QUIZ HOW SHARP IS YOUR BRAIN?

Read each statement below. If it sounds like something you would be likely to say or that generally describes your experience, tick 'True'. If it does not describe your experience, tick 'False'. Before you begin, try to remember these three words: tree, basin, dinner.

**1** My friends and/or colleagues joke about my forgetfulness.

☐ True ☐ False

**2** If I'm introduced to someone, the chances are I won't remember his or her name an hour later.

☐ True ☐ False

**3** When I'm having a casual conversation, I often find myself struggling to think of the right word.

☐ True ☐ False

**4** When reading a book or long magazine article, I regularly have to go back and reread passages because my attention wanders.

☐ True ☐ False

**5** It is not unusual for me to say, 'Could you repeat that more slowly?'

☐ True ☐ False

**6** I sometimes worry about my memory.

☐ True ☐ False

**7** My memory isn't bad; it might just take me a little longer to think things through.

☐ True ☐ False

**8** I often misplace items I use every day (keys, pens, mobile phone, shopping list).

☐ True ☐ False

**9** I don't trust myself to do even simple maths without a calculator any more.

☐ True ☐ False

**10** I find it very difficult to add numbers in my head.

☐ True ☐ False

**11** I couldn't function without a calendar or written schedule – I need something to remind me of important dates and appointments.

☐ True ☐ False

**12** I have a lot of stress in my life.

☐ True ☐ False

**13** It is not unusual for me to say, 'What were we talking about again?'

☐ True ☐ False

**14** More than once a week, I forget why I went into a particular room or cupboard.

☐ True ☐ False

**15** I do better if I focus on a single thing at a time – I don't like multi-tasking.

☐ True ☐ False

**16** I don't like adding new electronics to the house – I've barely learned (or didn't learn) how to work the DVD player.

☐ True ☐ False

**17** It feels as though the world is running at a much faster pace than I am – people seem to be constantly waiting for me.

☐ True ☐ False

**18** It is difficult for me to hold more than three numbers in my mind.

☐ True ☐ False

**19** My abilities in games of skill and strategy (for example, bridge or chess) would be better if my memory were better.

☐ True ☐ False

**20** I routinely take more than three prescription medicines per day.

☐ True ☐ False

**21** I have been diagnosed with Type 2 diabetes, depression or heart disease.

☐ True ☐ False

**22** I smoke.

☐ True ☐ False

**23** I quit smoking less than 20 years ago.

☐ True ☐ False

**24** I can't seem to find enough time to exercise – twice a week is a lot for me.

☐ True ☐ False

**25** I have a sweet tooth and eat sweets, cakes or desserts almost every day.

☐ True ☐ False

**26** I often get lost, probably because of my poor sense of direction.

☐ True ☐ False

**27** Thank heavens for speed-dial; I just can't seem to remember phone numbers any more.

☐ True ☐ False

**28** People often tell me that I've already told them the same story or joke before.

☐ True ☐ False

**29** When I go to the shops to get groceries or other items, I almost always forget something and have to go back.

☐ True ☐ False

**30** It feels as though I go through life with the notion that a name or fact is 'on the tip of my tongue'.

☐ True ☐ False

**31** I know what I want to do; I just have a difficult time working out how to accomplish my goals.

☐ True ☐ False

**32** Organisation is not a strong point for me.

☐ True ☐ False

**33** I often find it difficult to persuade people of my opinion, or to make a reasoned argument against someone else's opinion – my thoughts simply don't come out as organised as I want them to be.

☐ True ☐ False

**34** I frequently 'get lost' while I'm watching a film or reading a book – plots seem to be much more complicated these days.

☐ True ☐ False

# HOW SHARP IS YOUR BRAIN? Scoring

**1** **Do you remember the three words you were asked to note at the beginning of this quiz?** *(No peeking!)*

1 ...........................    2 ...........................    3 ...........................

Give yourself one memory point for each word you missed. If you got them all, your score for this question is zero.

*My memory points: ............*

**2** **Count the number of True responses for questions 1 to 34. Add this number to your memory points. This is your general** *Sharp Brain* **score.**

*My general Sharp Brain score: ............*

**If your score is 0:** Are you sure you answered all of the questions honestly? Everyone has mental blocks from time to time, regardless of age or mental capacity. Perhaps you should have another go at the quiz?

**If your score is 1 to 10:** Now is the perfect time to begin taking care of your brain – before forgetfulness and fuzzy thinking become a problem in your life.

**If your score is 11 to 20:** Your minor memory problems probably pop up as little surprises in your daily life. You can benefit from brain training, and from the lifestyle changes outlined in Part 2 and Part 3.

**If your score is 21 to 37:** You probably feel as though your brain is betraying you. It is possible to reduce or eliminate many of your memory problems with the exercises in this book, along with the lifestyle changes discussed in Part 2 and Part 3.

**Note:** If you get a very high score and find memory problems interfering with your life, it might be a good idea to ask your GP to check if you have an underlying problem that could be resolved.

● **ATTENTION AND FOCUS**
● **MEMORY**
● **PROCESSING SPEED**
● **VERBAL SKILLS**
● **NUMBER SKILLS**
● **REASONING SKILLS**
● **LIFESTYLE/HEALTH ISSUES**

## A clue to the colours

This quiz taps into six main facets of cognition: attention and focus, general memory, mental processing speed, verbal skills, number skills and reasoning skills. It also looks at some lifestyle habits that affect the brain. Keep your answer to each question handy; you'll look back at this quiz when you get to *Your Brain Fitness Programme* in Part 4. There you'll discover how to use the colour coding of the questions to learn more about your particular areas of strength and weakness.

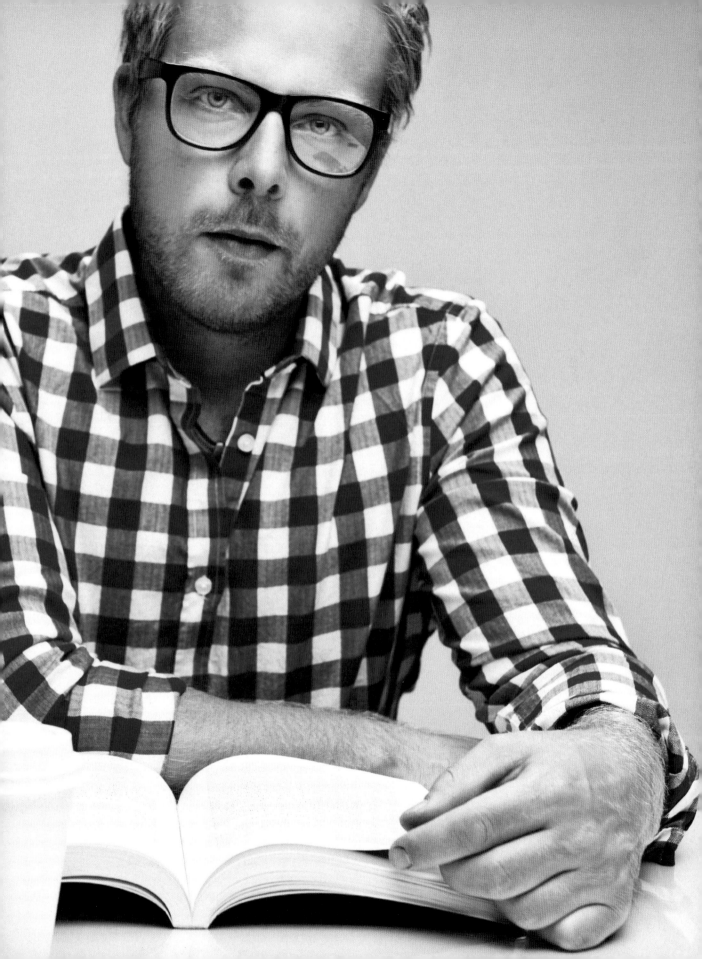

# IT'S RUBBISH!

Don't believe these three common brain myths.

**MYTH 1 Our ability to remember declines with age.**
**THE TRUTH** The older brain loses some agility, but still has plenty of storage capacity. Remembering a complicated set of directions or a long list of words will require more time and repetition. But if we put in the effort, we'll retain the information just as well as, if not better than, a younger person.

**MYTH 2 Memories are precise photocopies of information or events.**
**THE TRUTH** Memories are not stored. They are interpretations of events, reconstructed every time we call one up. They live in complex networks of nerve-cell pathways throughout the brain, which contain fragments of events and a lifetime of accumulated knowledge. Each reconstruction is a mixture of what actually happened and our brain 'filling in the gaps' based on 'what must have happened' from accumulated knowledge, so most recollections are not completely accurate.

When we commit something to memory, we are 'laying tracks' along a memory trail. Just like a woodland path, the more we walk down it, the more firmly established it becomes. However, we lose details of any one specific journey along the path, just as if, say, we go to the same restaurant many times. We may remember what usually happens there, but tend to forget details of individual visits.

**MYTH 3 Our brains are less sharp from our forties or fifties onwards.**
**THE TRUTH** Mental agility actually begins to slip from around the age of 24 for some skills, while others seem to get better in early adulthood, before starting to decline in middle age. The older we are, the harder we need to work to keep our brains functioning efficiently, but if we find ways to compensate by gaining expert knowledge and experience, or learning useful techniques, then our brains can outstrip even those of younger people.

What really happens is that most new brain cell growth continues until early adulthood, around the age of 18 to 20. Thereafter, new brain cells do grow, but more die off than are replaced, so there is a small and gradual but progressive overall loss of brain cells throughout the rest of adulthood.

The crucial point to bear in mind is that it's not the number of cells but the connections between them that count. Whenever you learn new things, you create new connections between the cells and thus increase the capacity of your brain. The activities outlined in *A Sharp Brain for Life* could even help to speed up that process.

## THE MORE YOU USE YOUR BRAIN, THE GREATER ITS CAPACITY

The second major new finding is equally encouraging. We used to think of the brain as if it were a fixed electric power grid, like the many that send electricity to our cities. When the system gets old or overloaded, the power decreases, which leads to, for example, flickering lights and dead appliances. We believed that age wore down memory and comprehension in a similar way and there was nothing we or anyone else could do about it.

Today, we know that the brain can continue to adapt and expand its capacity as needed. Not only does it generate new brain cells but it also creates new connections between those cells in the form of intricate nerve fibres called dendrites. The more connections in your brain, the faster and better you think. The advice, strategies and exercises in *A Sharp Brain for Life* are designed specifically to help you to expand your brain's power grid.

# USE IT OR LOSE IT

Whether you're balancing your accounts, learning salsa or playing gin rummy, your brain's 'electricity grid' lights up like Oxford Street at Christmas. Chemical messages zip along at speeds of up to several hundred miles per hour from one nerve cell to the next along 'cables' called axons. Waiting to receive all that information are the nerve cell 'branches' mentioned earlier, called dendrites. And guess what? You play the most important role in keeping this network humming.

'Learning new skills and new knowledge increases the number of connections in the brain, and the more connections there are, the more efficient the brain will be,' says Robert Logie, professor of human cognitive neuroscience at Edinburgh University. Forcing our brains to learn something new causes them to sprout more and more dendrites, expanding our capacity to think, decide, learn and remember.

On the other hand, being mentally lazy – getting stuck in a rut, never trying anything new – has the opposite effect. The brain, in constant clean-up mode, allows unused neurons to die and 'prunes' under-employed dendrites, just as a gardener prunes dying branches on a tree.

## RICH REWARDS

Keeping our brains in tip-top shape may even protect against the decline in mental functioning that tends to occur with age. Many studies have shown that higher levels of leisure-related mental, physical and social activities are associated with better cognitive health in later life. Of course, it could be that the people who choose a more varied and challenging

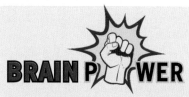

**BRAIN POWER**

A small number of people possess what memory experts call 'total recall'. They can remember every detail – what they wore, what they ate, what the weather was like, who visited that day and so on – of any specific day from adolescence onwards. Such memory feats highlight the vast potential of the human memory.

lifestyle are those who are more mentally active to begin with. But taking up or increasing your level of activity does seem to confer benefits. A 2008 review commissioned by the UK government's Foresight Project, 'Mental Capital and Wellbeing', noted that cognitive training in later life could improve memory, reasoning and speed of information processing, and that the gains could be long-lasting, for at least five years. A multitude of other studies have reached similar conclusions. Here are three simple everyday ways to boost brain power:

● **Talking.** A study found that chatting for 10 minutes a day improves memory and test scores.

● **Walking.** In a study published in the *Journal of the American Medical Association*, researchers looking at data from the US Nurses Study, involving more than 18,000 women, found that long-term regular physical activity, including walking, is associated with significantly better cognitive function and less cognitive decline in older women.

● **Playing video games.** A study of people in their sixties and seventies found that playing a strategy video game, one that focused on world domination, improved cognitive skills.

# YOUR SHARP BRAIN ACTION PLAN

What's the best way to nurture your neurological garden? In Part 2, *Five Brain Boosters*, you'll discover which small lifestyle tweaks can help you think more clearly, retain information more effectively and concentrate better. It can be something as simple as going for a brisk walk or taking an occasional class.

Your diet is especially important. A study published in *Archives of Neurology* suggests that following the Mediterranean diet can provide a powerful defence against mental decline. After five years, people who followed this diet – high in fish, fruit, vegetables, legumes and monounsaturated fats such as olive oil, moderate in alcohol and low in red meat and dairy products – had a 28 per cent lower risk of cognitive impairment.

Later in the book, you'll find advice on the best foods to eat for brain health – and what to avoid. You'll learn why gaining abdominal fat can be bad for your brain as well as your heart. You'll discover why exercise is good for your brain, not just your body, and how simply getting adequate sleep can almost magically clear up fuzzy thinking. (The ability of test subjects assigned to memorise lists of words improved by 30 per cent after a good night's sleep.)

## FIGHT THE FOES

In Part 3, *Five Brain Enemies*, there's information on the villains that can rob your brain of its power, and advice on how to protect yourself. Some are the usual suspects: smoking and drinking to excess are just as bad for your brain as they are for the rest of your body. But others are more surprising.

Muddled thinking? Many of us can blame it on stress. In one study, stressed-out medical students performed markedly worse on an important exam. Depression can also rob us of brain power. When the blues turn black, the symptoms can include foggy memory, difficulty with comprehension, even slurred speech.

In elderly people, these symptoms are commonly mistaken for dementia, but mental skills quickly bounce back when the depression is treated. Even high cholesterol levels and belly fat can wear down your brain. There's plenty of information on how to combat each of these 'enemies'.

## CROSS-TRAIN YOUR BRAIN

Finally, we've all heard the advice to take up crossword puzzles or play chess to keep the mind fit. That's a good starting point. It'll definitely make you better at crosswords or chess – but that alone won't help you find your car keys, says cognitive neuroscientist Robert Logie. Just as runners devote a portion of their

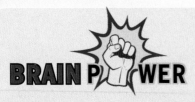

**BRAIN POWER**

A 'happy' brain can help to fight off infection. The body's immune system responds directly to changes in the brain. A sad event – such as losing a loved one – can produce a measurable depletion in the number of infection-fighting blood cells within four days.

## ... soon you'll find that your brain has recharged and rejuvenated, and is ready to learn and remember.

training to swimming and cycling, you'll need to vary your activities if you really want to keep your brain in prime shape.

Athletes call this cross-training. Part 4 of this book, *Your Brain Fitness Programme*, is designed to help you do just that. You'll discover a series of entertaining puzzles and exercises specially designed to challenge your brain in the six main cognitive areas mentioned on page 10: attention and focus, general memory, processing speed, verbal skills, number skills and reasoning.

Spend a few minutes on them every day, and you should notice improvements in your brain 'fitness' in no time. You'll also discover useful everyday strategies for everything from remembering phone numbers to recalling names that are always on the tip of your tongue.

There's evidence that intellectually curious people are more resistant to brain decline. They have what scientists call a cognitive reserve, which means they have more nerve cells and dendrites than others

to begin with. So if their brains eventually suffer damage due to a disease such as Alzheimer's, they're likely to function well for a longer period.

Bearing all this in mind, are you inspired to banish memory slips, chase away brain fog, sharpen up your concentration and focus, reduce your dementia risk and boost your self-confidence? You've come to the right place. This practical, comprehensive plan is based on the latest science, but promises to be an enjoyable challenge every step of the way. Try the puzzles and exercises, follow the advice, and soon you'll find that your brain has recharged and rejuvenated, and is ready to learn and remember.

As for losing your car keys, no one can guarantee it won't happen again. But you can rest assured that it's something we all do, regardless of our brain health. So instead of worrying, use your mental energies to find a designated spot to keep those keys. And develop a new habit of putting them back when you come home.

## AN ODE TO WISDOM

When we're young, the only kind of intelligence that is valued is the kind that results in high scores in school exams. But in older people, different types of intelligence become increasingly useful and garner respect. It's about the depth of knowledge that can come only from experience. 'Sixteen-year-olds think they know it all and reject the advice of their parents, but when they themselves get older, they recognise the knowledge that comes with life experience and are puzzled as to why the young do not want to listen to their advice,' says Professor Logie. Wisdom isn't just about having an evolved opinion. Think of it as being 'streetwise' – in other words, older people's broader knowledge and experience enable them to put together different pieces of information more effectively.

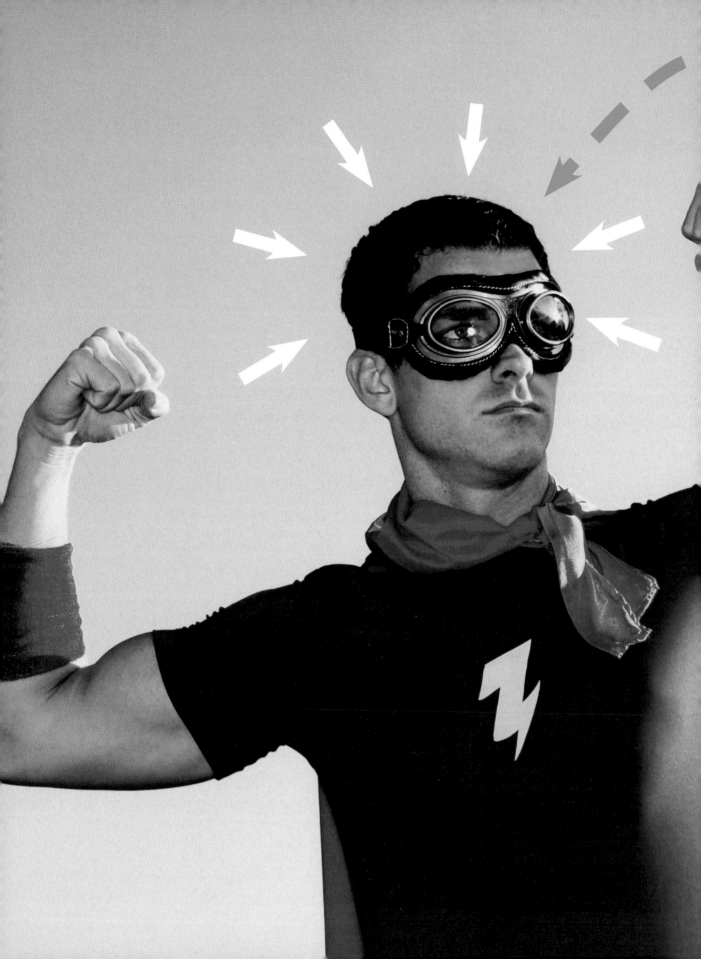

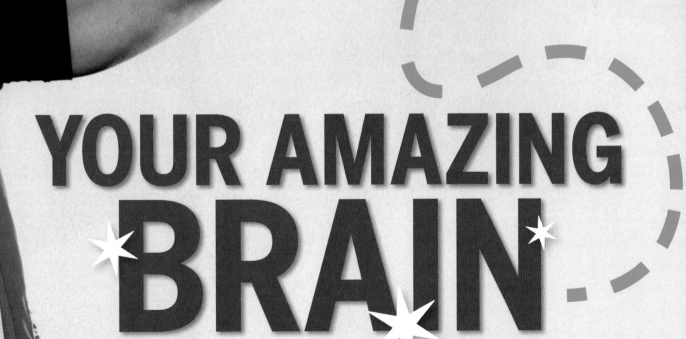

# part 1

# YOUR AMAZING *BRAIN*

# WHAT MAKES US TICK?

## a brief brain tour

**At first glance, the brain is less than impressive. It's a wrinkled grey mass whose surface resembles that of a walnut** (that's because the brain folds itself up – just as your intestines do – to fit more matter into a small space). If you were to poke it, it would feel like a mound of soft tofu. Not very promising.

Appearances are deceptive, though: your brain is astoundingly complex and perpetually active. Even while you sleep, it isn't entirely at rest, carrying on its vital role of maintaining breathing, heartbeat and other bodily functions, and dealing with bursts of increased activity as you dream. When you're awake, the brain has truly amazing multi-tasking abilities. In an instant, it controls all your physical functions, with your senses sensing on full alert, all while you drive a 2-tonne vehicle at 70 miles per hour down a busy motorway, watching the road signs, remembering your route, digesting your lunch and listening to the radio. Not bad for a wobbly mass of grey matter.

How does it get it all done? You'd never know by looking at it, but the brain contains distinct regions, each with its own job to do. Much of what is known about how different parts of the brain work came from observing how people act and react after damage to certain areas due to injury, tumours, seizures or stroke. Now fMRI scans, which highlight brain activity, complement this valuable work.

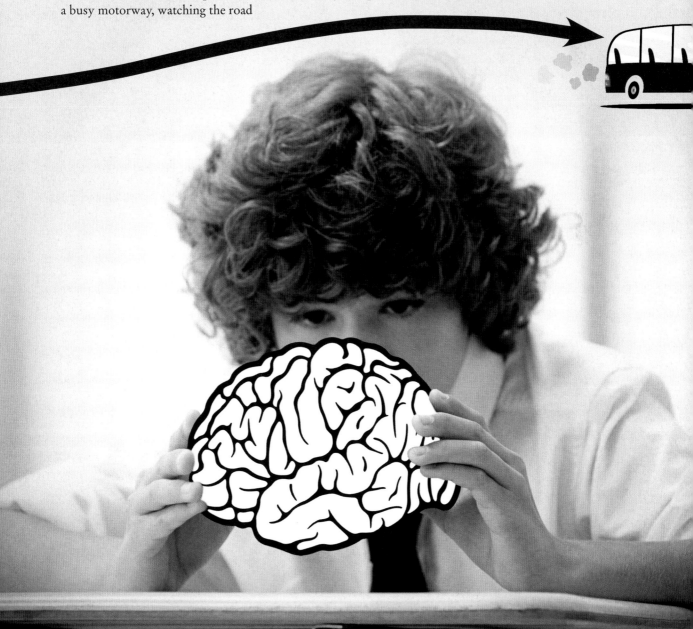

# GREY MATTER: WHERE IT ALL HAPPENS

The entire wrinkled outer layer of the brain is the cerebral cortex, also known as grey matter. Only a few millimetres thick, it contains 77 per cent of the total volume of brain tissue, much of it hidden in its many folds and convolutions. The cerebral cortex (see pages 22–23 for more information) is largely responsible for all forms of conscious experience, including perception, emotion, thought and planning.

The two sides of the brain – the left and right hemispheres – further divvy up these functions. Usually in right-handed people – and generally vice versa in left-handers – the left hemisphere controls language, while the right side controls art and spatial orientation skills. Writing a letter involves your left brain; painting a picture or finding your way back to your car in a crowded car park would be down to your right brain.

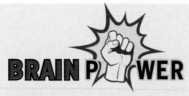

**BRAIN POWER**

The brain is able to alter almost any body function. Heart rate can be slowed, the bowel relaxed and blood vessels opened or closed, just through thought. Simply imagining being warm, for instance, can increase the temperature in a person's fingers by more than 1°C.

Because the body's nerves cross sides, the left hemisphere controls the right side of your body, and the right hemisphere controls the left. The two halves of your brain are connected by millions of nerve fibres bundled together in a thick cable called the corpus callosum. This 'bridge' allows the brain to merge and coordinate skills so it can act as a united whole.

An interesting aside: if the corpus callosum is damaged or severed, the two sides of the brain can't communicate. If an apple is placed in the left hand of a blindfolded person who's suffered this kind of brain damage, the right side of his or her brain would recognise it as an apple using smell and touch. But because the brain hemispheres aren't talking, the right side can't relay the concept to the language centre on the left side. It would be impossible for this person to come up with the word 'apple'.

## COMPLEX NETWORK

Grey matter is not a single material but a biological construct of capillaries (which carry oxygen and nutrients throughout the brain), nerve cells (also known as **neurons**) and glia, the cells that support, feed and communicate with nerve cells. Its **nucleus** contains genetic material (DNA) and generates proteins to maintain the neurons.

If you suck away the glia, you are left with a communications network wired from billions of nerve cells. This lacy structure underlies everything in your physical, mental and emotional life.

Life depends on neurons passing messages to other neurons. The messages from one neuron are transmitted along a single fibre called an **axon** and received by a multitude of short branches called

# YOUR BRAIN'S COMMUNICATION NETWORK

Every thought, idea and memory you have forges a unique electrochemical path among the billions of neurons in your brain.

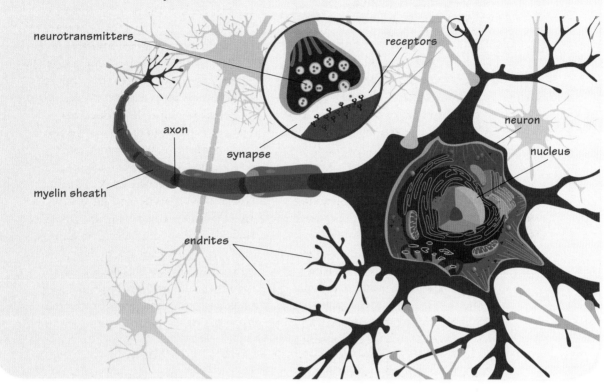

dendrites. As the information passes from one neuron to the next, it must jump across countless tiny gaps called **synapses**. This is where brain chemicals called **neurotransmitters**, such as serotonin and dopamine, come into play. When the information reaches the end of one neuron's axon, they carry it across the gap to **receptors** on the next neuron.

As with any communications network – think about your internet service provider, or mobile phone company and the satellites it uses to send information from one place to another – the better the network, the clearer the messages and the faster they are able to get through.

To transport information from one part of the brain to a more distant area, the brain uses special high-speed cables – bundles of axons coated by a fatty substance called **myelin**, which stands out from the rest of the brain and gives the brain's white matter its name. The coating insulates the bundles and speeds the transmission of electrical signals along this communication expressway, allowing for faster cognitive processing.

The brain can alter almost any body function.

# YOUR grey matter AT WORK

We call brainy people cerebral for a good reason: the cerebral cortex, also known as grey matter, is where complex thought, attention and memory take place. Different functions occur in different areas.

**1 SHORT-TERM MINI-STORAGE** The part of the frontal lobe closest to your forehead is the prefrontal cortex, the primary area for keeping short-term memories (also called working memory). Think of it as a temporary filing system that holds facts for just a few seconds – a phone number you are about to dial, for example. Thoughts or ideas reside here briefly unless you make the effort to commit them to long-term memory.

**2 DECISION MAKING, PLANNING AND PROBLEM SOLVING**
The large portion of the brain called the frontal lobe is the brain's command centre. It controls decision making, planning, organising and problem solving. It also creates our personalities, sharpens our attention and keeps us focused on goals. It allows civilised societies to exist by putting the brakes on some of our baser instincts.

**DAMAGE REPORT** *The 'caveman effect'* Damage to the frontal lobe can result in wildly fluctuating emotions and difficulty performing even simple tasks. Think about it: just brewing a cup of tea requires dozens of individual steps, including finding the tea, filling the kettle, switching it on, waiting for the water to boil, pouring it into a cup, adding milk and more. Without planning abilities, this would be impossible to pull off

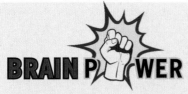

# BRAIN POWER

The human brain has a built-in awareness of the thoughts of others. An intuitive grasp of other people's thinking and their view of situations develops in children at around the age of four. Before this age, children usually assume that others have the same information and feelings as themselves. This 'mind-reading' ability is located in the frontal lobe of the brain.

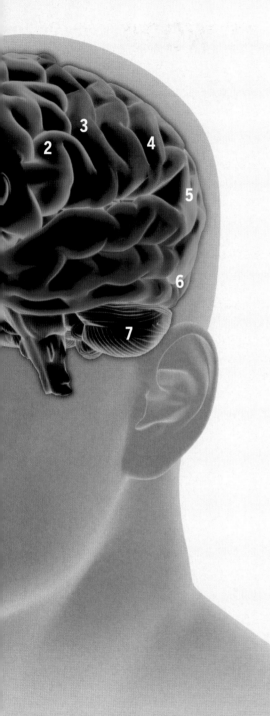

### 3 MOVEMENT

At the rear of the prefrontal cortex is the primary motor cortex, controlling all movement. Brain scientists can now identify the locations in the motor cortex associated with distinct patterns of movement, such as the hand motions of musicians. In fact, it's even possible to know what instrument a musician plays by looking at changes in this part of the brain.

### 4 PHYSICAL SENSATIONS

The parietal lobe, towards the back of the brain, is responsible for the body's physical sensations. A disproportionate amount of the parietal lobe is dedicated to some of the smallest – but most sensitive – parts of the body, such as the tongue, hands, face and genitals. The parietal lobe also plays a role in spatial recognition, language and our ability to focus attention.

**DAMAGE REPORT** *Half the story* Damage to the parietal lobe can distort the way a person perceives space and objects. If the damage is on the right side, the person may be totally unaware of anything on the left of his or her visual field, including the left side of a computer screen, the left side of someone's face or even his or her own left leg.

### 5 VISION

The occipital lobe at the back of the brain manages vision. It controls eye focusing, interprets the meaning of all the shapes and colours we see, and records short-term visual memory.

### 6 REMEMBERING NAMES

The temporal lobe, beneath the temples, connects to the ears and processes and interprets sounds. It also has a role in memory, particularly for words, ideas and names.

**DAMAGE REPORT** *Subtotal recall* If the temporal lobe is damaged, a person is unable to learn new facts or remember events. Life seems eternally new (and frustrating) because no new memories can be formed. A person with this type of damage could read the same newspaper over and over without getting bored.

### 7 COORDINATION AND BALANCE

The cerebellum (the 'little brain') is a small wrinkled area at the base of the brain. Don't let its small size fool you – it contains half of the brain's neurons. While the motor cortex is the area that sends messages to the muscles, causing them to move, the cerebellum acts like a conductor, coordinating all the movements that let you successfully swim a length in the pool, knit a jumper or walk down the street.

**DAMAGE REPORT** *Drunk while sober* Injury to the cerebellum can cause dizziness, slurred speech, nausea and uncoordinated movements. Affected people are often mistaken for being drunk.

# THE LIMBIC SYSTEM: BASIC INSTINCTS

Buried deep under the cerebral cortex is the limbic system, a set of primitive structures responsible for some of our most basic human instincts and drives. Craving a piece of chocolate cake? Blame, in part, the limbic system, which regulates our response to pleasure. Bolting down the street to escape a fierce dog? Thank the limbic system, which is largely responsible for our survival instincts. Terrified of bees after being stung badly as a child? The limbic system is the culprit, because it won't let you ever forget that event. Emotional memories are often subconscious, but they may suddenly pop up in the form of panic attacks or flashbacks.

The limbic system is also in charge of our most primal urges, including those of a sexual nature. Damage to this part of the brain leaves appetite, aggression and sex drive completely unregulated.

## DÉJÀ VU?

The limbic system may be involved in the unique phenomenon we know as 'déjà vu' (literally, 'already seen'). This sense of having been in an unfamiliar place or of having had a conversation and lived through the moment before has been regarded by some people as evidence of reincarnation. Others have explained it as the memory of a dream in which the person 'experienced' the moment in advance of it happening. Conversely, the sense of 'jamais vu' ('never seen') occurs when what is known and familiar becomes for a while strange and unusual.

Scientists now believe that both are caused by a momentary failure of the limbic system to react appropriately. When déjà vu takes place, information flowing through the limbic system is mistakenly tagged with familiarity. When this incorrectly identified information merges with information from elsewhere in the brain, it produces a puzzling sense of familiarity. Conversely, in the case of jamais vu, the information's true emotional significance is not recognised as it should be.

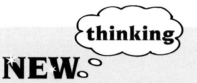

## NEW thinking

### A brain in your belly?

What sends and receives information along a complex neural circuit, communicates with the help of chemical messengers called neurotransmitters (such as dopamine and serotonin) and is capable of functioning independently? Yes, it's the brain – but it's also the stomach.

The brain and the gut are intimately linked. For example, when you imagine something fearful or exciting, your heart rate increases and you get butterflies in your stomach.

### Did you know that:

● An upset stomach can lead to a headache?
● Stomachs get their own form of 'migraines'?
● Antidepressants can calm the intestines of people with irritable bowel syndrome?

Some experts hypothesise that the brain in our stomachs may even hold sensory memories that we don't consciously recall, but which nonetheless guide us. Gut instinct? Maybe so.

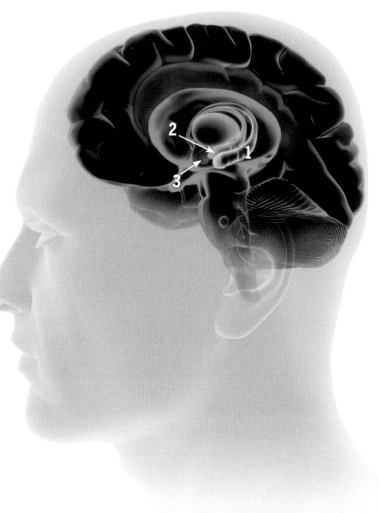

**① THE HIPPOCAMPUS** This tiny area of the brain, whose shape first reminded scientists of a seahorse (*hippocampus* is Greek for 'seahorse'), converts short-term memories into long-term ones. It shares responsibility with the hypothalamus for aggressive behaviour, sex drive and appetite. And it's largely responsible for spatial memory and navigation. It's one of the first regions to become damaged in cases of Alzheimer's disease, causing memory problems and disorientation.

**② THE AMYGDALA** This part of the brain helps to regulate fear, anger and sexual response. The old thinking was that it played a special role in processing emotional memory, taking highly charged events, such as a traumatic attack, a flunked job interview or a first kiss, and making sure they are stored permanently in your mind. The new thinking is that the amygdala may actually play a role in all long-term memory formation.

**③ THE HYPOTHALAMUS** Does your heart beat faster even when you just think about a scary upcoming event? Pehaps it's your driving test, an exam or an important meeting at work. That's the hypothalamus at work. About the size of an almond, this region has an amazing amount of control over what happens in our bodies, and even over our moods and actions. It not only controls sexual arousal and behaviour but also regulates hunger and thirst, sleep and wakefulness, responses to pain and pleasure, levels of anger and aggression, and even our body temperature, pulse, blood pressure and other physical responses to emotional events.

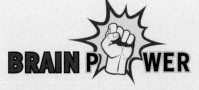

Some of our most emotional memories are triggered by scent. The olfactory system, which processes smells, has direct links to the amygdala – the group of brain cells now thought to help forge long-term memories. This may be why unusual scents from the past have such power to evoke vivid personal recollections.

# MEMORY & LEARNING

Do you remember the geometry equations you learned in school? Can you still recite a poem off by heart? Do you recall what you had for breakfast last Tuesday? Some bits of information just seem to slip away, while others stick in the brain with startling clarity and little or no effort.

how they work

It's a good bet that you remember the words to the theme song of your favourite childhood TV programme, the exact time of day your children were born, the name of your favourite primary school teacher and the price you paid for your first house or car. Yet, no matter how hard we try, we are never totally in control of our own memories.

Cognitive neuroscientists, however, are gradually learning exactly what happens in the brain to allow us to process and record our experiences – and why some ideas, facts and images stay with us while others are destined to dissolve in the mist.

## MEMORY: THE LONG AND SHORT OF IT

Certain kinds of information in our brains are captured and released without our even knowing it. Other types stick around very briefly, long enough for the knowledge to be used and forgotten – or, if we make an effort to learn it, transferred to longer-term storage.

### HERE AND GONE: BELOW THE RADAR

Memory begins with experience, and we're drenched in a sea of experience every second of every day. There's no getting away from it. If you close your eyes, you can still hear. Block your ears and you can nevertheless taste. Shut your mouth and you can still smell. Hold your nose and you can still feel. Registering these sensory experiences is effortless and automatic – it doesn't even require

your attention. Stop reading this book for a few seconds and look around the room. Without any conscious effort at all on your part, your brain is registering everything within the scope of your vision. This first level of memory is called sensory memory.

> Memory begins with experience, and we're drenched in a sea of experience every second.

So where does all that sensory information go? Pretty quickly, it vanishes. If you look out of the window and see a bird alight on a branch of a tree, then fly away again, within just 60 seconds you wouldn't be able to point out which branch the bird had landed on. You saw it, your brain registered the information, but the sensory memory (the visual image of the bird on the tree) melted away.

While you may not notice sensory memory, it's essential for navigation, not to mention safety. (For example, it reminds you that a loud crashing sound indicates danger.)

The only way to hold on to these fleeting memories for longer is to pay conscious attention to the sensory input you receive. In the example of the bird, if you knew in advance that you'd be asked which branch it had landed on, you'd pay more attention, focusing on that bit of information and taking it to the next memory level – working memory.

# brain HiCCUPS

## Twin vanishing act

One of my silliest 'senior moments' happened on the second day of a new school year. I was running around frantically trying to find the twins' books, and make breakfast and packed lunches, while also dealing with the girls' anxieties about their new class. They had gymnastics after school, so I sorted out their kit – shorts, T-shirts, socks and gym shoes – wrote a note to the teacher that the twins were not to come home on the school bus, and reminded the girls three times that they had gymnastics that day.

When 3pm came round, I went to meet the girls at the bus stop. The other children got off as usual, but not the twins. I screamed, 'Where are my children?' My heart was pounding. The bus driver calmly called the school to ask about them. The school responded, 'They are at gymnastics.' Of course! I walked away, thoroughly embarrassed.

## TEMPORARY STORAGE

Working, or short-term, memory, requires you to pay a bit of attention, unlike sensory memory. As you're reading this passage, you're using your short-term memory to remember the gist of the sentences that came before so that what you're taking in makes overall sense.

True to its name, short-term memory lasts for only a few seconds to a few minutes. Think of all the times you looked up a phone number, got briefly distracted before making the call, and had to find the phone number all over again. Not only is the storage time for working memory short, the storage space is small. For example, when scientists test working memory for numbers, they find that we can hold only about seven digits at a time – fewer, coincidentally, than the number of digits in many phone numbers. Of course, some people can remember eight or nine, but recalling more than that requires knowing and using specific strategies. (There's more about those in Part 4.)

## BRIEF BUT VITAL

With only a small capacity and short storage time, what's the point? Actually, short-term memory plays a vital role in our daily lives. Those slivers of temporary information allow us to write down doctor's appointments, make everyday decisions and even have a conversation. Think about it: you have to recall what someone said to you 5 seconds ago in order to respond, though you don't need to remember it for ever.

This is information you use and forget – and good riddance. 'If we were to remember everything that we experience, our memories would rapidly become cluttered with lots of irrevelant detail. This would make it very difficult to recall specific details that we need to remember,' says Robert Logie, professor of human cognitive neuroscience at Edinburgh University.

Of course, it would be nice if some details didn't disappear before we could make use of them. When people say that they feel as if they are losing their memories, they are usually talking about short-term memory. Do you forget where you put your glasses or lose your train of thought during a conversation? Blame your working memory for those brain

# WHY DO WE forget?

We all know lots of excuses for forgetfulness. When we say, 'I'm sorry I forgot your birthday because [insert reason here]', are we just making up a fake excuse? Here's a quick legitimacy check on the most common excuses:

| Excuse | Truth? | |
|---|---|---|
| 'I'm under too much stress.' | Yes | Chronic stress is like poison to the brain. Stress increases production of a natural steroid called cortisol, which damages the hippocampus– the brain's memory centre. Studies show that chronic stress reduces the efficiency of brain function and impairs attention, memory and thinking. |
| 'I'm pregnant.' | No | There is no evidence that pregnancy itself has any effect on your mental clarity. However, if you are anxious about the pregnancy or about impending parenthood, this may affect your attention or memory. |

## Pregnancy itself has no effect on your mental clarity.

| Excuse | Truth? | |
|---|---|---|
| 'I'm going through the menopause.' | No | With apologies to women who feel blitzed by the menopause, the decline of oestrogen that marks the menopause does not cause much – if any – change in memory or cognitive function. (If you're not getting enough sleep, that's a different story.) |
| 'I'm on a diet.' | Yes | People intent on losing weight quickly often put their bodies into a state of near starvation. Memory and thinking suffer as the brain is deprived of necessary glucose (blood sugar). Very low-carb diets can also make you feel tired, light-headed and headachy. |
| 'I'm having chemo.' | Yes | Cloudy thinking in chemotherapy patients is so common, there's even a term for it: chemobrain. The medicines themselves can act like a brain-rattling smack on the side of the head. Chemo side effects, such as anaemia, fatigue, insomnia and worry, can also make concentration difficult. And one often-neglected cause is poor nutrition, as patients frequently lose their appetite. |

hiccups. And yes, this function does tend to weaken with age. In fact, all of those so-called 'senior moments' may be related to a decline in working memory. But as you'll discover shortly, the more attention you pay in the first place, the better the information will stick.

## LONG-TERM STORAGE

To keep information for days, months or even years, we need to consolidate it into long-term memory. And here's the good news: our brains have an unlimited amount of long-term memory storage capacity. The filing cabinet never gets filled up.

Of course, long-term memories can and will fade with time if you don't revisit them every so often, but the potential is there to remember them for ever.

The brain stores three main types of information in the long-term:

● **Words, facts and numbers.** When you're struggling to recall the name of the star in a film, the number of feet in a mile or the author of *Treasure Island*, you're wrestling with semantic memory. In Part 4, you'll find some tricks for improving this type of memory.

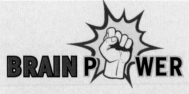

It can take up to two years for a memory to become permanent. Experiences that are being processed for storage as long-term memories may be replayed in the mind for up to two years. Once a memory is consolidated in this way, it has the potential to last a lifetime.

● **Events.** Episodic memory – think episodes – involves events or scenes from your life. Storing the general details of major events is effortless. You don't need to work at remembering what it was like to watch your daughter get married or how you felt the day you got your university place; you just do.

Certain exhilarating scenes, particularly around life milestones, such as a first kiss or the first day of a job, simply captivate us – and stick around. We also remember unpleasant experiences without effort. No one forgets being robbed, cheated or fired, for example.

But we do tend to forget specific details of even the most important events in our lives. You'll remember if you were robbed, but you might not remember the face of the thief, and there are numerous examples of mistaken identity, with, for example, an innocent bystander being identified as the criminal. The Alfred Hitchcock film *The Wrong Man* tells a true story of exactly this kind of event.

We also tend to forget details of more mundane events in our lives. What did you do on March 29, 2009? Unless that date was important in your life, it is unlikely that you will be able to remember more than where you were living and what kinds of activities dominated your life around that time.

● **Physical skills.** They say you never forget how to ride a bike, and it's true. You can thank a form of long-term memory called procedural memory, also called muscle memory. It's responsible for acquired habits and motor skills, such as the ability to play an instrument, drive a car or even tie your shoes (something else we never forget how to do). You acquire these skills through practice.

## PLAY BALL – BUT START YOUNG

When older people are asked to memorise lists of words or numbers, they often do as well as younger adults. But some things – especially those that involve muscle memory – are simply easier to learn when we're children. Encoding new physical memories becomes more difficult as we get older, which means that it's much harder to learn to play an instrument, take up a new sport or learn sign language. It can be done, but it will take longer and require more effort.

Learning to play an instrument is easier when you're young.

If you ever learned how to play the guitar, for example, you'll remember how difficult it was to get your fingers into position to play a chord. But finally, after hours and hours of practice, those subtle hand motions became second nature, and your fingers went straight to their proper positions. Even years later, without practising, the chances are that you could quickly find the G chord.

Muscle memory is stored throughout the brain, which makes it virtually immune to the factors that cause us to lose information memories. That's why Alzheimer's patients retain their basic motor skills even when the disease robs them of the ability to recall a family member's name.

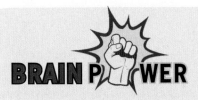

Consciousness steps in only when it is needed. A skilled tennis player does not consciously work out where to place her racquet or feet when playing a shot. Only when a ball presents a special problem does conscious decision making come into play.

### PROSPECTIVE MEMORY

Have you ever forgotten to post a letter, pass on a message or turn up for an appointment? Everyone experiences these everyday failures of 'prospective memory', or remembering to do things. It might be that you put a letter by the front door intending to pick it up on your way out but forgot to do so a few minutes later, or you might intend to make an appointment for the dentist later in the day but come the evening the appointment has not been made. Most of the time we do remember to do things – turn up for work, take our children to school, buy food for dinner or meet up with a close friend for coffee. But, without prospective memory, it would be very difficult to function in our daily lives, and might even have serious consequences: for example, if we forgot to take medicine or check the cooker when deep-frying chips.

# HOLD THAT THOUGHT – BUT HOW?

All this talk about memory storage makes it sound as though there is some kind of brain warehouse just waiting to be filled; the metaphor has even been used of a memory filing cabinet when describing the brain's capacity to keep information in the long term. Yet no such cabinet or warehouse exists. Cognitive neuroscientists have searched for decades to find it, with no luck. So where exactly do memories live – and how do they get there? Even more important, how do we make sure they stay there?

### CREATING A MEMORY

Science now suggests that long-term memories aren't stored in a single place but, rather, in vast networks of nerve-cell pathways. Every recollection begins as a 'spark' in the brain triggered when we receive input from our senses. This spark becomes an electrical signal as it travels from neuron to neuron. Each memory

# Ask the
# MEMORY EXPERT...

**My husband can drive or be driven somewhere once and remember the route months later, even if it's in a distant part of the country. I, on the other hand, continue to get lost in my own city unless I follow a known route. Is there a sense-of-direction centre in the brain? Or does he just have a better general memory (even though he can't remember to buy milk)?**

**PROF. ROBERT LOGIE:** Men do seem better than women at learning and recalling directions and orientation – which involves the right parietal lobe and other areas of the brain. Women tend to be more skilled at reading human emotional cues. But there are many exceptions to such general findings with, for example, outstanding female navigators and very empathetic men. Different people, different talents.

forges a unique pathway among the billions upon billions of neurons in the brain, as if blazing a new trail through a dense forest.

As the information passes from one neuron to the next, it jumps across gaps called synapses, with the help of neurotransmitters, such as serotonin and dopamine. Neurotransmitters are vital to memory – and, unfortunately, we produce less of them as we age. But by continuing to challenge our brains to learn new skills and information, we can create more and more dendrites, which help keep our brains young and sprightly.

Work hard enough or for long enough at a given type of memory and your brain will grow and adapt in other ways, too. In an astonishing 2000 study, London taxi drivers, who spend their whole careers learning to navigate one of the largest, most-convoluted road systems in the world, underwent MRI screenings of their brains. The cabbies

were found to have unusually large hippocampuses, an area of the brain that plays a major role in memory formation, particularly spatial memory. What's more, the longer someone had been driving a taxi, the larger their hippocampus – an association not found in bus drivers, who drive set routes, according to a later study. This suggests that acquiring a specific expertise, in this case complex navigational skills, can actually cause structural changes in the brain.

## MAKING IT STICK

Some memories naturally tend to persist better than others, but you can help any memory to stick by following these two simple strategies.

### 1 Pay attention.
The first step in remembering something is paying attention to it. Unless you seize information by focusing on it, it can slip right past you.

# HOW A fact IS LEARNT

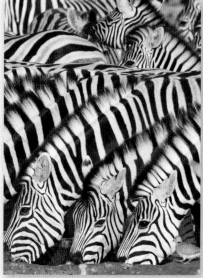

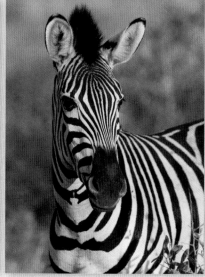

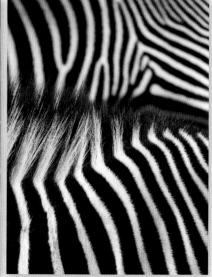

### Step 1

**We perceive** Sights, sounds, sensations, tastes, smells. Our brains take in this information whether we pay attention to it or not.

### Step 2

**We focus** If we focus on the information, it gets moved into the working memory. If we don't, the information fades within seconds.

### Step 3

**We rehearse** With enough repetition, study and review, the fact gets moved to the long-term memory. Otherwise, the fact placed in the working memory dissolves.

Can't recall the name of someone to whom you were just introduced? You probably weren't paying enough active attention to the name (maybe you were focused on smiling and looking friendly). Most people find it easier to remember faces than names, partly because even in a short conversation you spend, perhaps, 5 minutes concentrating on the face, especially one that you find particularly attractive or unattractive, compared with seconds to register the person's name. The trick is to link recognition of the face, which is generally easier, with the more difficult task of recalling the name.

You may notice that people who are good with names often repeat the person's name out loud. If they meet someone called John Robinson, for example, they may say, 'Good to meet you, John.' Silently, they may be making an association: 'John is from Switzerland: Swiss Family Robinson.' By repeating it, then making the effort to come up with a rhyme, a reference or an association, they create a nerve-cell pathway – a memory trail – in the brain for the name, so it doesn't vanish without a trace. You'll find more tricks for making names stick better in Part 4.

**2** Practise and repeat.

Consolidation is the process of making a nerve-cell pathway more permanent. Each time you review or revisit a fact, each time you repeat it, the pathway becomes a little stronger. This is what we typically think of as learning.

The likelihood of consolidating any particular fact or memory depends on a number of factors, including what you want to learn (whether it's a fact or a skill), your current knowledge base, your emotional state, and how well you take care of yourself. The work of consolidation is also easier if you have a background that relates to whatever it is you are trying to learn, just as it is easier to keep track of an invoice or important tax form if you have an existing file folder for this exact type of information than if you throw the paper on the desk and vow to remember its location later.

Inexperienced chess players who look at pieces on a chess board, for example, will find it very difficult to recall where all the pieces had been placed. But chess champions can remember the placement of the pieces quite easily because they have an excellent knowledge of the game. Rather than just seeing individual pieces set up randomly, they see the strategic challenges illustrated by the set-up of the board, and that puts the information in context, permitting better recall.

Similarly, a fascinating study by Robert Logie at Edinburgh University and his colleagues Richard Wright and Scott Decker at the University of Missouri, St Louis, USA, showed that thieves are more likely than others to remember the details of houses that might be relevant to a burglary, such as whether or not there is an alarm or a 'beware of

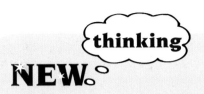

**NEW** thinking

**We remember useful information better.**

Information is easier to recall, especially as we get older, if it makes sense and seems useful. In typical tests of memory, researchers ask subjects to recall lists of random numbers or words. But psychologist Alan Castel, PhD, assistant professor of psychology at the University of California, Los Angeles, and an expert in memory and cognitive ageing, tried something different. He asked his human guinea pigs to memorise lists of grocery items as well as their associated prices. The pairings were either unlikely (for example, loaf of bread: £8.71) or likely (such as, loaf of bread: £1.50). Younger people outperformed the older people at remembering the unlikely pairings, but older folk redeemed themselves when the prices made sense. Implication: in effect, older adults have learned to compensate for the normal decline in working memory by not wasting time on useless information. 'They focus on information with high value and discard the rest,' says Dr Castel.

the dog' sign. Which all goes to show that if you take time to practise something (however dubious), your memory in that area of expertise will improve.

## MAKING IT STICK BETTER

In Parts 2 and 3 of this book, you'll learn about how certain emotional states (such as depression), lack of sleep and even certain medicines can make it harder to consolidate memories. You'll also read about strategies, such as getting enough exercise, keeping your social connections alive and eating brain-healthy foods, that can help you keep your brain skills at their peak.

## FLASHBULB MEMORY: PERMANENT SNAPSHOTS

Every so often, the daily routine of our lives is broken by the shock of an event so surprising, so monumental, that we remember every detail of where we were and what we were doing when we heard the news. Can you recall exactly where you were at the moment you learned about the September 11 attacks on New York's World Trade Center or the death of Princess Diana or Elvis Presley? Even years later, most of us have memories so vivid that recalling those tragic days can feel as if we are looking at well-preserved photographs. The same thing can happen to an even greater extent with very personal events, such as seeing a bad car accident or being bitten by a vicious dog. Psychologists call these intense impressions flashbulb memories.

As the name suggests, a flashbulb memory is the brain's way of taking a mental 'picture' of a significant emotional event. Because they are so vivid, accessible and durable, they become cognitive landmarks that allow us to place other, less dramatic events into a before-or-after context.

## WHY IT IMPACTS

The closer a significant event hits home, the deeper the memory is embedded. Researchers from New York University interviewed 24 people who were in Manhattan at the time the World Trade Center's Twin Towers fell, and watched brain activity light up on scans as the they recalled their experiences that day. Some participants were within blocks of the Twin Towers, some were about two miles away, and others were more than four miles away. All had strong recollections of the day. But the strongest flashes, indicating the deepest, most searing kinds of memory, appeared only for those who were at or near the World Trade Center.

In forming these flashbulb memories, the hippocampus (which plays a major role in long-term memory) gets help from its immediate neighbour, the amygdala, which leaps into action when triggered by stress hormones such as adrenaline to process the memory quickly. These hormones prompt the amygdala to send messages to the brain that this is important and you'd better remember it. What's more, with events such as major disasters, 'flashbulb memories' result not only from an emotional response at the time but also the effect of 'practice and repeat'.

'At the time of a major event, there is massive news coverage on television and in the newspapers,' says Professor Robert Logie. 'It is the major topic of conversation with friends immediately

**BRAIN POWER**

When we first view a scene or situation, we rely on memory to help us make sense of it. The eyes see only a tiny part of any visual scene clearly. They dart around taking in more and more information, and memory enables us to assemble this sequence of fragments into a scene.

# MEMORY TIPS FROM A
## police expert

How many times a week do you try to recall a fact that stubbornly eludes you, like where you put the car keys? If only you could push a button to access the information. It's not that simple, but you can help yourself remember better with techniques that Natalie Sweet, a police composite sketch artist, uses with crime witnesses. Every day she helps ordinary people remember enough physical detail to create a meaningful portrait of a criminal suspect. Here are her tips.

### Step 1 Try to relax.
**If you've lost your keys, don't panic. That will only makes things worse.**

Sweet takes the pressure off by telling witnesses that the purpose of a sketch is to come as close as possible to the person in their memory. It is not intended to be perfect, and no one will be arrested based on the sketch alone.

### Step 2 Cast your mind back, picturing any details you remember.
**Close your eyes and try to remember the last time you had your keys. Were you coming from a meeting? What were you wearing? Was it raining?**

Sweet gives the witness's brain a chance to 'warm up' by talking over everything about the day of the crime, except the crime itself. For example, she might ask a man to go back in his mind to that day and remember everything that happened before the incident. Does he remember what he was doing immediately before? What was the weather like?

Once the witness seems relaxed, Sweet asks him to close his eyes and start describing what he remembers about the environment during the crime. She asks him to look around the room and describe everything he sees, such as what's hanging on the walls, the type of lighting and the colour of the walls.

### Step 3 Pretend you were an onlooker.
**If you had your keys when you walked into the house, imagine watching yourself enter. Are the keys in your hand? Did you linger on the doorstep?**

Memories of any incident can be blocked by emotions, such as fear or anger. So Sweet gets witnesses to picture the scene as an onlooker would.

'I take them out of whatever position they were in, victim or witness,' says Sweet. 'I tell them to think of it as though they were standing outside looking in, as though they were filming what happened, or watching it on TV. It gives a different perspective.'

### Step 4 Be flexible as you try to remember.
**Replay the incident backwards and forwards until your mind finds a clue that leads to the critical image: where you put your keys.**

Our brains have remarkable abilities to revisit our memories, backwards and forwards, from above and in freeze-frame. The memories are there – but we have to be flexible in how we hunt for them. After the witness describes the scene and event, Sweet asks him to 'rewind' the 'mind movie' to the place where he has the clearest picture of the suspect. Then, she asks him to freeze-frame it in his mind.

### Step 5 Don't rush yourself. Let the memory come to you.
**You will eventually remember; have patience.**

Creating a sketch takes an average of 2 hours. Some take considerably longer. Mostly, you can't rush memory and expect good results.

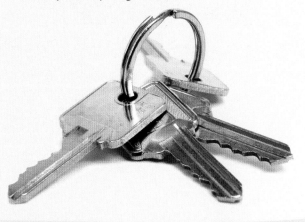

**Why does my mind sometimes go blank when I try to introduce people I know perfectly well? This happened once when I was shopping with my best friend, and met another friend. I looked at the two of them, realised I couldn't remember either of their names, and finally said, 'Would you two please introduce yourselves?' Why did this happen?**

**PROF. ROBERT LOGIE:** The information was encoded firmly in your brain; the problem was with retrieving it. It could be that spotting your other friend surprised you, or you worried about how to handle the situation, and the emotion temporarily jammed your retrieval system. This is totally normal.

Now, here's the bad news: because this has happened to you and the experience was embarrassing, any situation that requires introductions could become a source of anxiety. Then, the brain 'jam' could happen again and again. It is an everyday form of stage fright. Like any actor, try to rehearse your 'lines' as you see the scenario about to unfold, and you'll be fine.

following the event and for several days, if not weeks, afterwards. So there is a very large amount of repeated recall over an extended period, and this in itself can guarantee a vivid memory.'

Flashbulb memory is also influenced by expertise and interest in a subject. In a study Professor Logie and colleagues conducted with Professor Martin Conway (now at the University of Leeds, West Yorkshire), they found that interest in politics was a major factor in whether people had flashbulb memories a year after they heard the news that Margaret Thatcher had resigned as the UK's prime minister. People with a serious interest in politics, regardless of their political views, could remember very accurately what they were doing just before they heard the news, who they were with, and a host of other details normally forgotten.

People with a limited political interest didn't have these kinds of vivid memories, nor did people outside the UK.

# RECALL ON DEMAND

Once the new tracks of a memory are laid down and reinforced by focus and repetition, you still need a way to recall it. If memory is a path in the woods, retrieval is finding the correct path. But there are hundreds of billions of different pathways. Most people worry when they can't locate a specific recollection, but given the vast multitude of pathways in our heads, the real mystery is how we ever manage to remember anything at all.

'It's a matter of retracing our steps, and feeding in other general information that we have,' says Professor Logie. 'Recalling memories is basically "reconstructing memories". But the route to a piece of information you want isn't a straight line. We use cues and associations to help us navigate through the memory pathways. If you cannot remember the name of the actress who played Iris Murdoch as she progressed into Alzheimer's disease in the 2001 film, for example, the first thing that might come to mind is that Jim Broadbent was her co-star, then that Kate Winslet played the young Iris in the film. Next you might recall that the actress also played "M" in later James Bond films, and this finally – aha! – triggers the memory for the name Judi Dench. In the brain, that roundabout circuit could be completed in a split second. You'd probably not even be aware that it was a path-finding process at all.'

## WHY MEMORY IS FALLIBLE

As much as we would like to think that our recollections are accurate 'photographs' of events, they are more like impressionist paintings. Here's why.
● **Perception.** We all remember events differently because we perceive them in different ways in the first place. At your last family reunion, did you have a bad cold? If so, perhaps you remember the food as tasting rather bland, while your sister thought it was the best dinner she'd had for a while. Were you sitting at the end of the table, or in the middle? Your location affects which conversations you hear. Your sensory memory is unique and can never be replicated by anyone else, and it strongly colours your version of reality.
● **Interpretation.** If your uncle gave a long, impassioned political monologue, how you remember it will depend on whether you agreed with his viewpoint. If your cousin made an observation about a new exhibit at the museum, you're more likely to remember it if you believe your cousin knows what she's talking about. Your emotions, experiences and memories will all cause you to interpret events in your own unique way, and therefore skew how you remember them.
● **Recall.** Memories are not set in stone. The process of calling up the information from its disparate locations in the brain sometimes requires the brain to fill in blank spots. Consider this story: a woman was going through a family photo album with her mother. They came to a picture of a young girl on a pony, and the woman launched into her vivid memory of that day. 'But, darling,' her mother said, 'that's your sister. You weren't even born then.' The woman had seen the photo previously, assumed it was her, and her brain had filled in the details.

## brain HiCCUPS

### Missing the point – and the car

I needed to drop off my car at the garage for a minor repair in the middle of the day. My colleague Amanda offered to follow me to the garage, then take me back to work. Another colleague said she would come too. At the appointed time, we met at Amanda's office. Then we all got into her car and set out for the garage. When we were nearly there (gabbing the whole way), Amanda asked if I needed a ride back to the garage later to pick up my car. We both suddenly spun round and cried, 'We don't have the car!' We laughed so much that she nearly drove off the road.

# WISDOM, CREATIVITY & INTELLIGENCE

## the mechanics

**Chemical reactions, electrical impulses, grey matter, neurons – this is the language of neurologists.** They can explain the brain inside and out, from cells to lobes to hemispheres and back. But what about the elusive questions human beings have been asking for millennia about intelligence, creativity and wisdom?

What is intelligence? Where does creativity come from? What makes us truly wise? The answers don't lie in any single neuron or any single nerve pathway or any single place in the brain.

To understand these complex issues, we have to rely on psychology to make the connection between the physical brain and the intangible mind. While we may never be able to solve all of the brain's mysteries, experts are hard at work piecing together theories to explain these higher-order cognitions. In other words, they are thinking hard about the whole thought process.

# INTELLIGENCE: NOT JUST A NUMBER

In psychological circles, the nature and essence of intelligence has generated more theories than the origin of the universe. The debate didn't start with the invention of the infamous IQ (Intelligence Quotient) test, but that method of measurement certainly ramped it up. Since then, the discussion – who's clever? Who's not? Does intelligence come from our genes? – has become one of the most heated of academic disputes.

Over 100 years ago, the psychologist Alfred Binet devised a test of intelligence quotient, or IQ, as a means of identifying which students would benefit from extra help at school. Over the ensuing years, society latched on to IQ as a precise measure of overall intelligence. But, of course, there's much more to intelligence than one number could ever suggest. (Albert Einstein's IQ may have been estimated at 160, but it's well known that he failed his university entrance exams the first time he took them, for example.)

## NATURE OR NURTURE?

Researchers have theorised that intelligence is entirely inherited … entirely developed … 50 per cent inherited and 50 per cent developed. Some say intelligence is found all over the brain, others that it exists in specific brain locations only … that it includes more than 60 different abilities or is a single entity, or that cognitive intelligence is a subset within a more global general intelligence … that it is the single factor responsible for thought or that it is just one of many different cognitive abilities.

Whatever the truth, research does suggest that intelligence is relatively stable throughout someone's lifespan. One study by Professor Ian Deary and colleagues at the University of Edinburgh traced more than a thousand people born in 1936 whose IQ had been measured at age 11 as part of the Scottish Mental Survey in 1947. When they gave these individuals the same test at age 70, they found a strong correlation between childhood IQ and cognitive ability in later life.

This influence was far stronger than that of other factors, including people's own educational or occupational attainment and their fathers' social class. But neither intelligence nor background ensure either success or happiness. What also counts, it seems, is what we do with that intelligence and how much effort we put into exercising it during our lives.

As the researchers conclude, 'though social background may provide opportunities for educational and occupational attainment, the individual must embrace and pursue them in order for the effects of those opportunities to be realised. In fact, it may be that individual action has the strongest effects on late life cognitive function.'

This strongly suggests that learning new skills and knowledge, as well as using the various methods of improving your memory demonstrated in this book, can help your brain to work much more efficiently as you get older. There are many ways to develop and maintain your brainpower over the course of a lifetime.

## brain HiCCUPS

### Wrong number
I did something so stupid the other day when my friend left his mobile phone on my kitchen table. I knew he would miss it because it's the only phone he uses. So I called him to remind him that he had left it behind. It gave me such a scare when the phone on my table rang.

What's clear also is that there are different forms of intelligence, ranging from the erudition of a professor to the physical genius of the athlete. 'Not all intelligence is in the head,' writes Harvard professor Howard Gardner, explaining his mission to explore, identify and define its specific realms. After years of analysis, and using a strict set of criteria, Dr Gardner identified a total of seven intelligences. To find out what they are, see 'The Seven Intelligences' on pages 44-45.

It's a good bet that another sign of intelligence – one we could actually see, if ever a sufficiently sensitive method of brain imaging were invented – would be the number of neuronal connections throughout the brain. Given that neurons can increase their connections, theoretically, it should be possible to increase intelligence well into old age.

# FROM INTELLIGENCE TO WISDOM

Intelligence includes the capacity for understanding and reasoning as well as the ability to learn and to use what is learned to reach your objectives. Although we value intelligence, the real measure of a person lies in his or her wisdom. Intelligence is raw and unripened. Wisdom, on the other hand, has been called the epitome of human excellence, an ancient and virtuous quality. If intelligence is knowing how to build a bomb, wisdom is knowing how to build a bomb, understanding the ramifications of using it, and being able to solve problems in such a way that the bomb is not needed.

Cognitive neuroscientists distinguish what they call 'fluid intelligence' – our ability to solve problems, think creatively and deal with novelty – from 'crystallised intelligence', which applies to the knowledge and experience that we accumulate over a lifetime (what might be considered as 'wisdom'). Whereas fluid intelligence does reduce somewhat during adulthood, starting in the early 20s, crystallised intelligence generally improves with age.

*Continued on page 47*

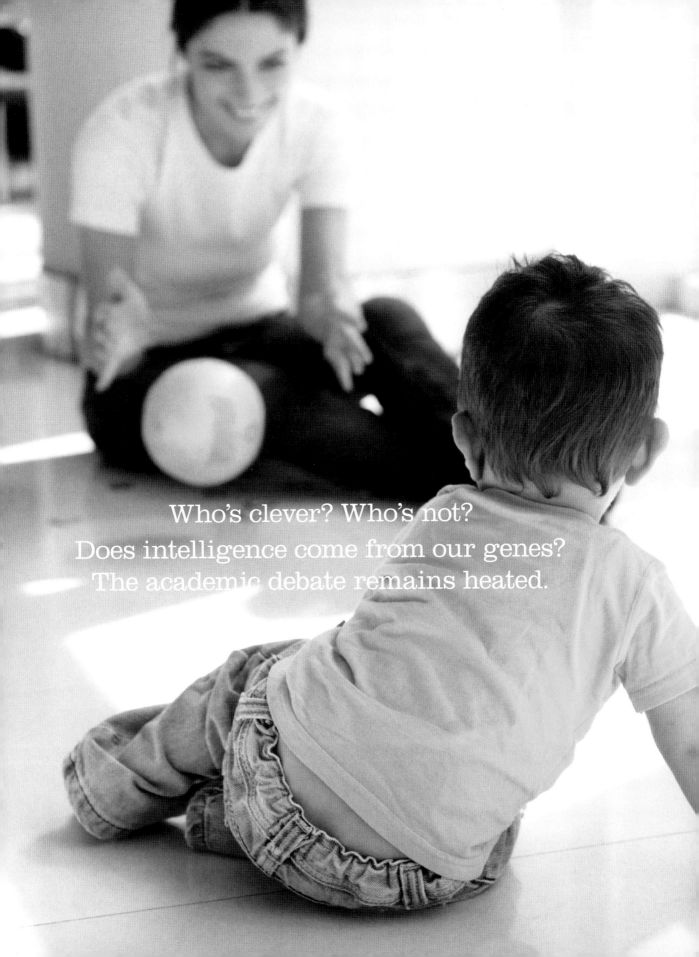

Who's clever? Who's not?
Does intelligence come from our genes?
The academic debate remains heated.

# THE SEVEN intelligences

To deconstruct what we commonly describe as intelligence is to recognise that every person's contribution to society is unique – and valuable. No one person has all the skills or the learning needed to accomplish society's tasks, but together we are complete. Think of the different intelligences as colours, which can stand alone or be combined, made stronger or lighter, intensified or subdued. It takes only red, blue and yellow to create the entire spectrum of colour. Just think what could be created by the seven intelligences.

## 1 LINGUISTIC intelligence

**Brain location** Left hemisphere in right-handed people (often the reverse in left-handers)

**Who has it most?** Poets, writers, orators, many lawyers

**What it's good for** Just about everyone can speak, but some people elevate language to an art. Some of Winston Churchill's speeches come to mind. This type of intelligence is also displayed by writers and every silver-tongued devil you've ever met. Shakespeare is arguably the ultimate genius in this category. The average English-speaker uses 4,000 words. Shakespeare had a working vocabulary of 29,000 words. He also coined more than 1,700 new words, including many we use today, such as 'amazement', 'gloomy', 'zany' and 'equivocal'.

**Recipe for improvement** Doing a lot of reading can definitely build your vocabulary and lift your linguistic skills.

## 2 LOGICAL-MATHEMATICAL intelligence

**Brain location** Frontal and parietal lobes

**Who has it most?** Scientists, engineers, statisticians

**What it's good for** Even our common expressions recognise the genius of the science whizz: 'He's a rocket scientist!' You might almost call this the classic form of genius; it's the kind of intelligence that would show up on an IQ test. People with high levels of logical-mathematical intelligence can gather and consolidate information quickly. They tend to be methodical and organised.

**Recipe for improvement** Many of the puzzles in Part 4 help to strengthen logic as well as number skills. Give them a try. And practise your everyday number skills by calculating in your head rather than on your calculator.

## 3 SPATIAL intelligence

**Brain location** Right hemisphere in right-handed people (often the left hemisphere in left-handed people)

**Who has it most?** Sculptors, airline pilots, architects, theoretical physicists

**What it's good for** At its most basic level, spatial ability means being able to get from your house to the supermarket and back without being confused. But people who are really gifted seem to possess an internal GPS system that tells them precisely where they are in the universe at all times.

**Recipe for improvement** Look for puzzles that ask you to envisage how a piece of paper with patterns on it will look when folded to form a box. Beyond that, your best bet may be to buy a GPS.

## 4 INTRAPERSONAL intelligence

**Brain location** Temporal lobes

**Who has it most?** Philosophers, psychologists, theologians, writers

**What it's good for** Intrapersonal intelligence is about self-knowledge, being fully in touch with your inner self – your emotions, beliefs and the precise tremor and bias of your moral compass. High intrapersonal intelligence allows us to navigate through the world without losing our sense of self, to rebound from setbacks, and to appreciate fully our fellow human beings.

**Recipe for improvement** Keep a diary. More important, look with a fresh eye back on pages you wrote long ago and reflect on what they tell you about yourself.

## 5 INTERPERSONAL intelligence

**Brain location** Frontal lobes

**Who has it most?** Salesmen, teachers, social workers, good managers

**What it's good for** People with strong interpersonal skills understand non-verbal communication and are able to read the character, emotions and desires of others. This is a unique form of problem-solving that is not as easily measured as other types of intelligence, but is critical to social success. All good leaders are interpersonal geniuses. These gifts can also be used for dark purposes by con artists.

**Recipe for improvement** Practise noticing other people's reactions to your words, your body language, your tone of voice. Then try reading other people by noting their body language and tone.

## 6 MUSICAL intelligence

**Brain location** Right hemisphere (or often the left in left-handed people)

**Who has it most?** Composers, musicians

**What it's good for** Music is a form of communication, crossing countries, cultures and even species – birds and whales are just two species that speak through 'song'. People with high levels of musical intelligence can find meaning in the rhythm, tempo, pattern, pitch and tone of music. They often show signs of musical ability early in life and seem to grasp intuitively the mathematics behind the notes. Some can pick up an instrument and play it with barely any training; it's as if they instinctively know how to speak the language of music. At the

other end are those who avoid karaoke bars like the plague, the ones you'll find silently mouthing the words to 'Happy Birthday' to keep from throwing everyone else off-key.

**Recipe for improvement** A talent for music is something you either have or you don't, so it's difficult to improve. But learning to play an instrument can't hurt.

## 7 PHYSICAL intelligence

**Brain location** Motor cortex

**Who has it most?** Athletes, dancers

**What it's good for** Although movement comes naturally to just about everyone, exceptional physical grace and athleticism involve their own kind of intelligence. Controlled movements are expressive and productive – consider that one of the common tests of intelligence in other species is whether they have the ability to use tools. We are fascinated by dancers and awed by superior athletes. Conversely, we often good-naturedly mock those who are lacking in coordination skills.

**Recipe for improvement** Some people are simply more physically gifted than others. But staying active will keep your sense of balance intact and improve your posture, which helps to impart physical grace.

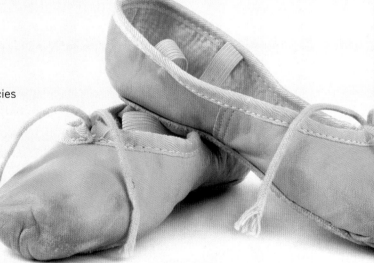

# How wise ARE YOU?

To get an idea of where you stand on the wisdom spectrum, read each statement below and check the appropriate response.

**1** I often reminisce about my past and am amazed at how far I've come.
☐ True ☐ False

**2** Teasing is never appropriate.
☐ True ☐ False

**3** Everyone is capable of dishonesty and hypocrisy.
☐ True ☐ False

**4** I wear my emotions on my sleeve – if I'm upset, anxious or sad, people know it.
☐ True ☐ False

**5** Before an election, I like to hear what all the parties stand for before coming to a decision about how to vote.
☐ True ☐ False

**6** When I think back to my most embarrassing moments, I still feel mortified.
☐ True ☐ False

**7** History is most interesting for what it can teach us about our lives today.
☐ True ☐ False

**8** I think it's important to form a strong opinion – waffling is a sign of weakness.
☐ True ☐ False

**9** I easily adjust my emotions to fit with the needs of the moment – it's not always necessary to let people know when I'm upset, anxious or sad.
☐ True ☐ False

**10** I make decisions effortlessly, often on gut instinct.
☐ True ☐ False

**11** I enjoy having religious discussions with people of different faiths.
☐ True ☐ False

**12** If someone told me a lie, it would change my opinion of that person for ever.
☐ True ☐ False

**13** I have experienced a lot of change in my life, and not all of it was positive.
☐ True ☐ False

**14** History is interesting as a story, but has little relevance to my life today.
☐ True ☐ False

**15** I have opinions, but I am always interested in hearing other points of view.
☐ True ☐ False

**16** When I try to express my emotions, I often lose control.
☐ True ☐ False

**17** I laugh easily and often.
☐ True ☐ False

**18** I quickly become annoyed when people challenge my opinion.
☐ True ☐ False

**19** I take my time before making a decision, often consulting many sources of information.
☐ True ☐ False

**20** I have lived a charmed life, without much conflict or many dilemmas.
☐ True ☐ False

**21** I've lived through a lot, and I've had to make some difficult and uncomfortable decisions.
☐ True ☐ False

**22** I'm a happy person – I never feel angry or annoyed.
☐ True ☐ False

**23** It's easy for me to laugh at my most embarrassing moments.
☐ True ☐ False

**24** I hate it when people have a laugh at my expense.
☐ True ☐ False

**25** Teasing can be a sign of affection.
☐ True ☐ False

**26** My life has turned out exactly the way I thought it would.
☐ True ☐ False

In some ways, wisdom is like beauty – we value it, we desire it, we know it when we see it, but it is nearly impossible to pin down such an ethereal quality. Yet researchers have tried.

In the late 1980s, the Berlin Wisdom Project at the Max Planck Institute for Human Development in Germany set out to define it. They came up with the following qualities, all of which a person must have to be considered truly wise.

✔ Intelligence and factual knowledge.
✔ A deep understanding of human nature, including an empathy for people who are different or from other cultures.
✔ Emotional resilience, or the capacity to rebound from a setback.
✔ Humility.
✔ The ability to learn from experience.
✔ Openness, or the maturity to be comfortable allowing the world to see you as you really are.
✔ Superior judgment and problem-solving skills.

Put this all together and what do you have? A portrait of someone who's been around the block. Wisdom accrues from experience, so it's fair to say, you need to be older to be wise. However, it should be pointed out: not all older people are wise. There are plenty who are painfully blinkered and set in their ways and their thinking.

In 2007, the psychologist Jeffrey Dean Webster, of Langara College in Vancouver, Canada, updated the work of the Berlin Wisdom Project, adding the notion that true wisdom could be measured only by what you did with it, both in terms of self-knowledge and the improvement of society at large. In other words, wisdom is there to be used. Webster's Self-Assessed Wisdom Scale (SAWS) on page 46 measures what he considered to be key traits of a wise person, including open-mindedness, the ability to control emotions, sense of humour, experience and the ability to learn from the past. How do you rate?

## PRACTICAL WAYS TO WISE UP

Almost everyone has the capacity to become wise, given the right mindset and a little effort. Wisdom requires a baseline of intelligence, but true wisdom is a mixture of balance (the ability to see all sides of an

## SCORING

Count the number of **TRUE** responses for **ODD-numbered** statements: ..............
Count the number of **FALSE** responses for **EVEN-numbered** statements: ..............
To get your Wisdom Score, add those two numbers together: ..............

## INTERPRETING YOUR SCORE

*0 to 4* Babe in the woods Best not to wander off alone
*5 to 9* Student Keep watching and learning
*10 to 14* Professor Wiser than most
*15 to 19* Leader People depend on your guidance
*20 to 26* Guru Consider setting up shop on top of a mountain

# MIND versus MACHINE

How does the human brain compare with a personal computer? See for yourself.

| | COMPUTER | | HUMAN BRAIN | |
|---|---|---|---|---|
| Processing speed | 60,000 million – or more – instructions per second | ✔ | About 100 million instructions – per second | |
| Work time | Unlimited, as long as plugged in | ✔ | Varies by person, but the brain tires relatively easily | |
| Memory capacity | A powerful desktop personal computer may have 1 million megabytes | | Unlimited | ✔ |
| Memory accessibility | Every megabyte is potentially accessible at any moment | ✔ | Can be difficult at times | |
| Computation | A 2GHz processor can calculate the value of pi to a million decimal places in 1 minute | ✔ | 30 million times slower than a computer | |
| Accuracy | Excepting a bug, computers are 100 per cent accurate | ✔ | The human brain makes many errors in all aspects of calculation and memory | |
| Adaptability | Once started on a processing problem, can't change unless redirected by a human | | Can change direction, task and action in an instant | ✔ |
| Creativity | Works on a binary system for processing information – either yes/no or on/off | | With at least 100 trillion neuron synapses, unlimited inventiveness is possible | ✔ |
| Energy efficiency | Computers use about a billion times more energy than the human brain | | Low energy needs – oxygen and glucose (blood sugar) | ✔ |
| Multi-tasking | Can work on multiple problems simultaneously and perform equally well on all | ✔ | Can work on several tasks at once – breathing, thinking, walking, chewing, etc. – but can focus directly on only one problem at a time | |
| Learning | Computers are programmed; they can't learn on the job unless the specific program enables them to do so, in a limited way | | Capable of learning from birth until death | ✔ |
| Free will and wisdom | No consciousness; no free will; can't learn, so incapable of wisdom | | Has consciousness and free will; can determine its own destiny; has vast potential for wisdom | ✔ |
| Imagination | Computers have no ability to dream or indulge in make-believe | | The human imagination knows no bounds | ✔ |

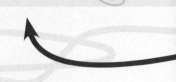

issue), open-mindedness, discipline and a concern for the greater good. There's no short cut to wisdom, but these strategies will lead you down the right path:

● **Read the newspaper.** You cannot make balanced choices unless you understand world circumstances and the experiences of others. If you don't already read a daily paper, start by going through a single front-page article, from start to finish, every day. Don't just scan or skip around it; read every word. Eventually, try to get through the main articles of a full newspaper every day. Most newspapers post their stories online, so you can have access to news from around the world virtually any time you want.

● **Find time for books.** While current events are important, both fiction and non-fiction books can help you expand your world view and allow you to explore new ideas and points of view.

● **Stay social.** Studies show that people who stay connected to others demonstrate higher levels of wisdom than those who are more isolated. Make an effort to join a club, sign up for Facebook, or invite an old friend or a new neighbour for coffee. And next time you're at a party or gathering, single out someone who's standing alone and start up a conversation. It's easy. Ask questions. ('Where are you from?' 'What kind of work do you do?') People generally love to talk about themselves. You, on the other hand, have the harder job: to listen closely.

● **Practise being more open-minded.** Wisdom is being able to understand all sides of an issue without letting emotions or personal feelings get in the way. Being open-minded means finding empathy and realising that everyone has a life story that influences their actions. During the course of every day, make a note of issues that get you hot under the collar, and take a moment to try to see the issue from the other side. No one needs to know.

● **Boost your self-knowledge.** You've learned a lot just by being alive, but have you taken the time to review all that you've learned? Try this exercise: write down your three biggest failures and your three greatest successes. For each, review the events that led up to it and what lessons you took away from the experience. Look for patterns. This is not a time for regret or pride; the goal is to learn to look at each experience, good or bad, as more fuel to enrich your wisdom.

● **Learn how to say these four important words: 'I could be wrong.'** A wise person understands that it is impossible to know everything and that life is capable of taking unexpected turns. Recognising your errors can lead only to greater wisdom – and admitting that there are times when you could be mistaken will go a long way in solidifying your reputation as someone whose advice can be trusted. As the Roman philosopher Cicero said, 'Any man is liable to err; only a fool persists in error'.

TOTALS... COMPUTER **6**     HUMAN BRAIN **7**

AND THE WINNER IS... **The human brain** – which also created and programmed the computer and harnessed the energy that drives it.

## Ask the
# MEMORY EXPERT...

**When I left home one morning, I set off on my usual route to work and when halfway there realised that it was a Saturday and I had intended to drive to the DIY shop instead as I needed to collect some paint for the bathroom we were redecorating. I obeyed all the traffic rules, stopping at junctions, signalling and allowing pedestrians to cross but could not remember doing any of this and was unaware that this was not the correct route today. How can the brain get us to carry out such complicated actions without us being able to remember or realise that we are going the wrong way?**

**PROF. ROBERT LOGIE:** You had completed the journey to work so many times that you were on autopilot. If we carry out the same actions many times over, we can do them almost without thinking. The network in your brain for the route is firmly established, and if the journey goes as normal, it does not use much of your conscious attention. If there had been a dramatic event, such as someone stopping very suddenly in front of you, or a diversion because of new roadworks, your brain would change to 'control' mode rather than 'automatic' mode. Being in automatic mode can be helpful for working efficiently, but it can also lead to everyday slips such as forgetting that you had actually intended to go to the DIY shop.

> We often overlook the importance of creativity in everyday life.

# EVERYONE CAN BE CREATIVE

Creativity is the most magical of the brain's skills. We trust that knowledge can be acquired and that wisdom will come to us with age. This seems to be true, according to Professor Logie. Fluid intelligence (see page 42) appears to be present at birth and has a major impact on how quickly we can learn. As people acquire skills and knowledge they gain new kinds of intelligence – or wisdom – linked to what they have learned. But creativity seems to be a gift bestowed upon only a few blessed individuals. It has proven more difficult to study than intelligence or wisdom.

Because creativity comes in flashes or floods, then dries up seemingly on its own, it is difficult to harness and nearly impossible to measure. As researchers from the University of Sydney, Australia, noted: ultimately, the only proven test for creativity is the creation itself.

Nevertheless, psychologists have uncovered some interesting facts about creativity. First, it's more evenly distributed than originally thought. Yes, some people are born with more creative gifts, but just about anyone can develop and nurture creativity at any age. Verdi, for example, composed his opera *Otello* aged 73 and *Falstaff* at 79.

Because creativity involves novel ways of thinking, it flourishes wherever originality is valued and individuals are encouraged to challenge traditional thoughts and styles. In other words, if you want to practise out-of-the-box thinking, you have to, well, step outside of the box.

## LETTING GO MAY BE KEY

What is the 'box' that often holds us back in our adult life? One view is that the primary limitation on creative expression is expectation. We expect or wish to be successful. We wish to make others laugh. We wish to please. But what if creativity surfaces only when you relinquish your expectations and start existing in the moment, like a child? Children play just to play, not to impress anyone. Consider then that creativity is simply about making a deeper connection with your creative force, surprising yourself, and letting go.

Creativity goes hand-in-hand with the arts – music, dance, theatre, film, writing, painting – but we often overlook its importance in everyday life. It is this ability that allows us to generate solutions to problems, to hold fresh conversations, and to plan for the future. For example, throwing a surprise party requires finding a creative way to spring the actual surprise. And plenty of us show remarkable creativity when it comes to talking our way out of a parking ticket or justifying to a partner why we simply had to buy yet another pair of shoes/set of golf clubs.

Creativity is just as strong in older people, but sometimes we have to be prompted to remember that it's OK to play the way we did when we were younger. Studies show that older people who are involved in creative activities are more likely to remain connected to the community, to suffer less debility over time, and to live generally healthier lives.

## FINDING YOUR CREATIVE SPARK

Creativity is about stretching your mind and coming up with solutions to unusual problems. To flex your creative muscle, try these exercises.

● Set a timer for 2 minutes and write down all the words you can think of that begin with the letter 'A'. Tomorrow, do the same for the letter 'B', and so on throughout the alphabet.

● For each of the following sentences, imagine what happens next. (There are no right or wrong answers.)

**1** A woman wearing a red hat knocks on the front door of a large, extravagant stone house. When the door opens …

**2** A man and a woman are out on a date, holding hands as they walk down a crowded city street. The woman looks up and gasps because …

**3** A young man moves to a new country with his family, but worries that he won't fit in and will never find friends. To his surprise, on the plane over, the person seated next to him …

# How your
# BRAIN AGES

**As we get older, our knees start to creak, our skin starts to sag, and our brains start to ... shrink?** That's right: between the ages of 20 and 70, brain weight and blood flow to the brain drop by 20 per cent. And the total number of fibres and nerves in the brain decreases by 37 per cent. Sounds scary?

Maybe, but the news isn't nearly as bad as you may think.

Many of these types of changes exert effects that are subtle, if they're noticeable at all. Most of us are still capable of learning – and remembering – most things at just about any age, though it may take us a little longer.

In addition, it's easy to compensate for any small cognitive losses that do occur. For example, just as wearing glasses can make up for a decline in vision, using the memory strategies described in Part 4 can compensate not only for declines in short-term (working memory), but also for declines in episodic memory and in prospective memory (remembering to do things that you had intended to do).

Do you want to take up the trombone at the age of 76? You can. Would you like, finally, to read the classics you always said you'd tackle some day? Go for it. Everything you learn to do in the rest of *A Sharp Brain for Life*, from spending time in the 'brain gym' to getting more exercise (which increases blood flow and promotes the formation of new brain cells and connections), will help you keep your brain as young as possible.

# AN HONEST ACCOUNTING

People over the age of 40 often worry about the state of their memory. We can be very hard on ourselves: one missed appointment, a forgotten phone number or two, and we panic. The truth is, most of us forget where we put things because our lives are too busy, we're trying to multi-task, we're too stressed or we didn't get enough sleep – not because we're losing our marbles. Some of us can also chalk up memory problems and dull thinking to a medical condition (see Brain Enemies: Medical Causes in Part 3).

We tend to expect a lot from our memory – maybe more than it actually needs to deliver. Page 13 of this book mentions a rare group of adults with total recall of every single day of their lives from adolescence onwards. Name a date, and these people can tell you what day of the week it was, what the weather was like, whom they met and what they ate that day. Would you want this kind of memory? Probably not. In fact, some of those who possess this talent describe it as more of an exhausting curse than a blessing.

Likewise, we may admire the sponge-like memories of children, but it would be a mistake to feel at a loss because we can't absorb new information as quickly as they can. Consider this: most of us don't worry that we can't turn cartwheels or jump over fences in a single bound any more. Children not only have amazing physical prowess, their little bodies, still malleable and forming, can do things most adults wouldn't want to try without a chiropractor standing by. Like our bodies, our brains have also

changed, becoming slightly less agile – but who really cares, as long as we can still perform the tasks we need to?

## WHAT GETS WORSE

So, what is normal for an ageing brain? Researchers tell us that we can expect slight declines in the following four areas.

● **Short-term memory.** For reasons that science has not been able to pinpoint, our short-term memory, also called working memory – the type that enables us to remember what we are doing from moment to moment – generally gets worse with age. Older adults have fantastic long-term memories, able to recall details about childhood friends, the town they grew up in, and films they saw during secondary school, but they may

## IT'S NOT ALL DOWNHILL

As with most things in life, getting older means you win some and you lose some. Here's the score card:

**Usually better with age**
● Long-term memory
● Emotional memory
● Untimed memory tests
● Wisdom

**Generally worse with age**
● Short-term memory
● Timed memory tests
● Speed of processing
● Reaction time
● Focus
● Multi-tasking

**Usually no change with age**
● Creativity
● Memory for important information

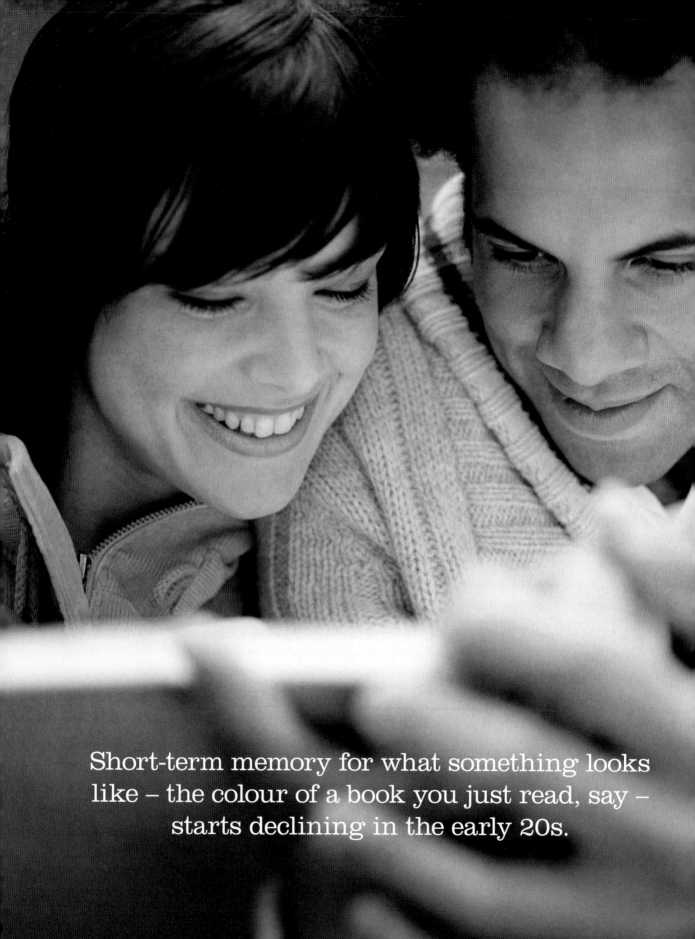

Short-term memory for what something looks like – the colour of a book you just read, say – starts declining in the early 20s.

forget whether they just swallowed the blue pill or the white pill, or whether the car that passed them a few seconds ago was green or red, or where they put down their glasses just moments earlier.

There are different kinds of short-term memory for visual and verbal material. Short-term memory for what something looks like starts declining in the early 20s – what colour was that book I just read, or where did my golf ball land? In contrast, short-term memory for verbal material – words, letters and numbers, for example, or remembering the sequence of a phone number until you dial it – tends to improve during adulthood and, assuming there is no underlying dementia or other problem such as depression, does not start to decline until well into retirement, when it drops off at a much slower rate.

Short-term memory is a temporary memory pathway that lasts only a few seconds and does not involve growth of dendrites, the connections between nerve cells. To grow connections in order to retain information, you need to pay attention to it and actively try to learn it. However, if you know a great deal about a topic, this will boost your short-term memory for information related to that subject. Professor Peter Morris at the University of Lancaster showed this in a study with soccer fans. When they were given the scores of real matches, they were extremely good at recalling them. But they were no better than soccer novices at remembering random scores.

So, while working or short-term memory capacity for information that is new and unrelated to something you know about may deteriorate with age, if you develop an expertise, your short-term memory for information related to that subject will improve. And the more expertise you gain as you get older, the better it will be.

● **Episodic memory.** When we have multiple memories of similar events or places, our brain creates related pathways that contain information specific to each particular event or episode. This is episodic memory and, in time, memories of each event merge to become part of our self-knowledge – for example, of the town we grew up in or the face of an old

We tend to expect a lot from our memory – maybe more than it actually needs to deliver.

friend. Such long-term memory for facts, known as semantic memory, is generally retained with age. But we are likely to remember specific details from a single occasion only if it was important to us – our wedding day, or the day we moved into a new house, for example.

Memories of other occasions tend to fade – you are unlikely to remember what happened on an ordinary weekend ten years ago or what you had for breakfast on the first Tuesday in June 1995. And such episode-specific information tends to get lost more often as we get older – so you may not remember what you had for breakfast yesterday. This explains why older people can usually remember events from their distant past, but often cannot remember what they did a few days ago.

The good news: although visual short-term memory and episodic memory tend to decline with age, as does prospective memory (remembering to do things in future), semantic memory – or knowledge – improves as we get older. This can often compensate for the declines in visual short-term and episodic memory.

● **Focus.** We also lose some of our ability to focus our attention, a problem that might mean it takes longer to read a book. We are more easily distracted by competing cries for attention, so reading a book with the television on can be challenging for some, impossible for others. Older adults also have a harder time multi-tasking.

● **Speed.** As we get older, our reaction time and the speed at which we process information both slow down. This means that not only do our brains sift through information more slowly, but our bodies also react more slowly.

It is important to be vigilant and make sure, for instance, that these normal changes don't affect your ability to drive or perform other tasks that require split-second reactions. In those cases, it's best to understand that slowness isn't necessarily an impediment. But most of the things we do are not potentially life threatening.

In timed tests of knowledge, younger adults do better than older adults, but take away the time factor and older adults do better. You can compensate for any slowdown by allowing more time to learn and remember things that matter to you.

## PACE YOURSELF

Most of us can deal with learning a little more slowly as we age or having to turn off the TV while we're trying to read. Our real fear is that the little brain hiccups we all experience are the first symptoms of Alzheimer's disease or another form of dementia. This kind of worry may be worse than the actual forgetfulness.

But these are the facts: only about 5 per cent of men and women aged 65 to 74 have Alzheimer's disease. The numbers do go up after 75, to 16 per cent, though experts are not sure why there is this increase with age. But dementia doesn't necessarily have anything to do with being old, and not everyone who lives until old age will develop dementia.

The brain changes that take place in dementia are quite different from those of normal, healthy ageing. This is one reason why the word 'senile' is a far from accurate term for memory decline, as the root meaning of the word literally refers to old age. Instead, scientific experts have divided memory decline into three broad categories: normal age-associated forgetfulness, mild cognitive impairment (MCI) and dementia.

● **Those annoying brain hiccups.** Age-associated forgetfulness describes the normal state of having brief 'senior moments', when your short-term memory becomes weaker and, well, shorter. By the age of 60, about 40 per cent of us will experience this problem.

What causes it? As mentioned earlier, neurons shrink and die off, which decreases the number of synaptic contact points – those all-important brain-cell connections. We also produce smaller amounts of the brain chemicals called neurotransmitters, which allow communication to take place, and reduced levels of the hormones that support healthy brain function. Blood flow is reduced in all portions of the brain, but most strikingly in the frontal cortex, which is where our thinking, planning and speaking abilities reside.

This is a normal part of ageing, no worse than that mild ache you may feel in your knees. These age-related brain changes explain why we forget that appointment or have trouble coming up with the right word during a conversation. Mild forgetfulness is all part of the normal wear-and-tear of ageing, much of which can be compensated for.

● **When it's more serious.** Unlike the everyday forgetfulness described above, mild cognitive impairment suggests

have memory problems that they simply can't cover up. These problems are serious enough to be noticeable to others and significantly change their ability to function in the world. They may forget how to cook, have trouble dressing themselves, and feel lost even in familiar surroundings.

Some dementias can be reversed, particularly if they have been caused by dietary deficiencies, a medical disorder (such as diabetes, depression or liver disease), or a side effect of a medication. Alzheimer's disease and similar types of dementia are irreversible today – though

Mild forgetfulness is a normal part of ageing, no worse than the mild ache you may feel in your knees.

a deeper problem. Typical symptoms include regularly forgetting things you really should remember, such as doctor's appointments or a weekly card game, frequently misplacing items and having difficulty following a conversation.

People with this condition are often aware that they're slipping, but possess the intelligence and social skills to cover mistakes so well that others may not notice. But this could be an early-warning sign of impending dementia and, like dementia, has a range of causes, some of which are reversible. Some people with MCI do go on to develop dementia but many don't. Elsewhere in the book, you'll find plenty of advice on memory techniques and aids to help symptoms, reducing their interference in your life.

● **When it's much more serious.** People who are described as having dementia

there's evidence that a combination of proper medication, nutrition and a fitness programme, can help to mitigate the symptoms.

# FOR MOST OF US, THE BEST IS YET TO COME

If the older brain is not quite as agile as it once was, it has just as much capacity as the young brain. Remember that although in timed tests of knowledge, younger adults do better than most older adults, if you take away the time factor, older adults do better. Plus, those lab tests of memory skill tend to ask subjects to study and spit back lists of words or numbers. That's a small part of the total cognitive picture.

# NORMAL or NOT?

The majority of us worry about the state of our brains at one time or another. But most of the time, our cognitive slips are perfectly normal. The main problem is knowing whether you should laugh it off or see a doctor. Here's how to tell a routine brain hiccup from a matter of serious concern.

| PROBABLY NORMAL | SEE A DOCTOR |
| --- | --- |
| You feel forgetful, but your family and friends don't notice it. | Your family and friends tell you that they are worried about your forgetfulness. |
| Sometimes you struggle to find the word you were looking for. | You often lose words and have to use substitutes or change the subject to avoid embarrassment. |
| You can come up with examples of times when you felt your forgetfulness was worrying. | You know that you've been forgetful, but you can't remember details – you forget what it was you forgot. |
| You enjoy seeing friends at your usual level. Socialising is fun and enjoyable. | You avoid social activities because you're afraid that you'll do something embarrassing. |
| You find it difficult to learn how to use new appliances or electronic devices. | You find it impossible to learn to use new appliances, and you even find it difficult to use the old ones. |
| You frequently lose your car keys. | You look at a key and can't remember how to use it. |
| You walk into a room and forget why you went there. | You forget how to find the kitchen in your own home. |
| You forget the name of a person you were just introduced to. | You forget the name of a family member. |
| You momentarily forget the name of a close friend. | You don't remember the person who says he or she is your friend. |
| You put the paper towels in the refrigerator and the milk in the cupboard and have a good laugh about it. | You frequently have no idea where things are supposed to go. |
| Mornings can be hectic, and you sometimes find it difficult to leave the house on time because you misplaced your belt or forgot to set the alarm clock. | People comment because you leave the house without showering or because your clothes are dishevelled. |
| You take a wrong turn on the way to your favourite food shop, or get momentarily lost in familiar territory. | You sometimes leave home and can't find your way back. |
| You forget to go to your dentist appointment. | You forget to go to your daughter's wedding. |
| If asked, you could give details about yesterday's dinner or your most recent phone call. It might take a while, but you can do it. | You have difficulty remembering recent events. Or you may not recall them at all. |

Older adults do much better on tests of semantic knowledge, such as vocabulary tests or general knowledge, than they do on episodic or working memory tests.

Also, studies led by Professor Louise Phillips at the University of Aberdeen and Professor Matthias Kliegel at the University of Dresden, Germany, have revealed a curious paradox. In laboratory settings, young people generally outperform older people in tests of prospective memory – remembering to do things. But when tested in more naturalistic settings, such as their own homes, older adults actually do better than younger adults, especially when there is emotional or social importance attached to 'remembering to remember'.

Why this is so is not entirely clear, but it may in part be because a familiar environment supplies more of the cues used for prospective memory. Also, older people more often spontaneously use reminders, such as Post-it notes and diaries – just the kind of memory techniques that you'll learn about in this book – whereas younger people tend to rely totally on their memory, which may be better but is still fallible.

Scientists can't even come close to measuring the true intricacy – and deep reserves – of the older brain. Cognitive neuroscientists who study memory not only in the lab but also in everyday real-life settings know a great deal about what the older brain is capable of as well as where its limitations lie.

'As people get older, their life experience and well-honed skills make them capable of so much more than many of them imagine. The trick is to gather experience and skills throughout life to make it interesting no matter how old we are,' says Professor Logie.

● **Give yourself credit.** The first step in fighting brain decline is applauding the amazing potential you already possess. Another way to put it: you're probably in better shape than you think. In fact, sometimes, what feels like deterioration is actually something much more benign: mental laziness. We forget a name because we've just not made the effort to learn it.

In timed tests of knowledge, younger adults do better, but take away the time factor, and older adults win.

● **Take action.** The single key lesson is this: use it or lose it. Flex those mental muscles in order to preserve your powers of attention, comprehension and recall. So, the all-important second step in fighting brain decline is to decide consciously to do something about it. By reading this book, you've already begun.

● **Apply some grit and determination.** The third step: use a little elbow grease. This book aims to arm you with the most up-to-date advice on keeping your brain fit, capable and ready for action. In Parts 2 and 3, you can read specific brain-improving lifestyle tips, then, in Part 4, use the Brain Fitness Programme, which includes specially designed exercises and strategies to increase your brainpower.

Yes, you're being asked to do some work, but this sort of work is more like play. It's time to get started.

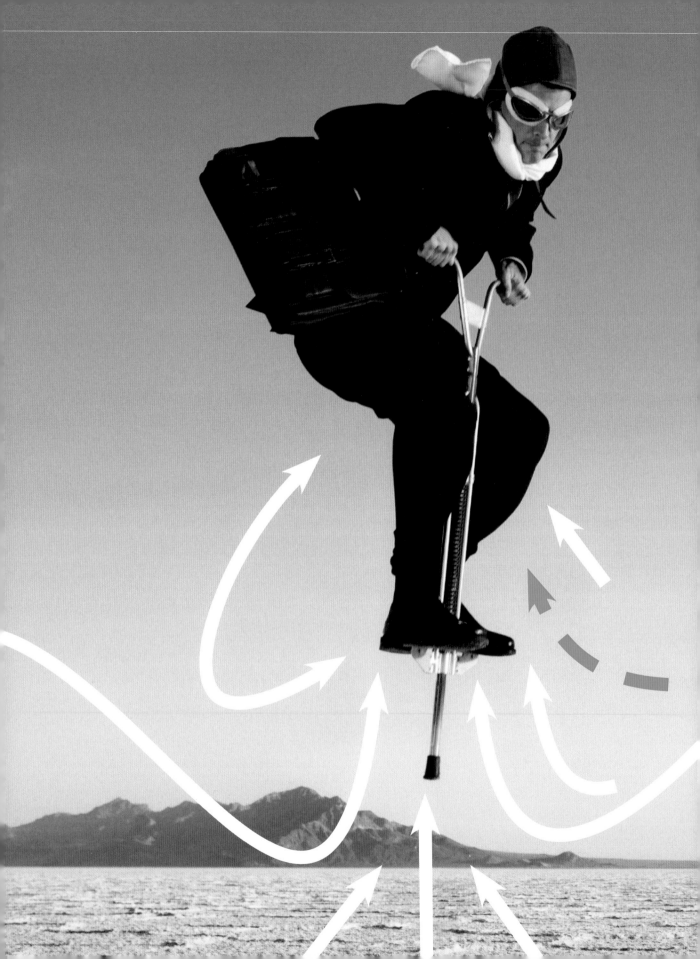

# FIVE BRAIN
# BOOSTERS

part 2

# BOOSTER 1

## Diet

Everyone knows by now that greasy burgers
are bad for the heart, while a meal of grilled salmon
and sautéed greens is just what the doctor ordered.
If eating heart-healthy foods, along with getting plenty
of exercise, can slash your risk of heart disease, imagine
what a brain-healthy diet can do for your brain.

You probably never give your brain a thought as you push your trolley down the supermarket aisles, but in recent years a stack of ground-breaking research has shown that eating more of certain foods and less of others can significantly improve your memory and thinking skills and even cut your risk of cognitive decline.

The ingredients for a healthy brain are as close as your kitchen. In fact, if you open your fridge or food cupboard right now, you may well see at least five foods that can help to keep your brain healthy.

## FOODS FOR THOUGHT

Every single thing your brain does – every thought and emotion it has, every calculation it performs, every memory it summons – requires energy and nutrition you can get only from food. That means your ability to feel good, think clearly and keep your memory sharp depends to a large extent on what you eat for breakfast, lunch and dinner.

To find the best brain-healthy diet, consider your heart. Blood pumped from the heart delivers vital nutrients and oxygen to the brain, so it's logical that foods which benefit the heart and blood vessels are also good for the brain. In fact, the surest dietary path to better brain health may start with an eating system that's well known for its heart benefits: the Mediterranean diet. Research shows that people who follow this traditional way of eating have a much lower risk of

The ingredients for a healthy brain
are as close as your kitchen.

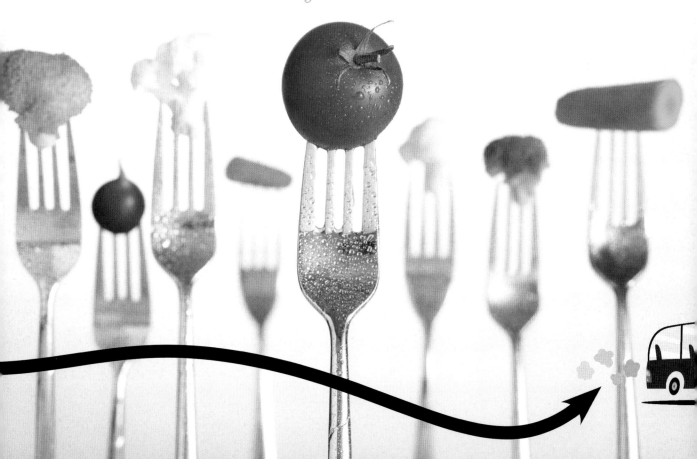

heart disease, heart attack and stroke. It helps control cholesterol, blood pressure and inflammation, all of which contribute to heart disease. But that's not all.

Neuroscientist Catherine Féart and colleagues from the University of Bordeaux in France examined the effects of a Mediterranean diet on the risk of age-related cognitive decline in 1,410 people all aged 65 or over at the start of the study. They scored each person from 0 to 9 depending on how well their food intake accorded with the Mediterranean diet. At the five-year follow-up, they found that higher adherence to a Mediterranean diet was associated with slower cognitive decline on a standard test of mental functioning, even after taking into account other factors including age, cardiovascular risk and physical activity.

What's more, strictly adhering to this type of diet has been linked to increased longevity and a lower risk of chronic diseases. Imagine living longer, keeping your mind sharp, your memory keen, your reasoning sound and your thinking clear – all because you ate the way you would on a holiday to the Greek Islands.

## Red wine contains flavonoids and other antioxidants with known health benefits.

### BOOZE FOR THE BRAIN?

Moderate red wine intake may contribute to the cardiovascular benefits of the Mediterranean diet – red wine contains flavonoids and other antioxidants with known health benefits. Some studies suggest that alcohol may also protect the brain, but results have been inconsistent – perhaps because both non-drinkers and heavy drinkers have a higher risk of cognitive decline than more moderate consumers. A study of more than 1,000 older people, carried out at the University of São Paulo, Brazil, found that those with mild-to-moderate alcohol use had the best cognitive function scores and lower rates of both cognitive impairment and dementia compared with non-drinkers. But heavy alcohol use was associated with increased cognitive impairment and dementia. Research by the University of Oslo in Norway suggests that the maximum benefit occurs with a wine intake of 75ml-100ml per day.

What this means in practice is consuming plenty of whole-grain foods, fruits and vegetables (picture a Greek salad made with tomatoes, cucumbers and onions), fish (often grilled), olive oil, nuts and low-fat dairy products, such as low-fat yoghurt. Meat, poultry and sweets are eaten only occasionally and are not a necessary part of daily meals.

## THE SHARP BRAIN DIET

We know the Mediterranean diet works, but is it enough to protect the brain?

It's certainly an excellent start, and a key part of the Sharp Brain Diet, which translates current research knowledge into a straightforward eating programme.

The Sharp Brain Diet is easy to follow because it works on a principle of add, switch, drop. That is, you get to add plenty of new foods to your menu selections, switch to brain-healthy choices instead of many of the less-healthy foods you currently eat, and drop the foods that are downright dangerous for brain health. And you can do it all in just a few simple steps.

# BOOST YOUR THINKING POWER WITH 'BRAIN FATS'

In the past 200,000 years or so, the human brain underwent a critical change: it grew larger in terms of volume and intelligence. Early human beings who lived near water experienced the biggest brain advances, and some scientists think they know why: seafood. Specifically, the fat contained in seafood, known as omega-3 fatty acids, nature's ultimate brain food.

Remember that your brain contains a high proportion of fat, not only in the membranes around the cells that regulate what gets in and out, but also in the myelin, an insulating layer around each of the nerve cells, the brain's high-speed communication cables.

Fat, therefore, is the single most important nutrient for protecting and preserving brain function. But it has to be the right sort of fat – omega-3s, which are crucial components of the cell membranes around our neurons.

Other dietary fats don't have the same effect. A steady diet of cheese-burgers, for instance, which are packed with unhealthy saturated fats, far from sharpening your cognitive skills could actually dull them by clogging up your arteries so that less oxygen and fewer nutrients reach your brain.

## 9 RULES FOR A SMARTER DIET

1 **ADD** foods rich in omega-3 fatty acids.
2 **SWITCH** to olive oil for cooking and in dressings.
3 **DROP** all foods that contain trans fats.
4 **ADD** more fruits and vegetables.
5 **SWITCH** to whole grains.
6 **DROP** sugary or artificially sweetened foods and drinks.
7 **ADD** small portions of nuts and seeds.
8 **SWITCH** to fish and poultry (without skin) instead of fatty red and processed meats.
9 **DROP** saturated fat-laden pies, cakes, biscuits and crisps.

Eliminating fats is not a good idea, either. Many people trying to eat a low-fat diet for a healthy heart are actually skipping omega-3s as well, which can be very bad for the brain.

### TOO MANY OMEGA-6S

Because dietary advice is often confusing, other people have followed recommendations to substitute supposedly healthier polyunsaturated vegetable oils, such as corn or sunflower oil, for artery-clogging saturated fats. But these polyunsaturated oils contain high proportions of a different type of essential fatty acid, omega-6s. So most people on a typical Western diet now eat far too many omega-6s and not enough brain-boosting omega-3s. Flooding your brain with omega-6s from processed vegetable oils isn't ideal either.

What the brain craves most are the omega-3 fats. They play a crucial role in brain development, as well as repairing and preserving brain cells and enabling

# RATE YOUR diet

Answer the questions below to help you rate your current diet. Answer honestly; no one's looking except you.

**1** I eat this many different types of vegetable a day, not counting potatoes:
- ☐ **0** 0 or 1.
- ☐ **1** 2 or 3.
- ☐ **2** 4 or more.

**2** I eat broccoli, cauliflower, Brussels sprouts, kale, mustard greens, watercress, dark leafy greens such as spinach, cabbage or Swiss chard:
- ☐ **0** Rarely.
- ☐ **1** Once a week.
- ☐ **2** Several times a week.

**3** When I eat bread, it's:
- ☐ **0** White bread.
- ☐ **1** Usually a fibre-enriched white bread (but not wholemeal).
- ☐ **2** Usually a coarse 100 per cent whole-grain variety.

**4** When I have meat for dinner, it's usually:
- ☐ **0** Burgers, sausages or other minced or processed meats, or fatty meat such as lamb chops, streaky bacon or pork with crackling.
- ☐ **1** A lean cut of meat such as pork tenderloin or sirloin steak with the fat trimmed off before cooking.
- ☐ **2** A small serving, more of a flavour enhancer, such as small strips of lean beef or pork in a stir-fry.

**5** I like my chicken:
- ☐ **0** Coated in batter or breadcrumbs, deep-fried or with the skin on.
- ☐ **1** Pan-fried or roasted with a butter or cream sauce, or a rich gravy.
- ☐ **2** Baked, grilled or roasted, without skin, sauce or gravy.

**6** I usually cook with:
- ☐ **0** Lard, butter or dripping.
- ☐ **1** Margarine or spread, or vegetable oils containing hydrogenated fats.
- ☐ **2** Olive oil.

**7** I eat salmon, fresh tuna, sardines or mackerel:
- ☐ **0** Never.
- ☐ **1** At least once a month.
- ☐ **2** At least once a week.

**8** With a meal I'm most likely to have:
- ☐ **0** Pastry, white rice, white bread, regular pasta.
- ☐ **1** Potatoes or corn, or long grain and wild rice.
- ☐ **2** Brown rice, whole-grain bread, whole-wheat pasta, oats, pearl barley, bulghur wheat, quinoa.

**9** From the following list of foods – flaxseeds (linseeds) or flaxseed oil, avocados, pumpkin seeds, walnuts, blueberries, apples, spinach – I regularly eat:
- ☐ **0** 0 or 1.
- ☐ **1** 2 or 3.
- ☐ **2** 4 or more.

**10** When I snack, I tend to eat:
- ☐ **0** Crisps, biscuits, sweets or chocolate bars.
- ☐ **1** Crackers or granola bars.
- ☐ **2** Fresh fruit or vegetables, nuts or seeds.

**11** My drinks of choice are:
- ☐ **0** Cola, lemonade or other fizzy drinks, fruit squash.
- ☐ **1** Pure fruit juice, sweetened coffee or tea with milk.
- ☐ **2** Water, black tea, fruit or herbal teas (without sugar).

**12** I drink alcohol:
- ☐ **0** Liberally (more than two drinks a day for women or three for men).
- ☐ **1** Never.
- ☐ **2** In moderation.

the cells to deliver signals efficiently; they may even facilitate the growth of new cells. Studies show that without enough of them, the brain can't function properly. Over time, lack of omega-3s may even contribute to the development of age-related cognitive decline.

The Sharp Brain Diet aims to redress the balance by increasing the amount you eat of foods rich in omega-3s, including fish, walnuts and flaxseeds (linseeds).

## THE POWER OF OMEGA-3S

Omega-3s come in three varieties: DHA (docosahexaenoic acid), EPA (eicosapen-taenoic acid) and ALA (alpha-linolenic acid). Brain cells need all three kinds to maintain their structure. These fats are concentrated in the frontal lobe of the brain and are critical for clear thinking, organisation, alertness, learning and reasoning. Low levels have been linked to memory and learning problems.

Omega-3s also help to prevent blood clots, reducing the risk of heart disease and stroke, two conditions that affect brain health. The vital fats may even help to improve brain function simply by boosting the brain's blood flow. Fish is the best source of the brain-boosting oils, but all fish are not created equal. So-called 'oily fish' (salmon, fresh tuna, mackerel, trout, sardines, pilchards and herring – think kippers) are packed with omega-3s, while white fish (cod, plaice, haddock) have much less. What's more, the type of omega-3s found in vegetable sources including walnuts and flaxseeds aren't as easy for the brain to use.

## Have fish twice a week.

### EAT WELL

● **Have fish twice a week.** You don't need to spend a lot of time, money or effort; even canned salmon, sardines, pilchards and mackerel count. Just make sure that at least one of your servings is an oil-rich variety (see above). But while fresh tuna is packed with omega-3s, most of the beneficial oils are lost in tinned tuna due to the processing involved, so a steady diet of tuna-mayonnaise sandwiches just

YOUR SCORE

Add up the scores beside your answers to find out how 'smart' your current diet is.

**0–6 points:** You have some real work to do if you want to maintain or recapture the brain power you had when you were younger.

**7–12 points:** You've stumbled on a few healthy foods, but, overall, your diet is probably doing more harm than good.

**13–18 points:** Not bad. You're making some smart choices, but there's still room for improvement in other areas.

**19–24 points:** Congratulations! Your diet is going a long way towards protecting your brain. Keep reading for more tips on boosting your brain power.

## SAFER SEAFOOD

Choose fish least likely to contain mercury and other contaminants. Here are some of the best and less good fish choices.

| Best choices | Less good choices |
|---|---|
| Wild salmon | Shark |
| Sardines | Swordfish |
| Organic farm-raised salmon | King mackerel |
| Tilapia | Tilefish |
| Haddock | Grouper |
| Anchovies | Fresh or tinned tuna |
| Mackerel (not King) | Chilean sea bass |
| Herring | Bluefish |
| Pollock | Marlin |
| Freshwater trout | Orange roughy |
| Mullet | Any farm-raised fish (unless organic) |

won't do it. Fish is a perfect week-night meal because it's ready in as little as 10 minutes, and frozen fish is an easy option. If you can afford it, buy wild fish; if you buy farmed, opt for organic farm-raised fish; it may contain fewer contaminants such as mercury (see above). Incidentally, canned salmon is made from wild fish – a bonus.

● **Expand your fish repertoire.** If you haven't visited a fishmonger or the fish counter in your supermarket for a while, you may be surprised to see how many varieties of fish are available. Experiment with a new type, say, once a month, until you find a few more that you enjoy.

● **Make a 'not-tuna' salad.** Tuna isn't the only fish that can be used in salads. Try this basic recipe, and add your own twist: flake or dice one fillet of smoked trout or smoked mackerel. Add 50g of any three chopped raw vegetables, such as carrots, celery, peppers, onions, tomatoes, cucumbers or broccoli. Add 1 tablespoon olive oil and 1 tablespoon reduced-fat mayonnaise. Season to taste with cracked pepper, chilli pepper, turmeric or fresh herbs. Mix well, and serve on a bed of lettuce or use as a tasty sandwich filling.

● **Add walnuts to everything.** They're terrific in salads, added to baked foods, and on top of cereal or low-fat ice cream.

● **Invest in a bottle of walnut oil.** It has a clean, delicate, slightly sweet flavour that is perfect in homemade salad dressings. Don't use it as a high-temperature cooking oil, though – as in pan-frying, grilling or barbecues – since it breaks down in heat and turns bitter. You can use it safely in baking or

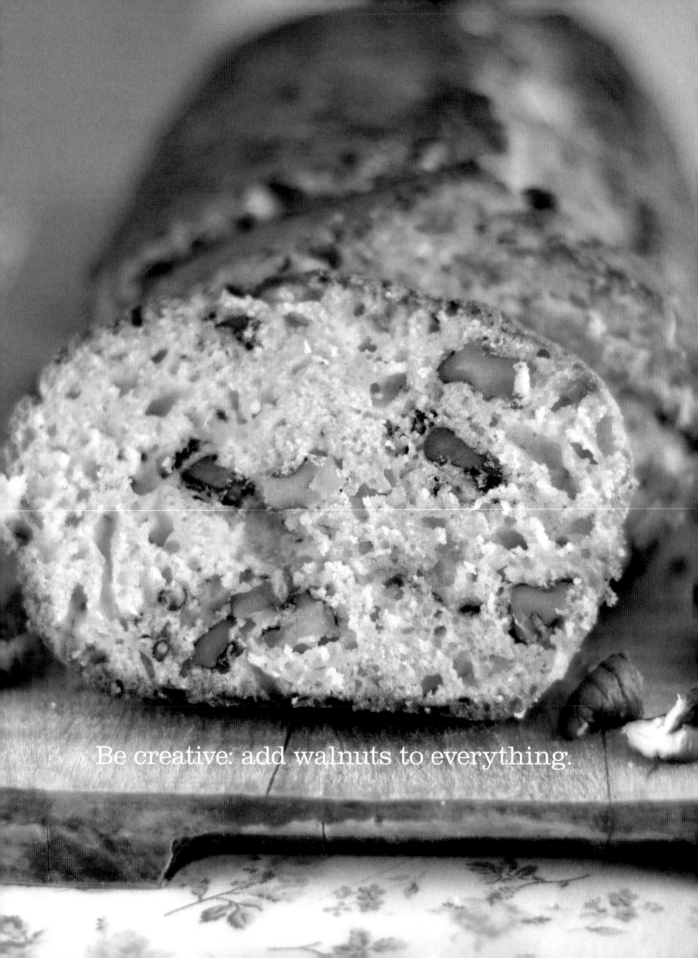

Be creative: add walnuts to everything.

slow roasting, or to toss pasta. Or halve a piece of fruit, such as a peach, and brush it with walnut oil and honey, then bake it in the oven and serve with yoghurt. Oils, especially nut oils, easily turn rancid when exposed to light, heat and air, so store them tightly sealed in a cool, dark place and discard after 6 to 12 months. Once opened, store in the fridge.

● **Keep a bottle of flaxseed oil handy.** The taste is powerful and slightly bitter; a little goes a long way. Also sometimes called linseed oil, flaxseed oil can be used as a nutty flavour enhancer, drizzled on veggie sandwiches and other raw foods, or added instead of margarine or butter to steamed vegetables and other cooked foods (but sprinkle only after the food is moved to a serving dish; heating flaxseed oil can create harmful compounds).

● **Put some flaxseeds in your grinder.** Buy whole flaxseeds (linseeds) from a health-food shop and grind them in a spice grinder as you need them. (Whole seeds keep longer than ground, but if you eat them whole, your body won't digest them so well and they may just pass through your system.) Sprinkle them on

your cereal, a salad or a smoothie. Or add to scone or cake mixes. If a recipe calls for 100g flour, use 75g flour and 25g ground flaxseeds instead. (Store the seeds in the fridge as they go rancid fast.)

● **Get seedy.** Seeds are packed with good fat, protein and vitamin E, and may even help lower your cholesterol. Here's one tasty way to enjoy them along with another brain-healthy food, fish: coat thin fish fillets (or chicken cutlets) with crushed sunflower and pumpkin seeds, then pan-fry or bake in the oven. Chopped seeds are also an interesting, crunchy addition to hot or cold cereal.

● **Use oils lightly in cooking.** Heating can reduce some of the health benefits of oils (never heat flaxseed/linseed oil as it can create harmful compounds). So cook with the minimal amount – as little as 1 teaspoonful may suffice – or use an oil spray. Omega-3 oils are best used in condiments, sauces or toppings.

## SWITCH TO OLIVE OIL

When you have the choice of eating butter (full of artery-clogging saturated fat), margarine or olive oil (which figures prominently in the Mediterranean diet), choose olive oil. It's a powerful antioxidant that also helps to reduce inflammation (see page 159) everywhere in the body, including the brain. Its powers against inflammation are so strong, in fact, that experts liken it to aspirin.

Olive oil also protects brain-cell membranes and may help prevent age-related cognitive decline. And it's good for your cholesterol (which in turn makes it good for your brain). One study

found that when 28 men and women added 2 tablespoons of olive oil a day to their diets, they saw a 16 per cent drop in LDL ('bad') cholesterol.

When you want a milder taste or an oil that survives heat better than olive oil does, go for rapeseed oil; it's a much healthier choice than corn, safflower or sunflower oil, all of which should be avoided because they can promote inflammation.

## EAT WELL

● **Choose extra-virgin olive oil.** Olives are crushed then pressed to make oil. The first pressing yields extra-virgin olive oil, which is fruity and full-bodied and contains the most antioxidants. The second pressing yields refined virgin olive oil, which is of lower quality and contains fewer antioxidants.

● **Find your favourite flavour.** Different brands and types of olive oil have dramatically different tastes depending on, for example, where the olives were grown and when they were harvested. Experiment until you find your preferred brand.

● **Store olive oil properly to avoid rancidity.** Like other oils, olive oil turns rancid when exposed to heat, light and air. Store it in a dark cabinet away from the cooker, and always kept tightly closed. Do not store it in the fridge; if condensation occurs in the bottle, it can ruin the taste.

● **Use a lower cooking temperature than usual.** Olive oil burns more easily than other oils. Plus, you don't want to ruin the healthy properties of your oil by overheating it.

Buy an empty spray bottle. You can find these in department stores or specialist kitchen shops. (Don't use a bottle intended for a different use or that came pre-filled with anything except

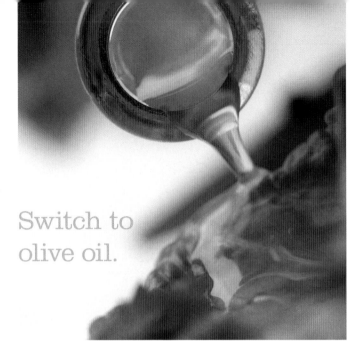

Switch to olive oil.

## WHAT ABOUT SUPPLEMENTS?

The ideal way to get your omega-3s is by eating oily fish at least twice a week, such as salmon, trout, herring, fresh tuna, pilchards and sardines. If you really don't like fish, omega-3 supplements could be the answer.

**Dose:** There's no official recommended daily intake of omega-3s, and the daily dose recommended on packets may vary. The key is to look for the DHA and EPA content and aim to get 1g.

**Type:** Look for algae-based (instead of fish-based) brands to avoid possible mercury contamination.

**Cautions:** Talk to your doctor first if you have any form of blood-clotting disorder, liver disease, depression, diabetes or weakened immunity (such as HIV/AIDS), or if you're taking anticoagulants (such as warfarin) or medications for high blood pressure.

**How to take:** Take with meals to avoid possible stomach upset. You can take the full dose at one meal. If you experience 'fishy' burps, try storing supplements in the freezer; many people say it helps.

cooking oil.) This gives you the option to spritz instead of pour, using much less oil. For instance, toast whole-wheat baguette slices in the oven with just a spritz of oil on each slice. When golden brown and crisp, remove and top with tapenade (olive spread), pesto (basil spread), chopped tomatoes or any topping of your choice.

● **Use mild, delicious extra-virgin olive oil in your homemade salad dressings.** Using olive oil 'raw' without heating it preserves more of its nutrients. You can also drizzle it over pitta-bread sandwiches and use it in place of butter to flavour your cooked vegetables (including potatoes).

● **Substitute olive oil for butter in baking.** Use light extra-virgin olive oil instead of butter or margarine in recipes for cakes, biscuits and breads. The flavour won't be exactly the same, but you'll be eliminating a lot of saturated fats. Keep this conversion information handy:

| Butter | Olive oil |
|---|---|
| 1 teaspoon | ¾ teaspoon |
| 1 tablespoon | 2¼ teaspoons |
| 50g | 4 tablespoons |
| 100g | 8 tablespoons |
| 250g | 300ml |

● **Substitute olive oil for butter at the table.** Instead of spreading saturated fats thickly on your bread, try dipping the bread in oil. Pour a small amount of olive oil into a saucer or shallow bowl, and dip the bread lightly (you don't want to come away with a dripping mess). Experiment with different flavours by adding a little balsamic vinegar, roasted garlic cloves, cracked pepper or anything else you fancy.

# AVOID 'BAD' FAT AND 'LAB' FAT

Our bodies use the fats we eat to make cell walls. Different fats create different types of cell walls, and the worst walls – stiff and rigid – are made from saturated and trans fats. Rigid walls can lead to insulin resistance and may interfere with how well cells function. In the brain, this means that brain cells with poor-quality walls have difficulty communicating.

To make matters worse, eating too many saturated fats can cause inflammation in the body and raise your levels of LDL ('bad') cholesterol. The result? Studies suggest that people who eat a lot of saturated fat (think meat, butter and cheese) have a raised risk of age-related cognitive decline compared to people who eat less saturated fat.

It's easy to reduce saturated fats – almost all are found in animal products. Some of the worst are fatty cuts of beef, pork and lamb, meat products (especially ribs, sausages, bacon, ham, mince and hot dogs), chicken skin, whole milk, cream, cheese, butter, full-fat ice cream and croissants. These foods should be eaten in very small quantities, and infrequently.

## TRANS FAT DANGERS

As dangerous as, or even more dangerous than, saturated fats are trans fats. These are found in nature only in infinitesimally small amounts. Most of the trans fats we eat are man-made. If you take a liquid vegetable oil into a laboratory and twist the molecules a little, you get a form of fat that is solid at room temperature, lasts for ever and is an enemy of the brain. Like saturated fats, trans fats make cell

membranes rigid and interfere with the neurons' ability to communicate with one another. Studies show that of all the fats, trans fats cause the most damage and carry the greatest risk of increasing impairment of brain function and age-related cognitive decline.

You can't cancel out the bad effects of trans fats – you have to eliminate them. If you simply add healthy fats to your diet without cutting out trans fats, the trans fats crowd out the other fats and bully their way into cell walls.

## EAT WELL

● **Buy a spread containing plant stanols.** These natural substances have been shown to reduce LDL ('bad') cholesterol, so in small amounts they're actually good for you. Examples include Benecol and Flora pro.activ.

● **Avoid all foods with the word 'hydrogenated' in the ingredients list.** Although all packaged foods in the USA must list the levels of trans fats on the nutrition panel on the label, in the UK there's no requirement for manufacturers to provide this information (although some products, most often spreads, declare that they are free from trans fats). It's therefore virtually impossible to know the precise amount of trans fats in a food product.

However, hydrogenated fats are usually included in the ingredients list, so if a product lists 'hydrogenated fat' or 'partially hydrogenated vegetable oils' in the ingredients list you can assume it contains trans fats and is best avoided. But there's no way of knowing what type of fat is used in takeaway foods and restaurant and café meals – so if you want to avoid trans fats, steer clear.

# Saturated fat
# CONTENT OF COMMON FOODS

| GRAMS/ML OF FOOD | SATURATED FAT |
| --- | --- |
| Quarter-pounder (115g) hamburger | 8g |
| 1 slice (200g) of pepperoni pizza | 8g |
| Fried chicken breast, with skin (150g) | 7g |
| 1 scoop (70g) vanilla ice cream | 6.3g |
| 1 sausage (50g) | 5g |
| 200ml whole milk | 4.7g |
| Sirloin steak (8oz/225g) | 4g |
| 25ml single cream | 3g |
| 1 roast chicken leg, without skin (150g) | 3g |
| 200ml semi-skimmed milk | 2.2g |
| 200ml skimmed milk | 0g |

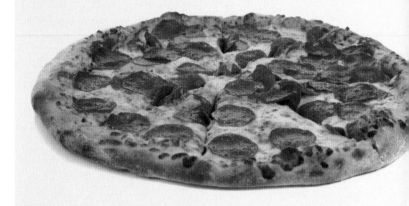

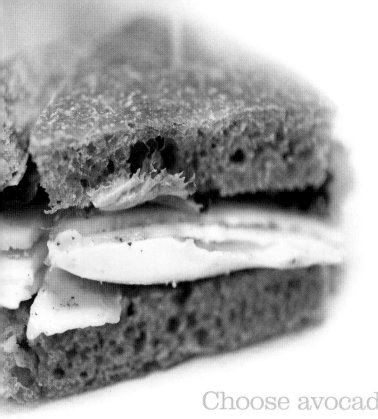

if you're on a diet of 2,000kcal a day. Switch to skimmed milk, which has 0g saturated fat per 200ml compared with 4.7g in whole milk – about as much as in a small grilled hamburger – and 2.2g in semi-skimmed.

● **Opt for lean and avoid processed meats.** Steer clear of processed meats, including sausages and burgers, and fatty cuts such as belly pork. Aim for at least three meat-free meals a week and when you do eat meat keep portions modest. Bulk out dishes like cottage pie with diced vegetables or brown lentils.

● **If you eat minced beef, choose extra lean.** There's 2g to 4g of saturated fat per

Choose avocado instead of cheese.

● **Add avocado to your sandwich instead of cheese.** You'll be trading saturated fat for brain-boosting mono-unsaturated fat that helps control blood sugar and protects your heart and brain.

● **If you eat pies, make them the one-crust version.** It's nearly impossible to make a good pie crust without either saturated fat (butter or lard) or trans fats (hydrogenated fat). The best advice: have pies only as a special treat, and if you make your own, opt for the one-crust variety.

● **Say goodbye to fried.** Many deep-fried foods are cooked in trans fats. Say no to chips, fried chicken, fried fish, crisps and anything else that leaves a greasy ring on a napkin.

● **Limit saturated fats to less than 10 per cent of daily calories.** Most of us should consume no more than 150kcal to 250kcal per day in saturated fats. If you're counting grams of saturated fat (see page 73), aim for less than 20g a day

100g in extra-lean (compared with 7g to 9g per 100g in standard minced beef).

● **Use unsalted nuts instead of meat in stir-fries.** Nuts contain fats that are actively good for your brain.

● **Choose lower-fat cheeses.** Go for tasty varieties that are naturally lower in fat. Good choices include Brie, Edam, goat's cheese and low-fat soft cheeses. Half-fat cheddar has 2.5g of saturated fat compared with the 5.5g of saturated fat in standard cheddar.

## LET FRESH PRODUCE SHINE

A study conducted by researchers at Heinrich-Heine University in Düsseldorf, Germany, showed that for healthy people of any age between 45 and 102, those with the highest daily intake of fruit and vegetables had better cognitive

performance than those consuming low amounts. In another study, scientists from the Rush Institute for Healthy Aging in Chicago showed that people who ate three servings of vegetables per day – any vegetables – slowed down the ageing processes in the brain.

Ageing anywhere in the body, including the brain, happens at the molecular level. Every day, our bodies naturally create destructive oxygen molecule fragments called free radicals. Left to their own devices, free radicals eat away at healthy cells, damaging them through a process of oxidation. The only way to fight back is with antioxidants, plentiful in fruit and vegetables, as well as other foods, most notably, beans.

## FRUIT AND VEG PHYTO-POWER

Every fruit and every vegetable contains not just vitamins but also natural disease-fighting plant compounds called phytochemicals. Although scientists have known of the existence of these compounds for decades, it wasn't until the 1990s that they began to understand their enormous disease-fighting potential. There are thousands of different phytochemicals; a single apple has more than 100. That's why it's important to eat a wide variety of foods. Just about all fruit and vegetables are good for the brain, but a few seem to be especially effective against brain decline.

● **Broccoli and its cruciferous cousins.** Sometimes called the odiferous cruciferous because of their tendency to cause gas, these veg include broccoli, cauliflower, Brussels sprouts, kale, mustard greens, watercress, cabbage and Swiss chard. Harvard Medical School researchers found that women who

frequently ate cruciferous veg – already known to have cancer-fighting powers – had fewer memory problems than women who rarely ate them.

A study at the University of Oslo in Norway that examined the effects of different dietary ingredients in more than 2,000 people aged 70 to 74 also showed that cognitive performance was best in those with the highest intake of fruit and veg and that the benefits were most pronounced for cruciferous vegetables, carrots, citrus fruits and high-fibre bread. If you don't eat many of them now, add them slowly to your diet to avoid gas or bloating.

● **Blueberries, apples and other polyphenol-rich foods.** This large class of antioxidants covers an alphabet soup of compounds including anthocyanins, quercetin, flavonoids and hundreds of others. You don't need to know the names, just the foods – for instance, blueberries, strawberries, cherries, grapes, red onions, apples, oranges, bananas, red cabbage, beetroot, grapefruit and lettuce.

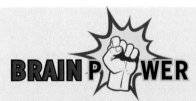

**BRAIN POWER**

In regulating the appetite, the brain can match calorie input to energy output almost perfectly. In practice, the brain region that controls food intake is frequently overridden by conscious desires for food created by social and other pressures. But left alone, the brain provokes hunger only when glucose levels fall below the optimum level. In this situation, a person's weight would vary by less than 5 per cent during his or her entire adult life.

*Continued on page 78*

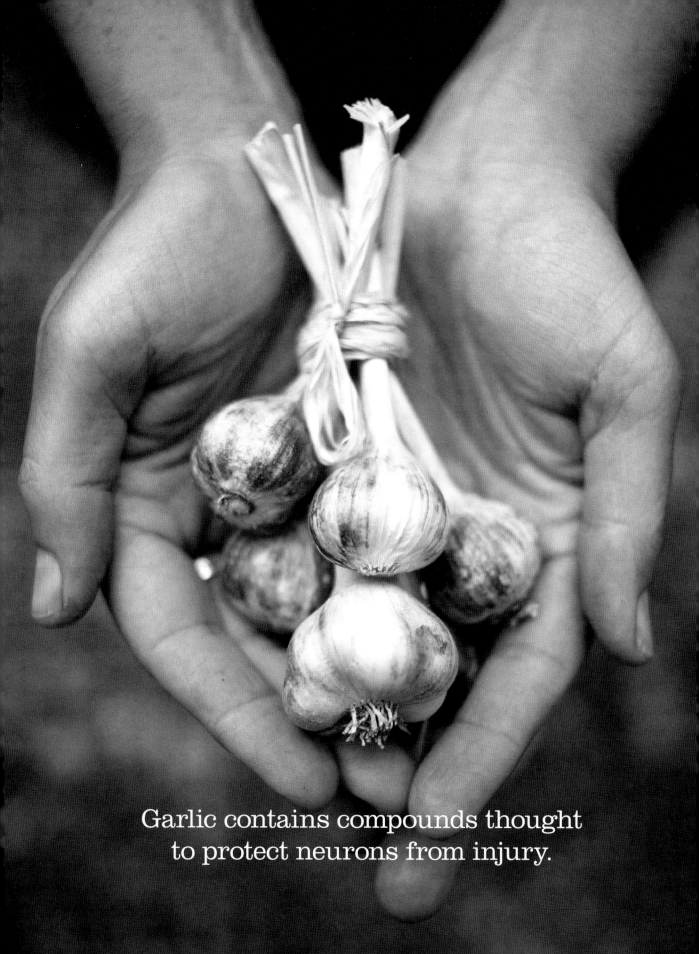

Garlic contains compounds thought
to protect neurons from injury.

# Best herbs FOR THE BRAIN

Many herbs and spices have medicinal benefits, and a handful are thought to boost brain health. Aim to get more of these four in particular.

## Turmeric

### Brain benefit

This mustard-yellow powder, often used in curries, is an antioxidant and a powerful anti-inflammatory. One study at the National University of Singapore of more than 1,000 people aged between 60 and 93 found that those who ate curry occasionally or often had significantly better cognitive performance than those who ate it rarely or never.

### Eat more

Add turmeric to any curry dish and to egg salad. Put up to a teaspoonful in pea soup or your favourite lentil dish. Use turmeric in casseroles and as an inexpensive alternative to saffron in paella and other rice dishes.

## Wasabi

### Brain benefit

Wasabi, a member of the mustard family, is the hot green condiment served with sushi. It's an excellent source of a compound (also found in horseradish and broccoli) known to help nerve cells grow extensions called dendrites and axons, which help cells to communicate with each other.

### Eat more

Good on fish of any sort. In specialist shops, buy wasabi in a tube or as a powder. Add a little bit to ginger, teriyaki, or peanut-based sauces, and to devilled eggs, salad dressing, coleslaw and crab cakes.

## Sage

### Brain benefit

A member of the mint family, sage is a known memory enhancer and may protect the brain against age-associated cognitive decline. It may work by protecting acetylcholine, a chemical messenger in the brain that's critical to memory. In an Australian study of 20 volunteers aged over 65, sage extract led to significantly enhanced performance on tests of memory and attention compared with a placebo.

### Eat more

Add to omelettes, tomato sauce, butternut squash, roasted chicken or pork. Steep 2 teaspoons of dried sage in just-boiled water for a strong cup of tea that provides a therapeutic dose.

## Garlic

### Brain benefit

Garlic thins the blood to help prevent blood clots and may slightly lower cholesterol. It contains compounds thought to protect neurons from injury and disease by stimulating the production of chemicals that help cells withstand stress.

### Eat more

Add lots of minced garlic or garlic paste to just about any marinade or salad dressing. Add sautéed garlic to chicken, beef, pork, tofu, pasta or vegetable dishes.

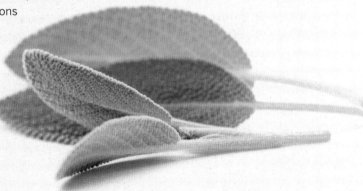

Blueberries have been celebrated as a top brain food because of studies conducted by researchers at the University of Barcelona. In the studies, older rats with memory problems were fed a diet of blueberries for eight weeks. Even after such a short time, the rats showed improved memory, as measured by their ability to find their way through a maze. But blueberries aren't the only food with brain-protective phytochemicals. Other studies show that neurons are protected by eating apples, bananas, oranges, strawberries, pomegranates and spinach.

● **Citrus fruits, nuts and seeds, and other foods rich in vitamins C or E.** Vitamins C and E are both powerful antioxidants, meaning that they help to combat free radical damage to cells. Several studies have found that people who eat plenty of foods rich in vitamins C and E have better memories and cognitive function as they move into old age than people who don't eat such nutritious foods. Also, if they do experience cognitive decline, it happens more slowly.

And the Düsseldorf study (see page 74) showed that the improved cognitive performance in subjects eating more fruit and veg was linked with higher blood levels of vitamin E and other antioxidants.

Good food sources of vitamin C include citrus fruits, bell peppers (capsicums), cantaloupe melons,

## THE BRAINIEST PRODUCE

All fruit and vegetables are good for you, but these are among the best for memory and cognition.

**Cruciferous veggies**
broccoli • Brussels sprouts • cabbage • cauliflower • kale • watercress

**Leafy greens**
lettuce • mustard greens • pak choi • spinach • Swiss chard • turnip greens • seaweed

**Legumes**
chickpeas • black beans • pinto beans • haricot beans • kidney beans • white beans • soya beans • peanuts

**Other vegetables**
onions • tomatoes • peppers • beetroot • avocados

**Berries**
blueberries • blackberries • raspberries • strawberries • boysenberries • cranberries

**Citrus fruits**
oranges • grapefruit • lemons • limes • tangerines

**Other fruits**
apples • bananas • cherries • persimmons (Sharon fruit) • pomegranates • grapes • kiwi fruit

strawberries, broccoli, kale and leafy greens. Vitamin E is quite difficult to get from food but is most abundant in wheat germ, sunflower seeds, almonds, avocados, olive oil and spinach.

● **Spinach, broccoli and other foods rich in B vitamins.** The B vitamins – especially vitamin B, vitamin $B_{12}$ and folate – are thought to help protect your memory by breaking down homocysteine, an amino acid involved in the inflammation of blood vessels. They are important for nerve health, and deficiencies can lead to sluggish thinking, memory problems and age-related cognitive impairment. Some studies show that people who get enough of all the B vitamins from food sources have better memories than those who don't. Beetroot is a good source of folate, while folate and vitamin $B_6$ are found in legumes, peanut butter, leafy green vegetables, broccoli and other cruciferous vegetables, strawberries, enriched cereals and whole-grain breads. Vitamin $B_{12}$ is found in foods of animal origin, and in fortified cereals and some yeasts. It is most plentiful in fish, shellfish, enriched soya milk, lean beef, cottage cheese, yoghurt, eggs and cheese. Vegans may need to take supplements to avoid a deficiency.

## EAT WELL

● **Have at least three servings of vegetables per day.** That seems to be the minimum number needed to maximise the brain-protective effects. The more you eat, the better. The exception is starchy vegetables – including sweetcorn, potatoes, sweet potatoes, yams and turnips – which cause a rise in blood sugar. Limit these to one serving per day.

● **Make leafy greens part of your day.** Aim to eat a salad or steamed greens every day. And mix it up a bit – experiment a little, combining a mild lettuce with a more tasty variety.

**Mild flavours:** Green leaf, Red leaf, Romaine

**Peppery:** Rocket

**Slightly bitter:** Belgian or French endive, chicory, escarole, radicchio

● **Start dinner with a salad.** It's a good way to squeeze in vegetables. Having salad before the main course ensures you fill up.

● **Eat your spinach.** It's an excellent source of folate, a B vitamin that helps lower homocysteine levels (see opposite).

● **Serve your meals on a bed of greens.** Simply steam some spinach, kale or Swiss chard, put it on your plate and place fish or chicken on top.

● **Dress bitter veggies in olive oil.** Some people find certain vegetables – especially cruciferous veg – too bitter. Instead of shunning these brain foods, dietitians recommend adding a little fat before serving to cut the bitter taste. And you're in luck – olive oil is a brain-healthy food. After cooking, top the veggies with a teaspoon to a tablespoon of olive oil for a double dose of memory-savers.

● **Shop often.** An apple picked off the tree is more nutritious than one bought at the supermarket, which may have spent weeks getting there. You may not be able to pick your own (though if you have a farmers' market, use it), but you can aim to eat fresh foods quickly. Shop European-style – purchase small quantities often rather than letting foods sit uneaten.

● **Fill the freezer.** If you buy frozen fruit and veg with no additives – no sugar, salt, butter, cheese, sauce or anything else – you'll have the convenience of frozen with maximum nutritional value. Because the produce is flash-frozen, nutritional experts say there is no difference in the quality of the vitamins and minerals; as it is usually frozen soon after picking it may even be nutritionally superior to fresh produce that has taken days or weeks to arrive in the shops.

● **Spend more for convenience.** Vegetables come in so many prepacked forms now, eating them has never been quicker or simpler. Look for pre-sliced or diced, pre-mixed or pre-washed. If you can stretch, the extra expense is worth it.

● **An apple a day …** Apples are rich in brain-protecting polyphenols. Keep them visible – say, on the counter on an attractive fruit plate – and you'll eat more.

● **Eat two to five servings of varied fruits per day.** But don't go overboard because though fruit's packed with nutrition, it's also full of natural sugar.

● **Experiment with colours.** Do you usually buy green peppers? Try red, orange or yellow. Different colours indicate different phytochemicals, and it's best to get the widest variety possible.

● **Shred and add.** Include veg – such as carrots, courgettes, peppers – in just about any dish by shredding them first with a cheese grater or in a food processor and throwing them in. They cook quickly, and you won't have to dirty an extra pan.

## An apple a day …

● **Have fruit for dessert.** When you eat dessert (no more than once or twice a week), try a roasted plum, 3 tablespoons of berries with low-fat yoghurt and a touch of honey, or a 'baked' apple (core it, sprinkle inside with cinnamon and a touch of sugar, and microwave until soft).

# SWITCH TO WHOLE GRAINS

Whole grains are a major part of the Mediterranean diet. While it's difficult to separate out the different dietary ingredients to look at individual effects, there is evidence that whole grains are important in themselves. In the Oslo study (see page 75), high-fibre (whole-grain) bread was linked with superior cognitive performance. Researchers also noted that the regular consumption of white bread was associated with decreased cognitive function.

In another study, scientists found that among older US people on a special diet to treat high blood pressure – the Dietary Approaches to Stop Hypertension or DASH diet – greater adherence to the diet was associated with better cognitive function and less decline in mental capacity over the next 11 years. Tests showed an independent association between cognitive function and the whole-grain component of the diet, as well as vegetables, low-fat dairy produce and nuts/legumes.

## PACKED WITH GOODNESS

What's so special about whole grains? Grains have three main parts: the bran (the protective skin, which contains most of the fibre), the germ (the unformed sprout, which contains most

## WHAT'S IN A SERVING?

| 1 Serving | Equals | Resembles, roughly |
|---|---|---|
| Chopped vegetables | 3 heaped tablespoons | What you can hold in a cupped hand |
| Cooked leafy vegetables | 3 tablespoons | What you can hold in a cupped hand |
| Raw leafy vegetables | 1 cereal bowl full | Two handfuls, packed |
| Legumes | 3 heaped tablespoons | What you can hold in a cupped hand |
| Chopped fruit | 4 tablespoons | What you can hold in a cupped hand |
| Whole fruit | 1 piece of standard fruit (such as an apple or pear) or 2 pieces of smaller fruits (kiwis or plums) or 1 slice of a big fruit, such as melon | About the size of a loosely clenched fist |

of the vitamins and minerals) and the endosperm (the starchy energy source). Whole-grain foods contain all three parts. When grains are refined, the most nutritious parts – the bran and the germ – are removed. All that's left is the starchy endosperm. Whole grains contain brain-protecting antioxidant vitamins and minerals that are largely stripped out when grains are refined, as well as fibre that promotes healthy functioning of the digestive system and may also help to defend against cognitive decline.

Researchers in one study that followed nearly 5,000 older French women for 13 years found that increasing the amounts of dietary fibre, omega-3 fatty acids and B vitamins in their usual food intake all had long-term brain-protective effects.

## EAT WELL

● **Ease into the whole-grain life.** If you find it difficult to let go of your 'refined' ways, make the transition slowly. In sandwiches, start with one slice of wholemeal bread and one slice of white.

Mix white rice and brown rice, gradually increasing the amount of brown rice you serve. In recipes for biscuits, muffins or quick breads, replace up to a third of the white flour with wholemeal flour.

● **Look for coarse whole-grain bread.** Don't simply buy bread with the word 'whole' in the first ingredient (such as wholemeal) as even whole grains are digested faster (raising blood sugar faster) if they are finely ground. Coarsely ground whole-grain bread, with specks of kernels, is your ideal choice.

● **Swap pearl barley for rice.** Even brown rice, while still good for you, raises blood sugar levels quite a bit. Once in a while, have pearl barley instead. It contains a good deal of soluble fibre, so its impact on blood sugar is minimal.

● **Make a whole-grain side dish on Sundays.** Most people have more time on Sundays than on week nights. Prepare extra, and enjoy it for lunch the next day. Try a pearl barley and black bean or chickpea salad, or quinoa with chickpeas and tomatoes.

● **Start with the right breakfast.**
Eating breakfast in the morning is a good way to keep your blood sugar on an even keel throughout the day. But forget toast and marmalade or croissants. Instead, choose hot oatmeal or a whole-grain cereal with at least 5g of fibre per serving. Top it with fruit and chopped nuts or ground seeds for extra brain benefits.

# DROP THE JUNK

Could a steady diet of processed food, takeaways, biscuits and crisps washed down with fizzy drinks be leading your brain down the path to slowdown and decline? It's entirely possible. The occasional over-indulgence is unlikely to do much harm, but making junk foods a regular feature of your diet could be hastening cognitive decline. In fact, researchers have demonstrated exactly how bad a junk-food diet can be for the brain. They studied rats, but it's not a huge leap to see how the results could apply to us too.

Scientists fed some rodents a healthy diet and others a high-fat, high-sugar diet. Some rats were allowed to exercise, some were not. Then they were all tested in a rat-size swimming pool to see how well they remembered the location of a platform. The junk-food-only rats who didn't exercise had virtually no memory and swam randomly around the pool. They were found to have a reduced level of a chemical known as brain-derived neurotrophic factor (BDNF), which stimulates the growth and proliferation of brain cells and is critical to long-term memory. The junk-food rats who exercised performed better, but the rats who ate well and exercised did the best of all.

One problem with sweets and sugary drinks is the effect they have on blood glucose. Most trigger blood-sugar swings that are toxic to brain cells. And, of course, they can lead to weight gain and contribute to the development of diabetes, stroke and cardiovascular disease.

## EAT AND DRINK WELL

● **Eat regularly.** If you leave too long between meals, you'll be more likely to reach for junk food that gives you a fast sugar high or satisfies your carbohydrate cravings and, as well as being laden with sugar or refined carbohydrates, may be high in saturated fat and salt. Try to go no longer than 4 to 5 waking hours without a healthy meal or snack.

● **Keep fruit handy at all times.**
Biscuits and sweets are available everywhere we turn. Surmount the problem by keeping a fruit bowl on your table, sticking an apple in your bag and stocking up on mini-boxes of raisins.

● **Keep junk hidden.** The saying 'out of sight, out of mind' is true when it comes

## THREE GREAT GRAINS

**Bulghur** This quick-cooking grain comprises wheat kernels that have been dried and cracked. To cook, boil 300ml water, add 150g bulghur, and simmer for 10 to 13 minutes, until all the liquid is absorbed.

**Quinoa** Quinoa is a sweet, light, fluffy grain with a slightly nutty flavour. Cook the same way as bulghur.

**Wholemeal couscous** Pasta-like couscous comes in spherical granules. To cook, boil 150ml water, add 125g couscous and turn off the heat immediately. Cover and let sit for 5 minutes, then fluff with a fork.

to junk-food snacks. You'll be more likely to stay away from junk food if you keep it stashed away inside a drawer in another room – or don't buy it at all.

● **Never buy junk foods in bulk.** Although you may pay half as much for a giant family-size packet of biscuits, food researchers have calculated that you'll eat them twice as fast. So basically, you're saving pennies to gain more pounds.

● **Never eat sugar on its own.** When you do eat sugary foods, eat them after a meal or with a food that contains fibre or protein to delay the sugar absorption and soften the effects of the sugar rise.

● **Avoid fizzy and sports drinks and other sugary beverages.** Read the ingredients label. If the drink contains sugar, dextrose, fructose, corn syrup or other sweeteners, avoid it.

● **Drink water with a twist of lemon or lime.** This may add just enough flavour and interest to keep you away from fizzy drinks or flavoured sugary waters.

● **Be wary of aspartame and similar artificial sweeteners.** Some people report side effects from certain artificial sweeteners, including dizziness and confusion. Even if this happens only in ultra-sensitive individuals, it suggests that artificial sweeteners have some effect on brain cells. In one study, rats who drank aspartame-flavoured water for four months appeared to develop memory problems – they took much longer working their way through a maze than rats who drank unflavoured water.

● **Indulge in tea.** Green and black teas are full of phytochemicals called catechins. Research has shown that green tea extracts can improve memory and learning in older rats, and may be helpful in reversing age-related deficits.

## GOOD NEWS FOR COFFEE LOVERS

For those of us who love coffee, there may now be good reason to forgo the decaf and stick with the caffeinated. A study involving more than 4,000 French women aged 65 or older found that those who drank three or more cups of caffeinated coffee a day scored higher on word-retrieval and spatial-memory tests than those who consumed one cup or less. The protective effect was found to increase with age, especially for those over 80.

Tea also contains powerful antioxidants called flavonoids, as does red wine and chocolate. In a study at the University of Oslo of more than 2,000 people aged 70 to 74, those who regularly consumed tea, wine or chocolate had higher cognitive scores than those who didn't – and people consuming all three did best. What's more, consumers of these items had the lowest risk of poor cognitive performance in tests. The researchers were

Start with the right breakfast.

even able to estimate the daily 'dose' needed for maximum cognitive benefit – 10g of chocolate and 75ml to 100ml of wine (see page 64), with the benefit of tea simply increasing the more you drink.

# BOOSTER 2

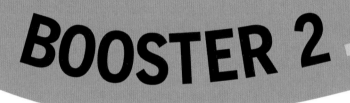

## Exercise

By now, you know that exercising your mind is one of the most effective ways to boost your brain and help stave off cognitive decline. Even a crossword a day can help you remain mentally active. But exercising your body may be every bit as important. In fact, just as physical exercise can make your biceps bigger, it can also increase your brain's size, strength and endurance.

The greatest neurological benefit of exercise: increased oxygen. The brain soaks up 20 per cent of all the oxygen in your body. Exercise increases blood flow to your entire body, including your brain, and that blood carries with it the oxygen your brain so badly needs. A sedentary lifestyle may lower the health of your cardiovascular system and is linked with an increased risk of cardiovascular disease. This could, in turn, lead to reduced brain function and a higher risk of cognitive decline with age.

One way that exercise increases blood flow is by encouraging the lining of your blood vessels to produce nitric oxide, or NO. Thought to play an important role in learning and memory, NO also dilates the arteries, increasing blood flow.

As critical as it is to get plenty of oxygen to your brain, exercise does even more to help you prevent age-related cognitive decline.

## HOW EXERCISE PUTS A SPRING IN YOUR MENTAL STEP

Many of the same health problems that lead to heart disease – high blood pressure, high cholesterol, diabetes – also increase the risk of cognitive decline. All of these conditions decrease blood flow to the brain, and they put you in danger of having a stroke, another major risk factor for cognitive decline. Yet all of them may be helped to some extent by exercise. Still, the advantages of exercise don't stop there. Here are a few more ways in which exercise can sharpen your brain power.

## 10 BRAIN BENEFITS OF EXERCISE

1 Faster processing speed
2 Sharper thinking
3 Lower dementia risk
4 Increased rate of cell birth and growth
5 Reversal of age-related cognitive decline
6 Improved recall
7 Faster decision making
8 Enhanced focus and decreased distractibility
9 Stronger multi-tasking ability
10 Faster reaction time

● **It spurs brain growth.** As we get older, the birth of new brain cells slows, and our brain tissue actually shrinks. Exercise may be able to reverse that trend. One brain-scanning study of 59 healthy but sedentary people aged 60 to 79 showed significant increases in brain volume after six months of aerobic fitness training, whereas no such changes occurred among controls who did only stretching and toning exercises. The researchers concluded that the improved cardiovascular fitness that comes with aerobic exercise is associated with fewer age-related changes in the brains of older people.

● **It increases your sensitivity to insulin.** When you eat, your body turns most of the food into glucose, or blood sugar, the main source of fuel for your body, including your brain. In order for that glucose to enter cells, it must be accompanied by the hormone insulin. Unfortunately, in some people, cells become resistant to insulin. The body has to pump out more and more of it, and still blood sugar levels rise, often resulting

in Type 2 diabetes. Even if you don't develop diabetes, insulin resistance is bad for your brain. When brain cells are flooded by glucose, it can adversely affect memory and thinking.

Regular exercise can actually reverse insulin resistance. In fact, your insulin sensitivity increases – stabilising your blood sugar after you eat – for at least 16 hours after a single exercise session. The better your blood-sugar control, the more protected you are against age-related cognitive decline.

● **It boosts brain-building hormones.** Much like plant food makes plants grow faster and lusher, the chemical known as brain-derived neurotrophic factor, or BDNF, stimulates the growth and proliferation of brain cells. This is especially true in the hippocampus, a region of the brain that is largely responsible for memory and which is particularly vulnerable to age-related cognitive decline. The more you exercise, the more BDNF you produce.

● **It fights depression and anxiety.** Depression slows the brain's ability to process information, makes it more difficult for us to concentrate and reach decisions, and causes real memory problems. For serious depression, your doctor may prescribe antidepressants. For milder cases, however, exercise has been shown to work wonders. It cranks up the body's production of serotonin and dopamine, two neurotransmitters crucial to upbeat, motivated moods. And it boosts levels of the feel-good chemicals called endorphins.

● **It reduces the effects of stress.** If some hormones make the brain younger, others age

Exercise is good for your body, but it's every bit as important for your brain.

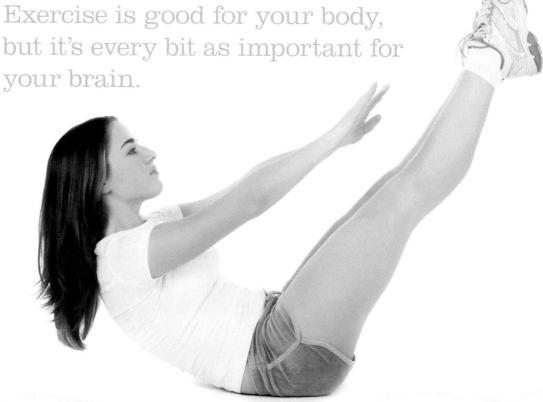

the brain. These include the so-called stress hormone cortisol. Slow, scattered thinking and forgetfulness are caused by stress more often than we may realise. Exercise lowers cortisol levels, helping you to think straight again. It is also believed to generate new nerve cells in the part of the brain called the dentate gyrus, an area of the hippocampus linked to the creation of new memories. Brain cells here are seriously depleted during times of stress.

● **It improves your brain's 'executive function'.** Executive function isn't reserved just for company directors; everyone uses it every day. Essentially, it's the cognitive abilities that enable us to act like grown-ups, including the ability to focus on complex tasks, to organise, to choose behaviour that's appropriate to a given situation, to think abstractly, to meet deadlines and to plan for future events. It also encompasses working memory, such as the ability to keep a phone number in your head while you dial.

When researchers set out to analyse the effects of exercise on executive function, they looked at 18 well-designed studies and found that, in men and women aged 55 to 80, those who did regular exercise (particularly a combination of cardio and strength training) performed four times better on cognitive tests than the studies' control groups, who didn't exercise regularly. They improved their individual scores by a solid 50 per cent regardless of the type of cognitive task. The effects were greatest among those who had exercised for 30 to 45 minutes each session for longer than six months, but substantial benefits were apparent after only four weeks of exercise.

# READY, STEADY, GO

We've all been there: even when you know all the good reasons to exercise, it can still be hard to get up and do it. You can't find the time, the motivation or the 'right' shoes or trainers to get out the door. Perhaps you haven't exercised in a while and you're afraid of looking or feeling foolish. There are a million excuses, but one bottom line: an active body encourages a sharp brain.

If you think about exercise as a chore, the chances are you'll never do it. So, the trick is to find ways to make it fun, easy and invigorating. Before you know it, being active will become an addictive habit that makes you happier, calmer and cleverer, not to mention thinner, healthier, stronger and more energetic.

● **Start with just 10 minutes.** One study found that overweight, post-menopausal women who exercised for an average of 10 minutes a day had more energy, less anxiety and were simply happier than they had been before they started their exercise programmes. And their bodies' ability to use oxygen during exercise increased by more than 4 per cent in six months.

In fact, there's increasing evidence that multiple short bouts of exercise accumulated over the course of the day may be at least as good for you as more prolonged workouts. In one study of older men with diabetes, researchers at Copenhagen University in Denmark found that three sessions of 10 minutes per day was just as effective in increasing cardiovascular fitness as one 30 minute session, and that blood sugar control was improved only in the group doing three 10 minute exercise sessions.

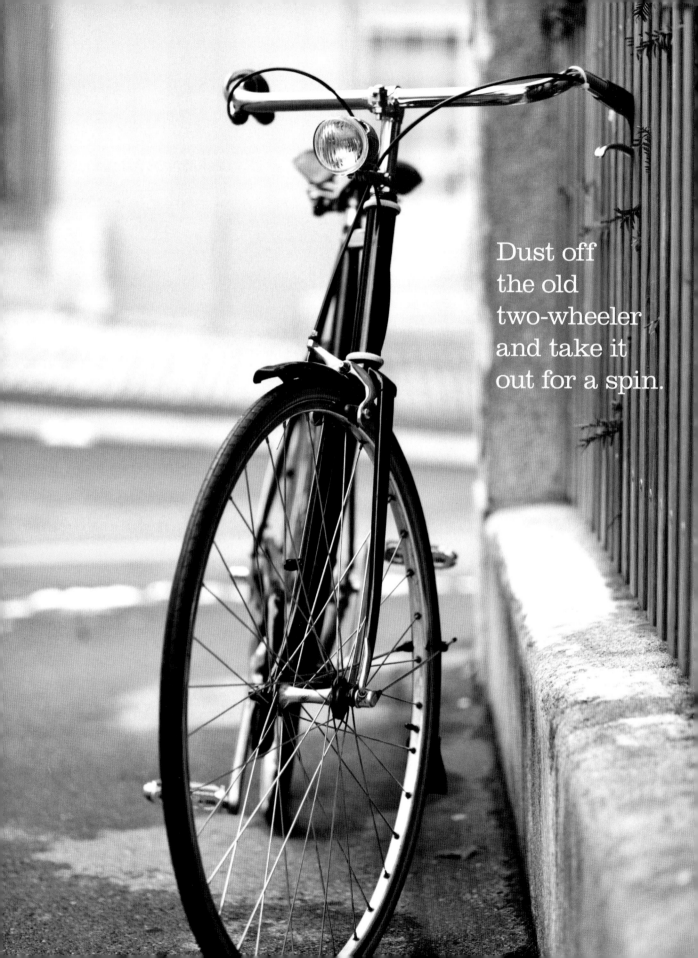

Dust off
the old
two-wheeler
and take it
out for a spin.

Put on your trainers, walk out the door, and head down the street for 5 minutes. After 5 minutes, turn round and come home. Repeat daily, adding a minute each day. There – you're exercising.

● **Burn calories any way you wish.** Don't like to exercise in a formal way? That's fine; anything you do to burn calories will yield benefits. One study found that for every extra 1,700kcal women burned in a week, they had a 14 per cent smaller risk of cognitive decline. That's the number of calories you'd burn playing two or three rounds of golf a week, or vacuuming for an hour or dancing around your living room for half an hour every day. As an added bonus, you'll lose half a pound each week without making a single change to your diet.

● **Do something you love.** The more you enjoy your chosen form of physical activity, the more you'll do it. If you have a passion for flowers, take regular walks around the botanical garden. If you used to love riding your bike as a child, dust off the old two-wheeler (or rent a bike for a week if you don't have one – see also page 90) and take a spin. If you discover you still enjoy feeling the wind in your hair, find a way to work regular bike rides into your schedule. Like to swim? Visit your local swimming pool; they may also run water aerobic classes which are fun and sociable. New activities like this delight and excite your brain.

● **Treat it like a daily prescription.** If you have pre-diabetes – and many people do without knowing it – your condition could trigger changes in the blood vessels in your brain and cause problems with thinking even before you are diagnosed with full-blown diabetes. But you can

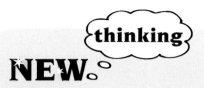

### thinking NEW

### Strength training or cardio?

What's better for your brain: lifting weights or cardio-vascular exercise? For optimal overall health, you want a mix of both, but aerobic (cardio) exercise is the clear winner when it comes to stopping brain decline.

One study randomly assigned 59 men and women to either an aerobics-focused or a stretching and strength-training programme. After six months, sophisticated brain scans showed that the aerobically fit adults had significantly more activity in the frontal cortex, the region associated with executive function (planning, long-term memory storage), and the parietal cortex (spatial orientation) – two areas often associated with age-related cognitive decline.

While cardio does increase blood flow to the brain, that's not the whole story. Researchers believe that many of the positive changes could be attributed to an increase in the brain hormone BDNF. The brain that enjoys cardiovascular training, the researchers say, is 'more efficient, plastic and adaptive', which translates into better learning and performance.

stop the progression with exercise. The Diabetes Prevention Program, a major clinical trial in the USA involving more than 3,000 people, found that people with pre-diabetes reduced their risk of developing diabetes by more than 58 per cent when they walked for 2½ hours each week (that's 30 minutes a day for five days), reduced their calorie intake only slightly, and lost 5 to 7 per cent of their body weight. The researchers actually had to cut the trial short by a year; the lifestyle intervention group was doing so much better than the drug intervention and placebo groups that it wouldn't have been ethical to continue.

● **Do chair squats when you stand up or sit down.** Doctors now classify the ability to get up out of an armless chair as one of the best markers of overall health and degree of functioning as we age. In fact, according to a review by researchers at University College London, older people with reduced performance on this test even have a higher mortality risk. Yet, as we get older, some of us tend to fall into chairs and then struggle to get out of them. Stay strong and in control with chair squats; they may not keep

walk, you're also talking, listening or recounting a story from last night – in short, many regions of your brain are being engaged at one time. Recruit a friend who's on a similar schedule and who lives within walking distance of your house; you can start each walk by meeting midway between your homes. If none of your closest pals is up for walking in your neighbourhood, become part of a walking club.

● **Join a club.** Simply having an active social network is highly beneficial to

## Try some chair squats when you stand up or sit down.

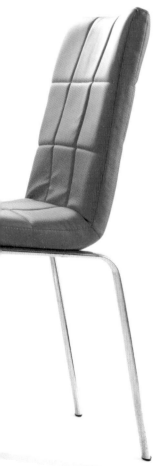

your brain sharp, but strengthening your quadriceps and stomach muscles will make other types of exercise more possible, safe and even fun.

To do a chair squat: stand in front of the chair, facing away from it. For safety, make sure you can feel the chair behind your legs, then, keeping your back straight, bend your knees and lower your body until the backs of your thighs hit the chair. Immediately straighten to a standing position and start over. When you've done a few, sit down. Repeat when you get out of the chair. Try this several times a day. .

### KEEP IT SOCIAL

● **Team up with a friend.** Exercising with a chum makes you more accountable, so you're more likely to stick to a regular routine; you may even challenge each other to walk farther or otherwise ratchet up your workouts. Your walking partner is more than just an exercise insurance policy: as you

the brain, and participating in group activities is one surefire way to cultivate yours. If you play tennis, join a tennis club or sign up at the local courts for a doubles partner. Prefer bowling? Have a ball with your friends. There's something for everyone, and evidence suggests that shared effort may even give your endorphin levels an extra boost. Research done in 2009 found that college crews who rowed in synchronisation had a greater rise in their feel-good hormones than those who rowed alone.

### MAKE IT CONVENIENT

● **Use a bike to get around town.** Put a basket on the front, buy a helmet, and you have an excellent way to get around town, save petrol and keep your brain and body young at the same time. If you don't want to buy a bike and you live close to or are visiting central London, try out the public bike-sharing scheme (referred to as 'Boris bikes' after the Mayor, Boris Johnson), which was introduced in 2010. If you're worried about traffic and other safety issues, many towns have safe-cycling classes where you can find out about the basics of handling traffic, signalling and changing a flat tyre. Bonus: learning the rules and tackling fears about navigating the roads will help you gain the confidence to take on other challenges, a brain-saving tactic with lifelong effects.

● **Do short workouts throughout the day.** If you can't devote a 30 to 45 minute block of time to exercise, don't. It's that simple. Instead, walk or do some other form of physical activity, such as riding a stationary bike or doing sit-ups and push-ups, for 10 minutes several times a day. Some research suggests that doing multiple workouts yields even larger releases of growth hormone and BDNF throughout the day.

● **Make a list of five active things you can do in your community.** Post it on the fridge and let it prompt you on weekends when you're bored. For example, you could walk or cycle to a local park for a picnic, stroll to the library and check out the secondhand-book sale, pick your own fruit, visit a museum or flea market, or volunteer with a local charity group to help less able people with decorating or gardening, or to muck in to clear up rubbish.

## MAXIMISE THE BRAIN BENEFITS

● **Don't be afraid of sweat.** If you've already started an exercise programme, don't be afraid to push yourself a bit, with your doctor's approval. When you increase the intensity of your workouts, you boost the amount of feel-good endorphins and growth hormone that

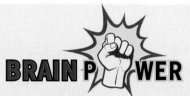

**BRAIN POWER**

You can respond to a stimulus before you are even conscious of it. It takes about a fifth of a second for you to become aware of a visual stimulus, such as a ball thrown towards you. But within a tenth of a second your brain has calculated what you need to do to catch it, and has started off the process.

your body releases. Growth hormone triggers the release of that brain-building, depression-fighting protein BDNF.

One way to increase intensity is to try a faster pace in brief 1 minute bursts during your workout. For example, you might increase the incline on your treadmill for a minute, then lower it again for 4 minutes, and repeat for the duration of your session. This kind of 'interval' training uses more calories and helps your body continue to burn more calories for several hours afterwards.

● **Do your exercise in the sun.** Using the treadmill is good, but if you can get outside, it's even better. Bright sunlight exposes you to 50,000 to 100,000 lux of light, versus the 400 lux of an average living room light. This natural light helps your brain create the chemicals that stave off seasonal blues and gives you more restful sleep; it also reacts with your skin to help your body generate vitamin D. Once converted to its active form, calcitriol, vitamin D binds to receptors in the brain and spurs the release of a powerful protein, known as glial cell line-derived neurotrophic factor, or GDNF, thought to prolong the life of several kinds of brain cells. Calcitriol may also reduce the production of inflammatory chemicals, called cytokines, that contribute to age-related cognitive decline.

● **Mix it up.** Variety is key to keeping the brain agile, whether that variety comes in the form of varied mental workouts or physical challenges. Novel exercises excite the brain in the same way that fresh experiences do; any time you surprise or challenge your brain, you build new and stronger connections between nerve cells. Games such as basketball or tennis, in which you have to react quickly, draw on both hemispheres of the brain and help improve your reflexes and reaction time. Your muscles love novelty, too, so switch your activities as often as possible – say, from walking to cycling to swimming to gardening. Look for an aerobics instructor who changes his or her routine often, or add a new class, such as yoga or Pilates, to the mix.

● **Learn to tango.** Or take up ballroom dancing, line dancing, belly dancing, disco … When you learn any type of dance, not only do you challenge your muscles in new ways, you also stimulate your brain to concentrate and count, remember the sequence of steps and how to do them, and react to your partner if you have one, all tasks that force your brain to stay supple and make new neural connections. Many community centres offer low-cost, ongoing dance lessons. As well as becoming fitter, you'll also meet a whole new group of people with whom to socialise, an extra brain-building draw that can be an added motivation to hit the dance floor.

● **Try some yoga or tai chi.** Chronic stress is toxic to the brain. Exercise of any sort helps reduce stress, but yoga and tai chi may be especially effective. Research has found that meditative exercises such as these help to reduce circulating levels of cortisol, a stress hormone known to hasten cognitive decline. And, of course, these exercise forms are good for you in other ways. In one small study published in the *British Journal of Sports Medicine*, participants who did tai chi and qigong (often described as moving meditation) three times a week for 12 weeks significantly lowered their body mass indexes, waist circumferences and blood pressure levels, all risk factors for cognitive decline. Their bodies became more sensitive to insulin and they reduced their circulating blood sugar, lowering their risk of developing diabetes, another risk factor for dementia.

# THE PERFECT SHARP BRAIN EXERCISE: WALKING

Walking is an ideal exercise for brain health. It's free, easy and can be done just about anywhere. The brain benefits begin virtually the moment you start and add up significantly over time. One study suggested that each mile walked per day is associated with a 13 per cent lower risk of cognitive decline – and every mile you walk burns 100kcal, so there's the added benefit of avoiding obesity.

In the US Nurses' Health Study of more than 18,000 women, long-term regular physical activity, including walking, was linked to significantly better cognitive function and reduced cognitive

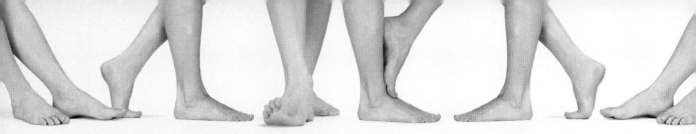

# Walk THIS WAY

You've probably been walking since you could say 'Mama', but, like most adults, your form may not have improved much since then. When you start your walking programme, follow these guidelines.

## Pretend you're a marionette.

Imagine that a string is holding up your head as you walk. Keep your neck elongated and your chin parallel to the ground, your shoulders down and back.

## Watch where you're going.

Many of us tend to stare at our feet as we walk, but that throws your neck and back out of alignment. Instead, point your nose forward and keep your eyes aimed about 3 metres in front of you.

## Keep your core solid.

Tuck in your belly and pelvis, and feel your tailbone pull under slightly. Don't arch your back – instead, think of your entire trunk as one solid block. This stance not only helps develop your abdominal muscles but will also prevent putting extra strain on your lower body.

## Pretend you're on skis.

Start with your feet shoulder-width apart and aim to maintain that distance as you walk. Consider using walking poles; they help absorb shock and deflect it from your joints, improve your balance and help you maintain proper form. Plus, you burn up to 40 per cent more calories when you use them.

## Think fast.

And small. Bend your arms at a 90-degree angle and pump them while you keep your stride short and quick – you'll cover more ground and burn more calories in the same amount of time.

decline in older women. The most active women were 20 per cent less likely to experience cognitive impairment than the least active women. Women who walked at an easy pace for just 90 minutes a week scored much higher than those who walked for less than 40 minutes a week. Even after the results were adjusted for all other factors – age, education, smoking status, antidepressant use – those who walked the most had cognitive performance equal to that of women three years younger.

Sold? Good. Now, how do you get started on a regular plan? Several different paths will take you to the same destination – a stronger, healthier, younger brain.

● **Just open up the door.** See 'The Sharp Brain Walking Programme' on page 95 to learn a simple strategy that starts with just 10 minutes of walking a day and builds up to 30 minutes. Or you can track miles or steps instead of minutes.

● **Do a little every day.** When you first start, consistency is more important than

## THE SOLE EQUIPMENT YOU NEED

Walking requires no equipment; you could go barefoot if you really wanted to. But having the right walking shoes or trainers can go a long way to keeping your feet happy as well as your knees and hips. To find the perfect pair, visit a sports or outdoors shop. Most shops that specialise in running and walking shoes have staff members who know a tremendous amount about footwear and feet in general. They'll measure your feet, look at your old shoes or trainers, watch you walk, ask questions and recommend shoes that are uniquely suited to your feet. Tell them about your walking plans as well as any special issues such as diabetes or osteoporosis. (Tip: it's best to shop in the afternoon as your feet expand during the day.)

Don't skimp. Your joints depend on your shoes to absorb much of the impact when you walk, so invest in a good pair. If you can afford to, spend at least £45. Regardless of how new they might look, trainers should be replaced at least once a year – more often if you walk at least five miles every day. Write a reminder on your calendar, perhaps timed to coincide with certain yearly bills or your car service.

time spent. Plan to do your 10 minutes at a set time when you'll be available each day, such as after breakfast or lunch or right before the evening news – and don't skip it. Your top priority is to make it a regular part of your day. Once you've established a solid routine, you can start adding on extra minutes.

● **Buy a pedometer.** Who doesn't love a new toy? These gadgets are fun and provide a good gauge of how much movement you get during the day. They count every step you take, and some track miles as well. Start a mini-contest with your partner or child to see who can pack the most steps into a day. Just a 2 minute round-trip out to the post box can net you 200 steps; a 10 minute walk with the dog, another 1,000. Why not set a goal to add at least 300 extra steps each day until you reach 10,000, the equivalent of 5 miles?

● **Start with 90 minutes' walking per week.** That's just three half-hour walks. One study showed that older women who walked for more than one and a half hours per week had higher cognitive performance and better memory than those who walked for less than 40 minutes per week. The women who walked for longer were also 20 per cent less likely to develop cognitive impairment. The researchers say that higher rates of physical activity, even if it's just frequent walks, enhance the brain's blood flow, and this may be one way to maintain cognitive functions with age.

● **Build up to two miles a day.** If the idea of a daily 10,000 steps seems overwhelming, start instead with about a quarter of a mile per day (measure it on a map or by driving the route in a car) and add another quarter mile each week until you get to two miles. If you live in a city, walking is easy – you probably have flat, well-lit pavements and plenty of choice of places to go. Use the opportunity to discover new restaurants or shops. The challenge is to turn in a different direction each time you leave the house and to try to discover a new route. One study of almost 6,000 women found that those who walked 14 miles a week were 35 per cent less likely to experience cognitive decline than women who walked only half a mile per week.

# THE SHARP BRAIN
## walking PROGRAMME

Several studies have found that a regular walking programme is all you need to cut your risk of cognitive decline in half. Tracking your progress is a proven motivator, yet everyone likes to note their walks differently – some prefer to chart the minutes, others the miles. No matter how you measure them, daily walks mean much less brain decline. The important thing is just to get out the door. Each of these three programmes gets you to add roughly two extra miles of walking to your standard day (most people already walk three 'base' miles) by the end of five weeks. Choose one of these measures (minutes, miles or steps) and stick with it, increasing your targets each day as shown.

| Week | Programme 1: Minutes of dedicated walking (per day) | Programme 2: Miles of dedicated walking (per day) | Programme 3: Total steps (per day) |
|------|------|------|------|
| 1 | 10 | ¼ | 2,000 |
| 2 | 15 | ½ | 4,000 |
| 3 | 20 | ¾ | 6,000 |
| 4 | 25 | 1 | 8,000 |
| 5 | 30 | 2 | 10,000 |

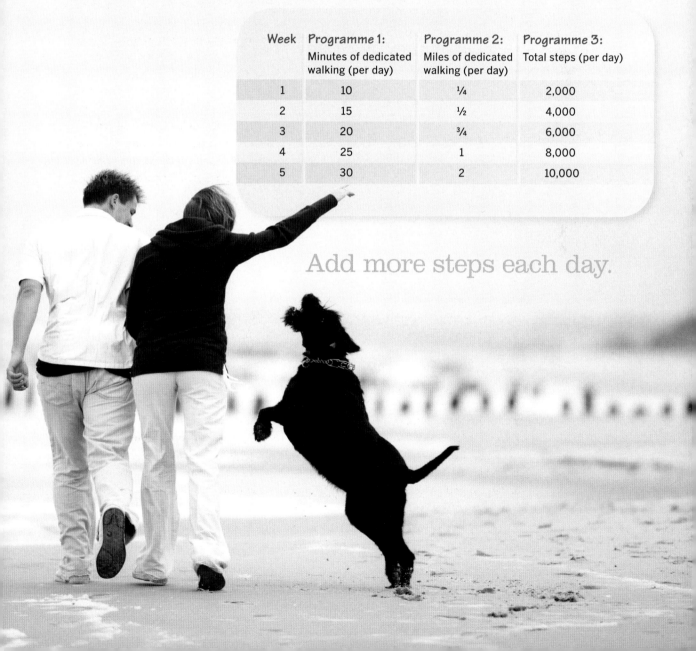

Add more steps each day.

# BOOSTER 3

## Social connections

**Next time you go to the zoo with your grandchildren, stand outside the chimps' cage for a few minutes.** Watch the animals for long enough and you'll see a complex social structure emerge, every bit as subtle as the one that governs the social lives of another primate: the human being.

No one is quite sure why humans developed big brains but scientists now know that there was a gradual increase in hominins (our ancestors) then a remarkable brain growth spurt as Homo sapiens evolved. Much larger brains than the creatures around us enabled humans to develop complex relationships with their peers. The earliest societies were born.

Right from our earliest beginnings, we needed to work out our place in the pecking order of the clan; brains that evolved to process social information were more likely to survive and pass on their genes to future generations. We process these particulars faster than other pieces of info and are more likely to remember details about people and relationships than abstract ideas or inanimate objects. Even while we dream, our brains are more likely to toss around images of people, not things. In other words, we are wired to be social.

Our brains get a good workout whenever we encounter another human being – even if it's just for a casual chat. To carry on a conversation, we have to pay close attention, respond to questions, interpret vocal tone and body language, and even use our short and long-term memory to access relevant facts. At the same time, we have to block out the other stimuli that compete for our attention. All of these are complex executive functions, demanding extra work from the prefrontal cortex, an area of the brain that is particularly vulnerable to age-related cognitive decline.

Every social encounter – even a casual 10 minute chat – gives our brains a good workout.

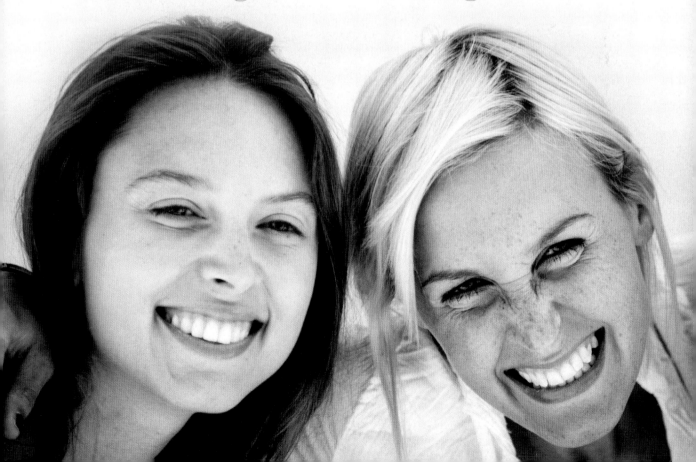

Countless studies have shown that people with more active social lives live longer, enjoy better health and are less depressed than those who go it alone – and they tend to suffer less cognitive decline later in life. No matter what your age, the mere act of spending time with friends or relatives can improve your working memory and processing speed, both immediately and over the long haul. Animal studies have shown that social contact encourages brain-cell growth and an increase in brain volume.

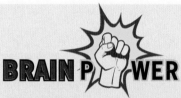

**BRAIN POWER**

Your brain remembers a face – even if you claim not to have seen it. If a photograph of a face is flashed onto the screen in front of your eyes for about one tenth of a second, it does not have time to enter your conscious awareness. However, if you encounter the same image later, your body will respond to it as though it is familiar.

### FRIENDS FUEL YOUR BRAIN

Now, there's one caveat: the relationships have to be positive ones. Fights with your partner and squabbles with your siblings can physically damage your brain by increasing levels of cortisol, a stress hormone believed to shrink the hippocampus, the seat of memory. Positive relationships serve the brain well, and the more diverse those relationships are, the better. Nurturing your social connections widens your support network

not only by increasing the number of people who can help you when you need help but also by boosting your confidence and your ability to help yourself.

In one study of people over 65 in Montreal, Canada, tests of cognitive function – orientation and memory – were carried out at the outset along with assessment of social networks, social integration and social engagement with friends, children and relatives. When they were re-tested four years later, researchers found that those with poor social connections, infrequent participation in social activities, and a lesser degree of social engagement with their friends, children and relatives had significantly increased rates of cognitive decline.

# CREATING A SHARP BRAIN SOCIAL NETWORK

Spending quality time with friends and family might just be the most enjoyable way to protect your brain. Don't worry; you don't have to become a social butterfly. If you're more of a mole, though, it's time to coax yourself out of your hole and into the world. Every little step counts. Not exactly the life and soul of the party? Start with a simple phone call to a friend, or a 'hello' to a neighbour, and take it from there. Researchers have concluded that even brief social interactions can have positive effects on memory and cognitive performance.

● **Deliberately widen your circle.** Many of us tend to have fewer relationships as we get older – the children move away, we retire, elderly friends and relatives start to slip away. We might not care so much about being with a hip crowd, but research shows that we should at least stick with the 'crowd' part. One 12 year study followed more than 2,800 adults aged 65 and older who lived in their own homes. Those who had five or six social ties had less than half the risk of cognitive decline of those who had none. The same results were shown three, six and twelve years after the start of the study.

● **Aim for daily contact with others.** Another study found that among women who were 78 or older, those with larger social networks were 26 per cent less likely to develop dementia or age-related cognitive decline. Of those women, the social butterflies – the ones with daily contact with friends and family – cut their risk in half. Researchers noted that they were the most likely to confide in their friends and ask them for help, not just go out for lunch, which may have been key to their retaining their independence.

● **See your best friends at least twice a month.** And talk on the phone once a week or more. The healthiest people maintain a core group of close friends over their life span. Studies that followed people from the age of 18 to 100 have found that, as we get older, we tend to 'prune' our social circle – we keep the people we're closest to but shed relationships that don't mean as much to us. Our close relationships provide the most emotional satisfaction, so make the most of them (but don't neglect adding new friends, too).

● **Turn off the TV.** As the song from *Cabaret* goes, 'What good is sitting alone in your room?' In fact, it may do harm, especially to older people. When we're alone for long stretches, especially in front of the television, we tend to switch

## MAKING 'ME' TIME

We often use the excuse that we're too busy to see other people, but it's vital for body and brain that you make time for yourself – even if it's just a few minutes every day. One of the easiest way is to create more order in your life. Here are four quick tips on how to free up precious minutes so that you can devote them instead to your social life:

**1** Think about ways to streamline your chores – could you make and freeze meals, or deal with emails or post only at certain times of the day?

**2** Take the time to put your affairs in order – file away documents, clear out messy cupboards. The time it takes will be repaid when you can find the things you need more easily.

**3** Consider getting up an hour earlier on certain days so that you get more done before the rest of the family wake up. Once it becomes part of your routine you'll hardly notice you're doing it.

**4** Find out how much it would be to have a cleaner for a few hours a week. The extra expense may be worth it if it gives you more time to spend with friends and family.

off. One researcher theorises that older people may have a hard time changing from that switched-off state to the more focused mode required to carry on a conversation or perform tasks. Therefore, the less time spent zoned out, the better. If you find yourself alone for a long stretch, walk outside and say hello to whoever's out and about, or pick up the phone and call a relative or friend.

## BREAK OUT OF YOUR RUT

● **Quiz your friends about their hobbies.** Tag along with friends or family to participate in their interests: music, theatre, art, even bingo. Ask them to help

*Continued on page 102*

# TAP YOUR RELATIONSHIP FOR EXTRA brain benefits

With your spouse or partner in the house, you have a built-in brain booster sitting right across the breakfast table. Get the biggest cranial lift from your relationship with these five tactics.

**Pair up with someone similar to you, perhaps a bit brighter.** The Seattle Longitudinal Study looked at 169 couples in seven-year intervals between 1956 and 1984 and found that the most stable relationships were those in which people were similar in intelligence, flexibility of attitudes, social responsibility and education levels. Researchers also found that after 14 years together, people with the better grasp of verbal meanings and word fluency had pulled the lower-functioning partners up to their level.

that when we kiss, we activate nearly half of the cranial nerves that affect cerebral function. All of the sensory information of a kiss – the smell and warmth of your partner's skin, the taste and feel of soft lips – shoots into your brain, delighting your neurons and forging new connections.

**Put pictures of your loved one on your desk.** Brain scans show that looking at a photo of your beloved, especially in the early stages of your relationship, activates a part of the brain associated with pleasure and reward as well as

> With your spouse or partner in the house, you have a built-in brain booster sitting right across the breakfast table.

**Hold hands whenever possible.** In addition to creating feelings of warmth and closeness, holding hands can help protect you from stress. One study using brain scans found that when married women were told they were about to receive an electric shock, just holding their husbands' hands minimised their brains' response to the threat. Women in the closest relationships experienced the greatest decrease in stress-related brain activity.

**Kiss at least once a day.** This intimate touch triggers the release of the bonding hormone oxytocin and lowers levels of the stress hormone cortisol – but that's not all. Researchers say

focused attention and motivation. This same area is triggered when a cocaine addict gets a fix – so you could literally get a healthy 'high' from looking at a picture of your new love. When you're in the throes of new love, your prefrontal cortex also gets in on the action, anticipating more time together and planning future events.

**Just be together.** One study found that average blood pressure was lower when people spent time with their partners than when they spent time alone or with other people. Even if you don't talk, just be together in the same room, reading, watching TV, surfing the web or doing crossword puzzles.

# Cuddling a baby encourages it to grow.

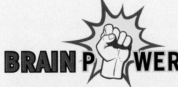

## BRAIN P WER

Cuddling a baby encourages it to grow. Physical affection causes the brain to secrete a chemical called dopamine, which in turn triggers the release of growth hormones. Babies deprived of close physical contact with others may therefore be slower to develop, psychologically as well as physically. In older people, physical affection also plays a vital role, chasing away brain-sapping depression and loneliness.

explain the nuances of each new discipline: What's so good about this piece of music? What's your favourite painting? How do you manage five bingo cards at once? Get them to introduce you to their hobby-related acquaintances, too. Hanging out with new, interesting people usually provides terrific stimulation for the brain.

● **Draw courage from friends to try new things.** Take part in a water aerobics or yoga class with a friend, or join a hiking group together. Experimenting with new activities in the safety of a close relationship helps you manage your anxiety (and prevent a negative stress reaction) while you get the brain benefits of new environments. One study asked three groups of volunteers to give a presentation – a standard way of measuring stress. Those in one group brought a friend for support, one group gave the presentation alone, and a third group had a critic present during the talk. All of the participants were found to have raised blood pressure, especially those in the presence of a critic, but the group supported by a friend showed the lowest rises. Having a friend to support you helps to reduce the amount of stress during a stress-inducing experience.

● **Make a date for something different.** Mixing novelty with love is a win-win situation for your brain and your relationship. Novel and adrenaline-pumping experiences switch on your brain's reward circuits and increase your levels of noradrenaline and dopamine, neurotransmitters associated with increased attention span as well as pleasure – the same brain chemicals released when you first fall in love. Act like children and go to a games arcade to play air hockey. Get out the ping-pong table or play badminton in the back garden. Take a day trip to a town or city you've always wanted to see, and seek out a restaurant with a cuisine you rarely try. It's no surprise that when committed couples spent 1½ hours each week for ten weeks doing something together they both find exciting (as opposed to merely pleasant), they experienced greater marital satisfaction.

● **Plan an exciting getaway together.** Organise a holiday with your partner or best friend to a place neither of you has ever visited. Make each person responsible for planning one full day of the trip, and surprise the other person with every activity and meal that day.

## COMBAT SOCIAL SHRINKAGE

● **Create a call list.** Write down all the people in your social life, along with their phone numbers. In addition to your closest circle, include the people

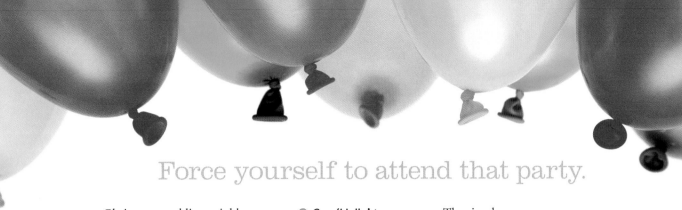

# Force yourself to attend that party.

on your Christmas card list, neighbours and friends you're less close to, such as people from work/religious organisation/aerobics class, and so on. Organise them into two lists: one local, one long distance. Then, make a point of reaching out to at least one person on each list every week, if you're not very social, or once a day if you are. But don't just phone. One four-year study of Spanish men and women over the age of 65 found that those who had a high frequency of visual contact with loved ones had a lower risk of cognitive decline.

● **Throw one party every season.** Connecting your friends to one another isn't just fun, it may help your brain, too. One study found that people at the centre of their network clusters – in other words, who had a lot of friends – were the most likely to be happy, especially when their friends also had a lot of friends.

● **Force yourself to attend that party or social event.** Shy people or those who're unused to socialising can find a million reasons not to go to social events. Instead of thinking of these social 'obligations' as chores, regard them as opportunities to grow your brain. Bonus: just as every personal interaction increases your brain power, it also strengthens your social skills. As those skills increase, you'll feel more comfortable spending time with others. Voilà! A positive brain feedback loop.

● **Say 'Hello' to everyone.** The simplest possible way to get yourself in a more social frame of mind is to say hello to everyone you meet. Make small talk – about anything at all – with the cashier at the supermarket as you pack your bags or the neighbour down the road who passes you while walking his dog. Get coffee at the same café every day, and learn the

## EMBRACE CHANGE

It's natural to feel alone or abandoned following a divorce or bereavement, and to want to withdraw from the world for a while. Don't take on any unnecessary change at this time, such as moving house, unless you absolutely have to. Once you feel ready, though, try to embrace aspects of your situation and see it as a liberating new stage of your life. There are many opportunities, and you may be able to please yourself for the first time in a long while. Think about what you'd like to do, whether it's:

● Taking the sort of holiday you've always dreamed of, such as a cruise or a tour of historical sites.

● Redecorating the house, or rearranging the furniture – it sounds simple but it can stop you feeling that you can't move forward.

● Starting a new exercise regime or developing a whole new look.

● Getting a pet – caring for an animal takes your mind off yourself and can be very calming.

name of the person who serves you. You may be surprised at the positive greeting you get the next time you go.

● *Get back out there.* If you've been widowed or divorced, it can be hard to start dating again. But your brain would love you to love again. One study of over 6,000 adults whose mental functioning was tested over nine years noted that widows and widowers, and those who had never married, experienced faster declines in cognitive status compared with married individuals. And a 2010 study by the Royal College of Surgeons in Ireland, in Dublin, found that among people aged over 65 living in the community, those who reported being lonely or prone to boredom – who were most likely to be people with low social activity, no leisure exercise or who had never married – were the most likely to have reduced cognitive function in older age.

Not sure how to get out there again? Check out online sites such as www.uk.match.com or www.eharmony.co.uk. (Choose a public place for your first meeting.) Screen carefully, but be reassured that online dating has become an efficient and socially acceptable way to meet people with common interests. You could also investigate the website www.friendsreunited.co.uk; who knows, you might reconnect with a long-lost flame from teenage years.

If you prefer to meet your dates the old-fashioned way, visit places frequented by like minds: go to social events at your local theatre or community centre, volunteer at a music festival or local museum, sign up for trips to see plays or attend cultural events in nearby cities. And, yes, get ready for that school, college or university reunion; you never know who's been pining for you all these years.

## PRETEND YOU'RE A CHILD: SOCIALISE IN GROUPS

Form a cinema gang. Gather a group of people with diverse interests and take turns selecting a film to see each month. Include movies that at least two of you wouldn't normally consider. Go to dinner afterwards, rather than before, so you can discuss the film's high and low points. Why not select the restaurant based on the film's setting? If the action takes place in India, for example, go to an Indian restaurant; if it's based in England, choose an old-fashioned tearoom.

● *Start a cooking club.* Get together with four or five other friends to share the cooking once a month. Ask each person to bring a new recipe centred around a certain theme, such as Italian food, or a seasonal vegetable, for example, asparagus or tomatoes. Join together to create a meal for everyone to take home, or ask each person to bring one course (starter, soup, salad, main course, dessert) and enjoy the meal together.

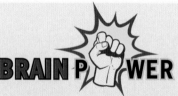

**BRAIN POWER**

A capacity for spiritual experience is wired into the human brain. Certain areas of the brain's temporal and frontal lobes produce feelings of transcendence (like experiences of religious ecstasy) when they're stimulated. This suggests we may be drawn to explore the religious and spiritual dimensions of life because of the way our brains are constructed.

# HOW SOCIABLE are you?

There is now ample evidence from numerous studies around the world that people with more social connections and a higher level of engagement in community activities are less likely to succumb to age-related cognitive decline. Check your own social network score:

**1** Do you live with your spouse or partner?
Yes = 1; no = 0

**2** How many close relatives do you have that you see more than once a month?
0 or 1 = 0; 2+ = 1

**3** How many close friends do you have?
0 or 1 = 0; 2+ = 1

**4** How often do you see work colleagues or neighbours socially?
Never or less than once a month = 0;
1+ times a month = 1

**5** How often do you attend regular meetings of clubs or societies (for example, amateur dramatics, choir or orchestra, chess or bowling club, political group)?
Never = 0; sometimes or frequently = 1

**6** How often do you undertake voluntary activities or attend group meetings such as parent-teacher or neighbourhood associations?
Never = 0; sometimes or frequently = 1

YOUR SCORE
Add up the scores associated with your answers to determine your Social Network Score. A score of 4 or above ('Medium–High') should mean a dramatically lower risk:

Low 0–2; Low–Medium 3; Medium–High 4; High 5–6

● **Trade tasks you don't like.** Maybe you love to garden, and your friend loves to sew. Why not trade those tasks and relieve each of you of the thing you most hate? Studies have shown that those people who ask for and accept help from others can slow their cognitive decline in later years. Learn from societies with a more communal approach to life, such as many in Asia: having more help with household tasks keeps people independent for longer, increases their time spent with others, and decreases brain-damaging stress.

## ADOPT THE RIGHT ATTITUDE

● **Start a 'happiness virus' in your neighbourhood.** Happiness truly is contagious. Harvard University researchers found, when looking at a group of 5,000 people over a period of 20 years, that even a total stranger's happiness can make you happy for up to a year afterwards. When you become happy, your next-door neighbour has a 34 per cent greater chance of becoming happy, and even your friend who lives within a mile has a 25 per cent greater chance of feeling good.

## COMMUNITY BRAIN BUILDERS

Joining a group of people who share common interests or values brings countless benefits to your brain. Not only does the activity itself let you challenge yourself mentally or physically but also the supportive environment makes it far easier to form bonds and to receive and give help – both ends of an equation that benefits the brain.

Consider this list of groups you might join:

- Book club
- Bus trips to cities, theatres or museums
- Choir
- Church or other religious committees
- Exercise class
- Farmers' market association
- Health club
- Social club
- Non-profit-making action group
- Political campaigning organisation
- Residents' association
- Town council
- University alumni association
- Walkers' club

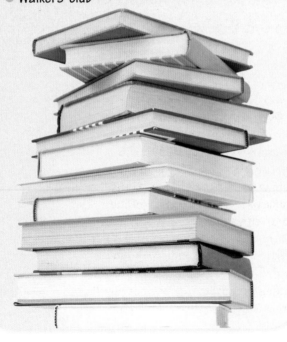

The tradition of bringing a cake or a plant to a new neighbour is an excellent starting point. Encourage neighbours to share good news, even if it's about people you don't know. Host an annual street party. Note people's names as soon as you learn them – the reminder will come in handy in the spring, when you haven't seen them during the long winter months. When you're out in the front garden, smile at anyone who walks past – who cares if they think you're crazy? They probably won't and your social circle will grow. You're starting a brain-building epidemic here.

- **Try to assume the best.** Simply imagining that someone has rejected you socially can negatively affect your performance on lab tests designed to assess cognitive function. When you experience social rejection, your brain registers it in an area of the brain that records physical pain. You're also less likely to be able to empathise with the person who 'rejected' you or to see things from his or her perspective – high-level cognitive functions associated with what we call wisdom.

If you're an anxious person who tends to feel fear or suspicion, try to work on trusting others. Before you react to a neighbour 'ignoring' you on the street, ask yourself, 'Is this really happening? What evidence do I have? Could I be imagining it? Perhaps she has other things on her mind?' Give people the benefit of the doubt by presuming the best in their intentions – and approach them with the best of intentions yourself.

- **Refrain from judging.** In one study, people who were concerned about being judged, or who were judgmental themselves, had a more difficult time concentrating and ignoring outside stimuli during a mental task.

● **Discard the whiners and the critics.** Every happy friend increases your chances of being happy by 9 per cent, but every unhappy friend decreases those chances by 7 per cent. High-maintenance friendships or interpersonal conflicts also cause people to do worse on standardised tests.

Check your feelings after visiting friends. Energised or depleted? Confident or insecure? Get closer to people who make you feel good and minimise time with people who make you feel bad.

## GET INVOLVED

● **Usher at concerts, events and lectures.** Get on the list of volunteers by calling your local theatre. Many places have a list of people they call on – stick with it and, over time, you can become part of the theatre's community. You'll help a theatre that can't afford to pay its staff and get to see events for free.

● **Volunteer for a soup kitchen or other community service on the same day every week.** If you keep the same schedule or route, you'll create mini relationships with each person you feed, and those connections help both of you equally. You'll also bond with fellow volunteers and may even find more interests in common with them than with friends you've had for years.

● **Help out your adult children.** They may be going through one of the most challenging periods of their lives: stressful but rewarding work combined with the exhaustion of parenting. By helping them with child care, shopping or other household tasks, you'll help yourself as well – and maybe even lengthen your life. Research shows that strong emotional

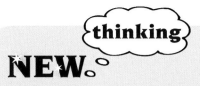

**Becoming a volunteer boosts your brain.**
Volunteering can help give you a sense of belonging within your community, which is good news for your brain. It's also an enjoyable way to learn fresh skills and meet new people. Think about what would suit you best and how much time you have free, then get searching (see www.volunteering.org.uk, www.csv.org.uk and www.Do-it.org). Here's how to get started:

● Find out what's available in your area by visiting your library or checking through local newspapers.

● Consider becoming a mentor to a young person (see www.mandbf.org).

● Contact BTCV, an organisation that arranges for volunteers to carry out practical environmental conservation work (see www2.btcv.org.uk).

● Consider joining a wildlife organisation such as The Wildlife Trusts (www.wildlifetrusts.org) or the National Trust (www.nationaltrust.org.uk).

● If the idea of volunteer work abroad appeals, and if you have a useful skill, contact Voluntary Service Overseas (VSO, www.vso.org.uk).

bonds between parents and adult children predict longer parental survival.

● **Bond with your grandchildren.** Never underestimate the power of time spent with grandchildren to keep a brain young. Depending on their ages, read them Harry Potter books and try to keep track of the characters; ask them to show you how to play the Nintendo Wii if you don't already know; find out what subjects they're studying at school and consider reading about them yourself so you'll have a new topic of conversation.

# BOOSTER 4

## Learning

**Human beings are creatures of habit.**
We often eat the same breakfast every morning,
drive the same route to work, watch the same TV
programmes at night. All of this sameness makes it easy for
our brains to operate on autopilot, which has its benefits
– but growing new neural connections and protecting the
brain from decline aren't among them.

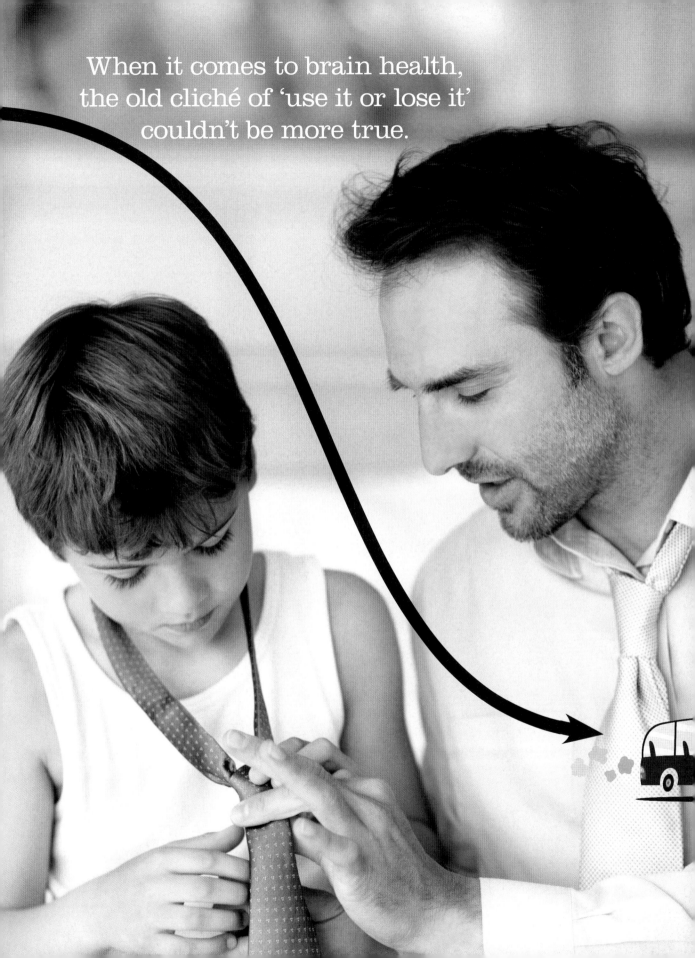

When it comes to brain health,
the old cliché of 'use it or lose it'
couldn't be more true.

Research shows clearly that mental activity benefits the brain and keeps it strong. When you learn, you grow new neurons as well as fresh and bigger connections between those neurons, creating more storage space for memories. You've already learned that long-term memories are stored in vast networks of nerve-cell pathways. The richer those pathways, the more permanent – and accessible – the information in your brain will be.

Remember the story from Part 1 about the London taxi drivers? When some of the drivers, who spent their careers learning to navigate the complicated London street system, underwent MRI scans of their brains, they were found to have an unusually large hippocampus, an area that plays a major role in memory formation, particularly spatial memory. You don't need to study maps of London to grow your hippocampus, but learning something – anything – will make your brain bigger, stronger and better able to resist age-related changes that can slow you down.

Challenging your brain is perhaps the best thing you can do to keep it young. One study looked at the degree of cognitive stimulation a group of older people experienced over a period of five years. Those who experienced the most had 35 per cent less decline in their cognitive abilities than those who experienced the least.

## WHAT COUNTS AS LEARNING?

'Learning' comes in many forms. Of course, challenging your brain with books, crossword puzzles, card games and classes is important. But so is brain stimulation of almost any sort. Any new experience you have, especially when it is very different from your normal routine, is a learning experience. Some of the most effective experiences are those that involve your senses.

Imagine walking through a botanical garden, surrounded by colours of every shade and hue, a gentle breeze on your face, and suddenly the smell of lavender transports you back to playing in the park as a young child. Or you attend a wine-tasting in a villa in Bordeaux, and you gaze at your partner in the fading sunlight as you drink a glass of amazing claret and think about the first time

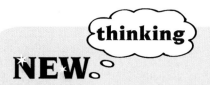

### NEW thinking

**Education: your brain's rainy-day fund?**
Intellectual experiences throughout your entire life, no matter when they happen, build your brain reserve. Think of it as cognitive cash in the bank; it's the 'money' that will cushion you against any shortfalls and delay 'bankruptcy' should you run into trouble.

Researchers from the universities of Aberdeen and Edinburgh looked at 92 people born in 1921 whose cognitive function had been tested at age 11. They were re-tested again at age 79, and their brain volume was measured on a brain scan. The findings were remarkable – educational level at age 11 was associated with memory capacity at age 79, and both education and occupational attainment during working life were related to reasoning ability in old age. Brain volume made no contribution at all. Researchers conclude that the intellectual challenges experienced during life, such as education and occupation, accumulate cerebral reserve and allow cognitive function to be maintained in old age.

you shared a bottle of wine together. Your brain is on the alert, absorbing and analysing the new sensory information and processing it together with stored memories to consider all this data in the new context. And most of this happens just by remaining in the moment and noticing details around you.

## SURPRISE YOUR BRAIN

To challenge your brain, you don't have to memorise the periodic table of elements or calculate pi to a thousand digits. All you really need to do is, well, anything other than what you've been doing. The best way to start is to think of a few things you've always wanted to try, and jump in. Here are a few suggestions to get your brain in gear.

● **Develop your alter ego.** When we like something, we tend to do it a lot. Readers read; knitters knit; computer programmers program. From now on, the old Monty Python line is your personal mantra: 'And now for something completely different!' During your leisure time, do whatever you perceive to be the complete opposite of what you normally do. If you're a carpenter, join a reading group. If you're a book editor, take a kayaking class. If you're an information technology expert, take up watercolour painting.

● **Shake up your environment.** If you spend 8 hours a day staring at a computer screen, ban all screens (computers, BlackBerries, TVs) for one day of the weekend and go off somewhere green instead. If you spend your days tending to others' needs – as a nurse, a volunteer,

a teacher, a caregiver – switch to total self-indulgence: go to a spa and get a massage or pedicure, or ring a friend and go to watch a film together. If you tend to spend quiet evenings at home, try out a lively bar. Any time you experience new, radically different sensations, your brain is shocked out of its stupor and undergoes a change that builds new connections, associations and memories – the exact process involved in learning. Your brain will not only thrive on the change of pace, you'll reduce stress (another drain on the brain), and be refreshed and ready to go on Monday.

● **Choose an activity you have to practise to master.** Most of us reach a point of competency in our jobs and hobbies, and then coast along on that competency. But in some ways, being a novice is better for your brain than being an expert. You get the biggest cognitive boost when you pick up a new skill: start with the basics, then practise, practise, practise until you master it. That thrill of mastery, and even the tiny victories along the way, creates a flush of pleasure chemicals that reinforce the learning and motivate you to continue.

If you're just learning to cast your rod, practise in the paddling pool in the garden until you feel confident, then take it to a riverbank. Or read up on the card game bridge, then play it online until you feel ready to join a real live bridge game. Progressive

*Choose an activity you have to practise to master.*

learning like this causes specific brain cells to specialise for the demands of your new task. Just like strengthening your abdominal muscles helps to improve your posture, as these individual regions of your brain get stronger, they fortify the brain as a whole.

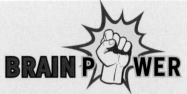

**BRAIN POWER**

Actions as well as thoughts can be involved in memorising. Learning is faster if the body as well as the mind is engaged in the task. For example, it's easier to remember the layout of a town by walking the streets than by learning it from a map.

● **Learn to play a musical instrument.** Playing an instrument physically strengthens the brain. One Canadian study found that children who took music lessons experienced a seven-point boost in their IQs. Another study showed that drumming helped adults reduce cortisol levels (high levels are toxic to brain cells). Still other research has shown that mastering an instrument leads to a better facility with numbers and an enhanced sense of spatial relations. At higher levels, music training may help improve our ability to manipulate information in both short and long-term memory, benefits that can help us in many areas of life. Even if you don't fancy learning an instrument, consider joining a choir or taking singing lessons. Singing is an aerobic activity that's

known to increase oxygen levels in the bloodstream and reduce stress – all of which is good news for the brain.

The type of music you listen to or play is very much a matter of personal taste, but researchers have found that the most natural tempo is 80 beats a minute – about the same as the average human heart rate. This suggests that music is appealing because it tunes in to our natural body rhythms.

● **Keep a journal.** Get into the habit of writing down your thoughts and feelings every day and you could well improve your physical and mental wellbeing. The trick is to write what comes to mind – don't edit yourself or worry about the quality or content of what you're writing. You'll find that it gets easier the more you do it, and you'll have an interesting record to look back on – it might even trigger the beginnings of the book you've always felt you wanted to write. If you discover that you enjoy writing, find out about creative writing or book groups in your area so that you can meet like-minded people and swap ideas.

● **Launch, or continue, a career.** Fewer and fewer people plan to stop working entirely when they retire. Continuing to work, even on a freelance or part-time basis, is an excellent way to line your pockets and protect your brain. It can even prevent the brain-draining depression that often results from having too much idle time.

● **Stay productive.** You don't have to have a job to produce, say experts – you could also pitch in at the soup kitchen, knit hats for babies at the hospital, teach your grandchildren how to read or tend a local community garden. While surveys have found that paid work drops sharply

Get into the habit of writing down your thoughts and feelings every day.

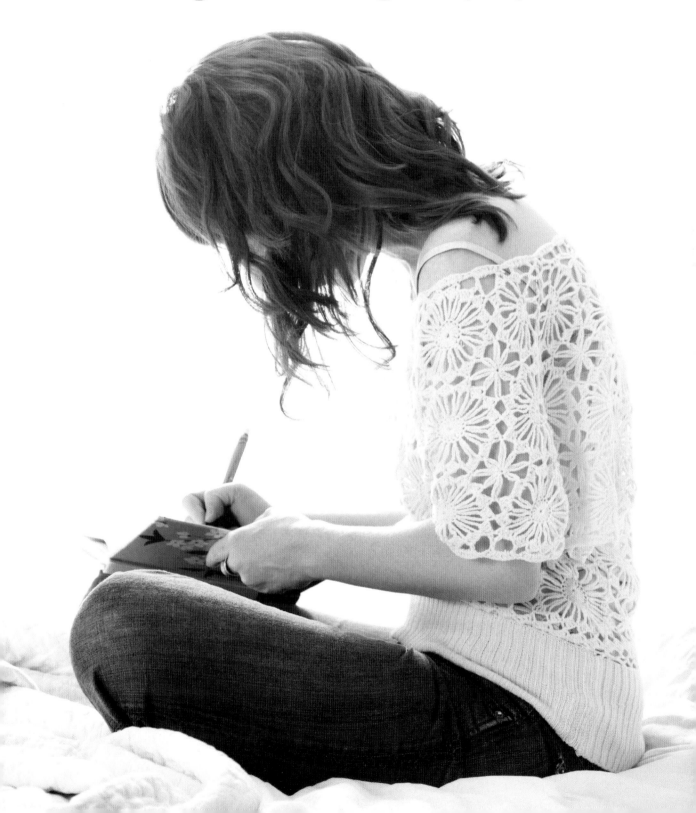

# THE POWER OF POSITIVE THINKING

The doddering old widow. The lonely, forgetful neighbour. It turns out these negative perceptions of old age can be self-fulfilling prophecies. Researchers at Yale University in the USA checked on the mortality rates of more than 600 people who answered survey questions some 20 years earlier, when they were aged 50 or older. The researchers discovered that those who'd agreed with such statements as 'Things keep getting worse as I get older' and 'As you get older, you are less useful' were more likely to die early than those who'd agreed with such statements as 'I am as happy now as I was when I was younger.' People with a more positive outlook on ageing lived an average of 7.5 years longer than the negative bunch.

The more negative the vision of old age people held when they were younger, the more likely they were to experience the very types of physical and mental decline they envisioned – in other words, they turned into their own stereotypes. What's more, psychologists have shown that if you think your memory will get worse with age, then it probably will. Senior citizens who believe that older people perform poorly on tests of memory actually score much worse than those who do not buy in to negative stereotypes about ageing and memory loss.

Other studies have found that when researchers used word prompts such as 'wise' versus 'senile' before older people engaged in specific tasks, that vocabulary alone led to enhancement or decline on a wide array of cognitive and behavioural results, including memory performance, handwriting and mathematical performance.

The moral? Think young. Any time you find yourself saying 'I don't do that', write 'that', whatever it is, down on a list. Show yourself you can do it, and you'll build up your belief in your brain's abilities, a key strategy for prolonging your life and avoiding cognitive decline.

after the age of 55, volunteer work peaks then. And informal help to friends and family peaks thereafter (between the ages of 55 and 64) and can continue until age 74 or later.

When older people continue to stay productive, they are not considered old by their families or friends, or by themselves – and, apparently, their brains agree. A study of more than a thousand Chinese adults aged 55 and older found that useful, constructive activities, such as painting, gardening, preparing meals and even shopping, lowered the risk of dementia, presumably because those activities demand complex thought and planning.

## TURN CHORES INTO BRAIN BOOSTERS

● **Learn a useful new skill.** Choose learning opportunities that help you in real life. Lots of libraries and local education establishments run introductory computer courses. Having trouble keeping your banking and investments straight? Take a financial-planning course, or learn how to use money-management software. You'll find your bills and savings fall into place, decreasing the stress that can sap motivation and atrophy your brain. These activities tap into a well of deeper attention because their relevance – the degree to which the information matters to you personally – is so high. Best of all, you'll break negative thinking patterns such as, 'I can't manage my money', which can accelerate cognitive loss.

● **Swap chores.** A survey of more than 20,000 Scottish men and women found that doing just 20 minutes of weekly housework or gardening was enough to increase their mental health markedly. But here's the twist: swap jobs. Let your

# 9 FUN, EASY WAYS TO LEARN something new

1   Buy a word-a-day calendar and try to use the word in conversation at least once during the course of the day.

2   Go to the zoo and actually stop to read all the signs and learn about the animals.

3   Look every day at 'Today's featured article' on Wikipedia (www.en.wikipedia.org), to find out more about a whole host of new and interesting subjects.

4   Take a one-day first-aid class.

5   Go to a beginner's wine tasting (free at many wine shops) and learn how to smell, taste and spit like a pro.

6   Pick a random topic – how to grow tomatoes, improve your petrol mileage, open a flower shop – Google it, and follow the links for 20 minutes and see where they take you.

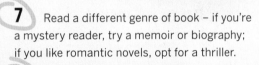

Hang out a bird feeder …

7   Read a different genre of book – if you're a mystery reader, try a memoir or biography; if you like romantic novels, opt for a thriller.

8   Learn to say 'hello', 'please' and 'thank you' in a new language every week.

9   Hang a bird feeder by your window and keep a bird book handy to help you identify feathered visitors.

partner pay the bills or send out birthday cards while you pull out weeds, change light bulbs or walk the dog. Trading chores not only challenges your brain in new ways but also helps you to see things from your partner's perspective – a higher-level thinking process that exercises multiple parts of your brain at once. Bonus: your relationship can only improve the more you appreciate each other.

● **Time your task.** If you're going to tackle a difficult cognitive challenge, such as reviewing changes in your insurance policies or energy providers, set a timer for 20 minutes and really focus. The combination of committed attention and a focused time period stimulates the nucleus basalis, an area in the forebrain vulnerable to Alzheimer's disease. Once you've finished, reward yourself – spend a few minutes watching a TV comedy or just sit quietly in the garden and let the sun warm your face – this will stimulate your brain's reward system, reinforce the benefits of the effort you've made and motivate you to do it again.

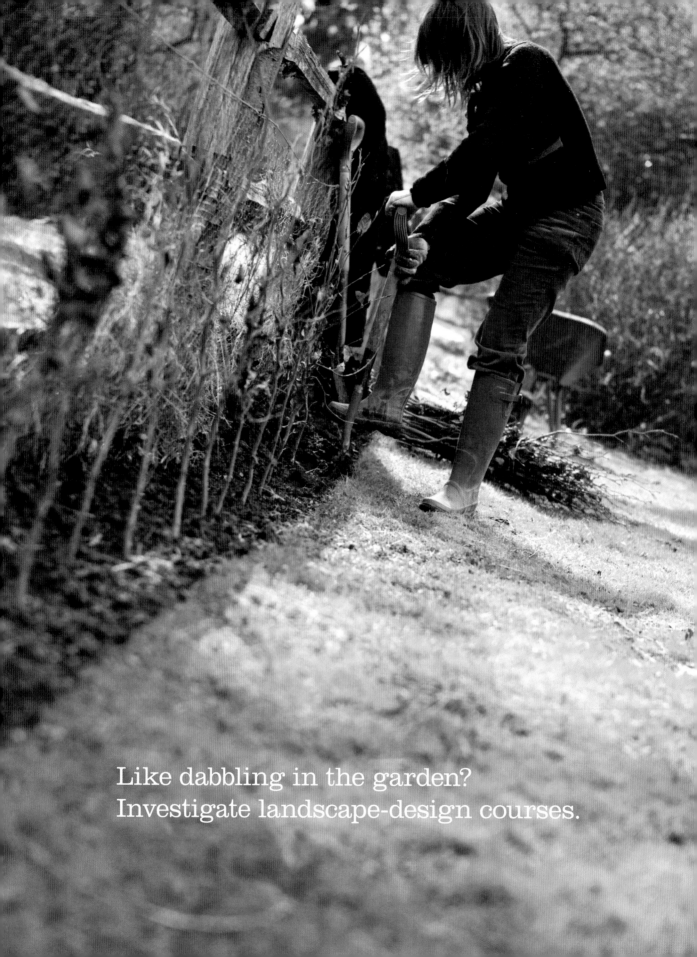

Like dabbling in the garden?
Investigate landscape-design courses.

## STIMULATE YOUR SENSES

● **Go to a rock concert or an amusement park.** Have you ever gone to an event and thought, 'I'm too old for this?' That's exactly where you need to be – at least for a little while. You needn't be a regular at rock concerts, video arcades or noisy bars, but occasional visits could do you a world of good. These experiences assault your brain with new sensations and nudge you out of your comfort zone, reawakening your senses. A word of caution: be sure to take earplugs if you're attending a noisy concert.

learn all you can about it. Maybe it's an upcoming election, an environmental issue (such as recycling), or something larger, such as an ongoing war. Many people find that getting involved in a cause they believe in helps them tap into a reserve of energy and excitement they didn't realise they had. If there's an issue you feel particularly passionate about – such as taking care of stray dogs or cleaning up your local area – go online to search for a local group that's working in your community (try www.volunteering. org.uk or www.csv.org.uk).

## Choose foreign films. Reading the subtitles while watching challenges your brain.

● **Indulge in small thrills.** Another reason fresh experiences benefit the brain is because they stimulate the release of dopamine, a neurotransmitter associated with attention and planning. Older brains release less dopamine, which may in part explain our dwindling attention spans as we age. Here's the fun part: you get dopamine surges from lots of very enjoyable things – eating chocolate (make it dark chocolate for its antioxidants), getting a foot massage, having sex.

● **Watch foreign films.** Reading the subtitles while simultaneously watching the actors challenges you to keep up. You won't be able to lie back and vegetate; you'll be actively involved in the film.

## FIND LIKE-MINDED PEOPLE

● **Gen up on a cause you care about.** There's a lot wrong with the world, and much you can do to help set it right. Choose a cause that interests you and

● **Join the WI.** The Women's Institute, the UK's largest women's voluntary organisation, is enjoying something of a resurgence. Members can try diverse activities and build new skills, as well as joining in with a number of campaigning issues (for more information go to www.thewi.org.uk).

● **Develop your art.** If you have an interest such as cooking or playing tennis, raise the bar. Sign up for a cookery course with a chef who'll show you how to use fresh, local ingredients, or take lessons with a tennis pro. Like dabbling in the garden? Investigate landscape-design courses in your area. Challenge yourself to rise above your current level – if you have to struggle to keep up, all the better.

● **Hit the stage.** If you've harboured a secret dream to be an actor, head to your local theatre and see if you can audition, even for a non-speaking part, in the next production. Or help behind the scenes to

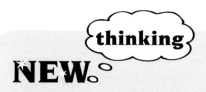

# NEW.

## Learn, don't memorise.

Don't bother to remember names – just tell yourself to learn them. One study found that when people were told to 'learn' statements from a list, they did much better than when they were told to 'remember' them. In fact, when adults between the ages of 60 and 75 were told to 'learn', they did as well as participants aged 17 to 24. If you, consciously or unconsciously, believe that memory gets worse with age, anxiety over remembering names and facts can prevent you from remembering them. Think in terms of learning instead and leapfrog over your own self-doubts.

create sets, write, produce, do make-up or sew costumes, other creative tasks that will tickle your brain. Actors also employ clever tricks to learn their lines, which can help hone your memory skills.

● **Walk and talk.** You know that exercise and social connections – Boosters 2 and 3 – help sharpen the brain. Combine them with mental stimulation and you'll reap maximum rewards. Try these tactics:

● Walk with a friend and discuss politics or a book you've both read.

● Learn to waltz, tango or swing dance – you'll memorise the steps and socialise with other students as you move.

● Cycle to your bingo game or to a friend's house to play Scrabble.

## WORK TOWARDS A FINISHED PRODUCT

● **Alternate difficult and easy craft projects.** Don't just knit a load of single-colour, one-stitch scarves while staring at the TV – really work at creating something you've never done

before. Challenge yourself to learn new patterns. Try intricate work that requires careful attention, counting and memory. Alternate these brain-intensive projects with more 'mindless' scarves, the creation of which can help manage anxiety and decrease blood pressure, protecting your brain from degenerative stresses.

● **Help your parents or relatives organise photos and memorabilia.** Or sit down and do it for yourself. Most of us have boxes of photos we never look through because they aren't in albums. Or we have electronic photos scattered on several different photo-sharing websites. (If you need help organising photos online, look for an internet class that covers photo management.)

Take time to sit down with your parent or relative and their boxes of photos, chatting and reminiscing. Recalling pleasant memories engages your nucleus accumbens, a part of the brain involved in memory consolidation that's also awash in dopamine, a brain chemical associated with pleasure and reward. A bonus: as you help get the memorabilia organised, you'll strengthen your own ability to classify and arrange, skills that can falter somewhat with age.

● **Create an audio scrapbook.** If your budget allows, buy an electronic voice recorder and voice-recognition software. The combination allows you to turn conversations into digital files that you can copy to CDs and share with the rest of the family, or turn into text. Go to a self-publishing website (such as www. lulu.com), turn your text into a book, and order copies for everyone in the family.

● **Take a class on using the internet.** You'll learn how to do everything from filing taxes electronically (faster returns) to shopping and paying bills online. There really is no limit to what you could learn. Remember, while TV makes you a passive receptacle, the Web puts you in control.

## GO BACK TO SCHOOL — AS A STUDENT OR TEACHER

● **Sign up for a class.** Have you always wanted to get your degree but never had a chance to finish? Maybe you'd like to learn more about art history or world economics. If you live near a university, ask what courses they run for the local community, or check out the Open

and can draw on their vast vocabularies for raw material. A 2004 study at York University in Canada found evidence to suggest that people who regularly use two languages perform better at complex tasks. So why not take a class in Spanish, French, Italian or any other language you love. If you're still as enthusiastic after a few months, consider taking a long holiday and, perhaps, an intensive course in the country of your choice. You'll help your brain connect real-world experience to each word, something you just won't get in a classroom.

> Take time to sit down with a parent or relative and their boxes of photos, chatting and reminiscing.

University (www.open.ac.uk). The rigour of a class will be infectious. You'll also be able to gauge your wisdom against that of younger people, and you may find that you have a certain edge.

● **Head back to school — on your kitchen table.** If you'd like to experience academia from the comfort of your home, investigate some of the thousands of online distance-learning programmes available from accredited universities around the country, and the world (start with the Open University – see above). Typically, you'll interact with your tutor by email or phone. Some courses also require you to attend an on-campus weekend, another mind-stretching experience.

● **Finally learn Spanish.** Do you think children are the only ones who can learn a new language? Hardly. Adults understand how grammar rules typically work,

● **Let your ears fill up your brain.** Listen to lectures whenever you have the time. The Great Courses programme (www. greatcourses.co.uk) collects lectures from some of the finest professors in the world on subjects ranging from Albert Einstein to opera appreciation to Zen Buddhism. Pop the CDs into your portable player and take them into the garden, or listen on long train or car journeys

● **Offer your expertise.** Sometimes the best way to learn is to teach. If you have a special talent or skill – a flair for science or computers, for example – you could try mentoring a young person who's struggling with these subjects. You'll boost your own self-confidence and self-worth at the same time as supporting others (go to www.mandbf.org.uk to find out more). Or offer your services to a local community centre or project.

# BOOSTER 5

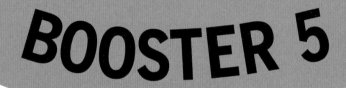

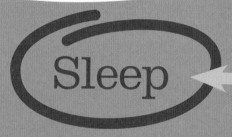

## Sleep

**Some Sharp Brain Boosters require a bit of work
on your part –** tweaking diet and exercise habits, signing
up for a class, making an effort to get out and see people. But
Booster 5 is defined by doing nothing at all. Zero. To reap its
tremendous brain benefits, simply pull back the sheets on your
bed, slide in and allow yourself to drop off to sleep.

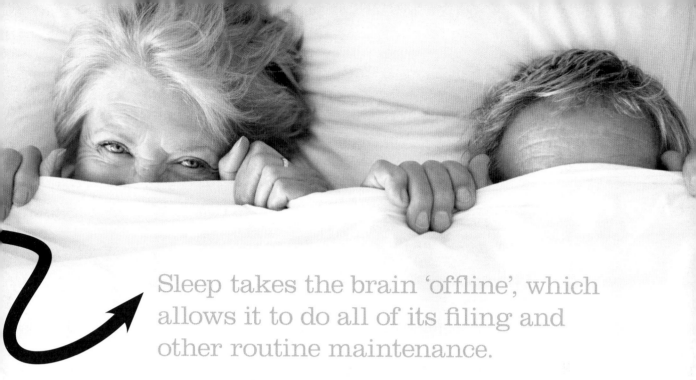

Sleep takes the brain 'offline', which allows it to do all of its filing and other routine maintenance.

**W**hile you sleep, your body may be still, but your brain is busy. It sweeps out all the detritus left behind by daily brain-cell activities – biochemical clutter that can interfere with normal brain functioning. It also repairs and regenerates tissues critical to memory and other cognitive processes. Indeed, high-quality sleep improves your ability to make plans, solve problems, concentrate and remember things. Want to get smarter overnight? Take a nap. Our IQ is actually higher when we are well rested.

Sleep takes the brain 'offline', which allows it to do all its filing and other routine maintenance. During the first hour-and-a-half after you fall asleep, you drift into the first of several nightly cycles of slow-wave stage 3 and 4 sleep, the deepest forms. This dreamless slumber helps you solidify long-term retention of declarative memories – the facts you have learned or situations you have experienced during the day. In order to reach this state, your levels of the stress hormone cortisol must be very low, a big reason why relaxation is key to a good night's rest – and good memory. (When levels of cortisol are too high, storage of memories in the hippocampus suffers. Over time, the cortisol slowly erodes this critical memory centre, and brain cells in the hippocampus waste away, considerably slowing your access to facts and memories.)

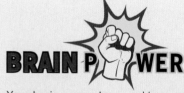

**BRAIN POWER**

Your brain never stops working, even when you are asleep. Even in deep sleep, there is activity in parts of the brain, including the cortex. Overall, there is practically no difference in total brain activity during a period of sleep and one of wakefulness.

## WHAT HAPPENS WHEN YOU SLEEP

- Brain cells are repaired.
- Experiences are processed into memories.
- Memories are solidified and put in places where they can be accessed more quickly.
- Health-promoting growth hormone is released.
- Connections between nerve cells multiply, increasing your brain's 'plasticity'.
- Decision-making skills, reaction time and hand–eye coordination are sharpened.

more good. Just 1 or 2 hours of additional sleep can help you perform much better on tasks that require sustained focus. Sleep can even help your brain shuffle newly developed ideas together and solve problems more creatively.

## OLDER PEOPLE DON'T NEED LESS SLEEP

Many of us don't get enough shut-eye, and that's bad, especially considering that sleep deprivation increases brain inflammation, which can prevent new brain cells forming. Researchers have even found that chronic sleep deprivation ages the brain at an accelerated rate, setting us up for

## Often, we don't even realise we're sleep deprived.

### REM – THE DREAM STATE

Towards the early morning, cortisol levels naturally rise, preparing to wake you up. Before you are thoroughly awake, you'll cycle through several stages of rapid-eye-movement, or REM, sleep. This dream-filled sleep allows your brain to rehearse skills you learned during the day, such as notes you played on the piano or a difficult dance step you finally mastered.

This rehearsal, which activates the same neural circuits as actually performing the activity, helps the brain store these 'procedural' memories for good.

During REM sleep, you also process and sort through emotional memories. High levels of cortisol can hurt here, too: while excess cortisol degrades long-term memory stored in the hippocampus, it actually enhances the storage of disturbing emotional memories in the amygdala, the seat of our most primal emotions.

If getting adequate sleep benefits your brain, a little extra on occasion can do even

early cognitive decline. Yet we often don't even realise we're sleep deprived. A study published in the journal *Epidemiology* found that when more than 650 adults were asked how much they slept, they regularly overestimated their sleep hours.

But don't we need less sleep as we age? No, say the experts, though it may seem that way because of a natural process called sleep phase shift. Basically, as we get older, we tend to go to sleep earlier or nap during the day and wake up earlier. We still need as many hours as ever.

## SUREFIRE STEPS TO BETTER SLEEP

Getting more sleep can be achieved by something as simple as going to bed earlier. It also helps to perfect what sleep experts call your sleep hygiene, that is, your sleep habits. What doesn't help much? Sleeping pills. People who take

# ARE YOU sleep deprived?

If you feel drowsy during the day, you probably didn't get enough sleep the night before. The Epworth Sleepiness Scale, developed by Dr Murray Johns of Epworth Hospital in Melbourne, Australia, is a test used by sleep specialists to judge a person's level of daytime sleepiness. To find out your level, ask yourself what the chances are that you'd doze off in the situations below, and give yourself the appropriate number of points.

**1** Sitting and reading

☐ **0** None
☐ **1** Slight
☐ **2** Moderate
☐ **3** High

**2** Watching TV

☐ **0** None
☐ **1** Slight
☐ **2** Moderate
☐ **3** High

**3** Sitting inactively in a public place, such as a theatre or a meeting

☐ **0** None
☐ **1** Slight
☐ **2** Moderate
☐ **3** High

**4** As a passenger in a car for an hour without a break

☐ **0** None
☐ **1** Slight
☐ **2** Moderate
☐ **3** High

**5** Sitting quietly after lunch (without alcohol)

☐ **0** None
☐ **1** Slight
☐ **2** Moderate
☐ **3** High

**6** Sitting and talking to someone

☐ **0** None
☐ **1** Slight
☐ **2** Moderate
☐ **3** High

**7** Lying down to rest in the afternoon (not intending to nap)

☐ **0** None
☐ **1** Slight
☐ **2** Moderate
☐ **3** High

**8** In a car while stopped for a few minutes in traffic

☐ **0** None
☐ **1** Slight
☐ **2** Moderate
☐ **3** High

YOUR SCORE

**Less than 8 points:** You're in good shape. You probably get enough sleep.

**8–11 points:** You're getting a little less sleep than you need; your brain probably isn't quite as fast or sharp as it would be with more sleep.

**12–15 points:** You clearly aren't getting enough sleep. This is an issue you need to address.

**16–24 points:** You get so little sleep that you shouldn't be behind the wheel of a car, responsible for balancing your household budget or working out your income tax.

them don't get as much extra sleep as they think – sometimes only a few minutes more. And once you start taking sleep aids, including over-the-counter products, you could become trapped in an addictive cycle.

If you are having trouble sleeping, you're not alone. Experts reckon that 30 to 45 per cent of people worldwide suffer from insomnia. You may find the following strategies useful.

## COMBAT STRESS HORMONES

● **Hit the gym.** One of the best ways to get a good night's sleep is to exercise. Most researchers think exercise reduces insomnia because of its effects on stress hormones. People with insomnia tend to have abnormally high levels of stress hormones, or release the hormones with very little provocation. Exercise initially increases stress hormones, but then a few hours later, seeking to return to balance, your body sends out signals to reduce them. That's why you shouldn't exercise in the evening. Try to get in your workout at least 6 hours before bedtime.

● **Try abdominal breathing.** Anxiety and tension often lead to fast, shallow breathing, which makes dropping off more difficult. To combat this, try a few minutes of abdominal breathing, which focuses your mind and provides feedback to your brain that you're relaxed and ready for sleep, as part of your winding-down routine. It may take a few attempts to perfect it, but you should quickly notice the difference.

To begin, lie down, with a light book on your chest – which helps you gauge that your muscles are moving correctly – and inhale slowly through your nose. Feel the book on your chest rise as you do so. Then, when your breath reaches your stomach, push your abdomen upwards, letting your abdomen rise slightly higher than the book (due to your diaphragm expanding). Hold for 1 second, then do the reverse: exhale and allow your muscles to relax, then let the air flow out of your chest and nostrils, relaxing your jaw as you do so.

● **Read – don't watch – the news, and only in the morning.** Try to get your news before noon, either in the form of a newspaper or online. Television news often sensationalises stories about child abductions and other crimes and makes them seem more common than they are. If you read your news instead of passively watching it, you're in control of the type of stories you consume.

● **Wean yourself from afternoon coffee.** A morning cup of coffee is very good for your brain indeed – caffeine increases brain activity in your hippocampus, and it may also increase

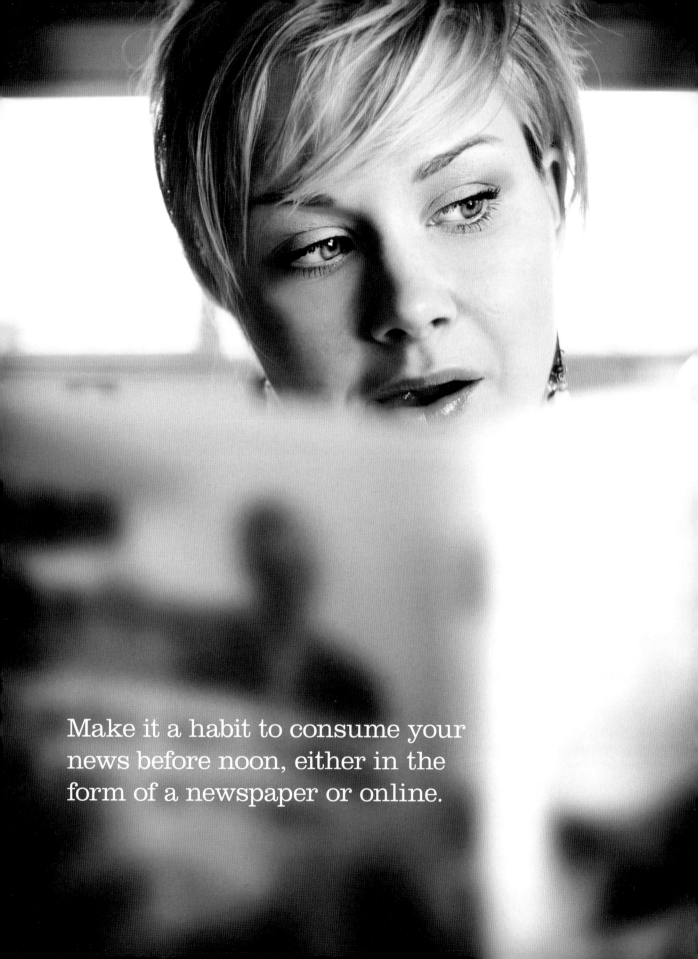

Make it a habit to consume your news before noon, either in the form of a newspaper or online.

levels of a key neurotransmitter. But make sure that you've finished your last cup of the day by lunchtime, since it can take as long as 10 hours for caffeine to leave your system. Until then, caffeine keeps your cortisol levels elevated, which can interfere with your ability to fall asleep.

## STAY TRUE TO YOUR BODY CLOCK

● **Get some bright light and outdoor sun during the day.** If you expose your eyes to bright light in the morning, you'll help reset your internal clock, making it easier for you to sleep at night. Light enters your eyes and triggers your suprachiasmatic nucleus – your brain's 'circadian pacemaker' – which regulates several biological rhythms during the day and night. One of these rhythms is the rise and fall of melatonin, a hormone that makes you more sleepy and less mentally sharp. Bright light depresses melatonin; the lower your melatonin during the day, the higher it tends to climb at night, which allows you to fall into a deeper sleep.

The day-to-night shift in melatonin levels is extreme when we're young but much less dramatic as we age. One

reason is that our eyes become less able to transmit light to the pineal gland (which produces melatonin) as we age. Less of a rise and fall in melatonin can result in more fatigue and decreased speed of thinking during the day, while also making it difficult to sleep at night. To combat this phenomenon, expose yourself to as much daylight as possible – the intensity of light is measured in lux, the amount of light you receive at a specific distance from the light source.

● Walk the dog in the early morning (400 lux).

● Use a light-therapy box for 15 minutes to 2 hours a day (2,500 to 10,000 lux).

● Take a stroll at noon or sit outside with the bright sun on your face (50,000 to 100,000 lux).

● Put all the lights on in your workspace or sitting area during the day (500 lux).

● **Keep lights low in the evening.** Bright light in the evening can disrupt melatonin release, so put dimmers on your switches and keep your lights lower after dark. Have just one small bedside lamp on for the half-hour before you go to sleep. Install blackout blinds to guard against

Don't drink coffee after lunchtime.

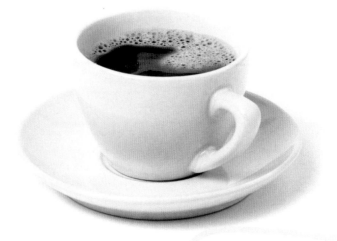

any exterior light entering your bedroom during the night. This is especially important if you have blue, green or light-brown eyes – one study found that, compared with people with dark-brown eyes, those with light-coloured eyes experienced 20 per cent lower melatonin when exposed to light at night.

● **Establish a strict bedtime and wake-up time.** When it comes to sleep, the body loves routine. Going to bed and getting up at the same time every day, even at weekends, is one of the surest ways to help yourself fall asleep at night. Working backwards from when you need to be up in the morning, choose a bedtime – such as 11pm – and make sure that you're in bed with the lights off at that time. Work backwards from there to create your set pre-bed routine, such as:

**10.25** – Shower and brush teeth.

**10.35** – Slip into pyjamas, soft bathrobe and socks.

**10.40** – Read something relaxing or write in journal.

**11** – Lights out.

At 7am, it's time to wake up. Having a sleep routine minimises circadian rhythm disturbances, which can become more prevalent as we get older.

● **Go to bed 15 minutes earlier every week.** Do this until you're getting the amount of sleep you need, then set your new bedtime in stone. A recent study found that one additional hour of sleep a night can lower your risk of developing calcified coronary artery plaque – hardened calcium deposits in the arteries of your heart – by up to 33 per cent, the equivalent of lowering your systolic blood pressure by 16.5 points. The result? Better blood flow throughout your entire body, including your brain.

## SNOOZE TO REMEMBER

Concerned that you'll draw a blank on names at tomorrow's wedding or reunion? Study the guest list the night before, then get a good night's rest. During sleep, new memories are strengthened within their own neural circuits and are also distributed throughout the brain to be filed in and among pre-existing long-term memories. This makes the information more solid and easier to access. Also plan to get a good night's sleep after the event. If you go to bed remembering Mary's name but you don't sleep enough, studies suggest you're likely to get the name wrong the next day. You might call Mary 'Margaret' at breakfast.

● **Buy an electronic enforcer.** If you're having trouble sticking to a set bedtime, buy a timer for the lights in your living room and even for the switch to your TV. Set it to turn off at 10.45pm or earlier. Turning them back on will be a hassle, and you'll find it easier just to go to bed. Or set an alarm clock to ring at 10.30pm – an alert that time is almost up. If you tend to surf the web at night, programme a reminder to alert you: '10.45 – bedtime.'

## MAKE BEDTIME A PLEASURE

● **Buy some high-thread-count sheets.** Then change them regularly, at least once a week, so they're always soft and fresh. And why not splash out on a down pillow? There's nothing like an inviting bed to lure you away from the TV.

● **Add a white-noise machine.** Or a fan, air-conditioner or earplugs – anything to block out noise and help you stay asleep. The longer you sleep (up to a maximum of 8 or 9 hours), the more cycles of restorative stage 3 and 4 sleep

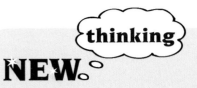

## NEW thinking

### Coffee or nap?

**Take the nap.** A study published in the journal *Behavioural Brain Research* looked at the performance of three groups of people: one group that napped from 1pm to 3pm, one group that got the caffeine equivalent of two cups of coffee at 3pm, and one group that took placebo pills. The caffeinated group thought themselves the least sleepy but, in fact, they performed the same as the placebo group, or worse, on several cognitive tests. The nappers did the best, outscoring the other two groups significantly on the sensory and verbal tests.

you'll have. Your body doesn't get to REM sleep until you've gone through several cycles of stage 3 and 4, but REM is essential for creating new neurons in the areas of the brain associated with long-term memory.

● **Choose the right mattress.** Use your own judgment when it comes to picking a mattress that suits you, but ask your GP or back specialist for advice if you have back problems. Consider buying a mattress topper, which can be used to alter the level of support – some differ on each side of the bed, which is ideal for couples with different preferences. To keep your mattress in tip-top condition, air it daily, turn it frequently and replace it every ten years.

● **Make your home safe.** You'll sleep better if you know that your home is secure and you have adequate, working smoke alarms.

● **Keep it cool.** When it's time to sleep, your body temperature drops, usually starting 60 to 90 minutes before you fall asleep and reaching its lowest point about 2 hours before you wake up. Help it along by turning down your thermostat before you go to bed, especially if you have trouble sleeping. Researchers at the University of South Australia have found that insomniacs have a higher core body temperature than sound sleepers.

wrong. It may help you fall asleep – if you don't drink regularly, that is – but as the effects wear off, you may wake up again.

● **Comedies only at night.** If you enjoy murder or crime shows, tape them and watch them early in the evening. One dream study found that people who watched more coverage of the terrorist attacks on the USA on September 11, 2001, experienced a dramatic change in the features of their dreams, even when they lived nowhere near Ground Zero or the Pentagon. Researchers said these results proved a direct association between watching images of violence on television and increased stress and trauma. Remember that high levels of

## If you have trouble dropping off, try a hard-boiled egg or a handful of peanuts with a milky drink before bed.

### PERFECT YOUR BEFORE-BED ROUTINE

● **Watch your bedtime snacking.** We know that eating some foods such as cheese before bedtime can disturb your sleep, as can indulging in heavy late-night meals or sugary snacks. But some foods are positively sleep-inducing – anything containing the amino acid tryptophan, which boosts levels of brain-calming serotonin. If you have trouble dropping off, try a hard-boiled egg, a handful of peanuts, sunflower or pumpkin seeds, dates or a small slice of chicken or turkey, along with a milky drink.

● **Skip the nightcap.** You might think alcohol helps you sleep, but you'd be

stress hormones rob us of deep sleep. And as we get older, our bodies become even more vulnerable to stress hormones.

● **Turn off the TV before you nod off.** Many people keep the TV on at night, especially if they live alone, for company. But you may squander the important stage 3 and 4 sleep that comes within the first hour-and-a-half by dozing off and waking with a start to gunshots or news bulletins. Several studies on children have found that television and computer time before bed decreases their quality and length of sleep and increases overall tiredness. It also causes children to perform worse on tests of verbal and cognitive skills.

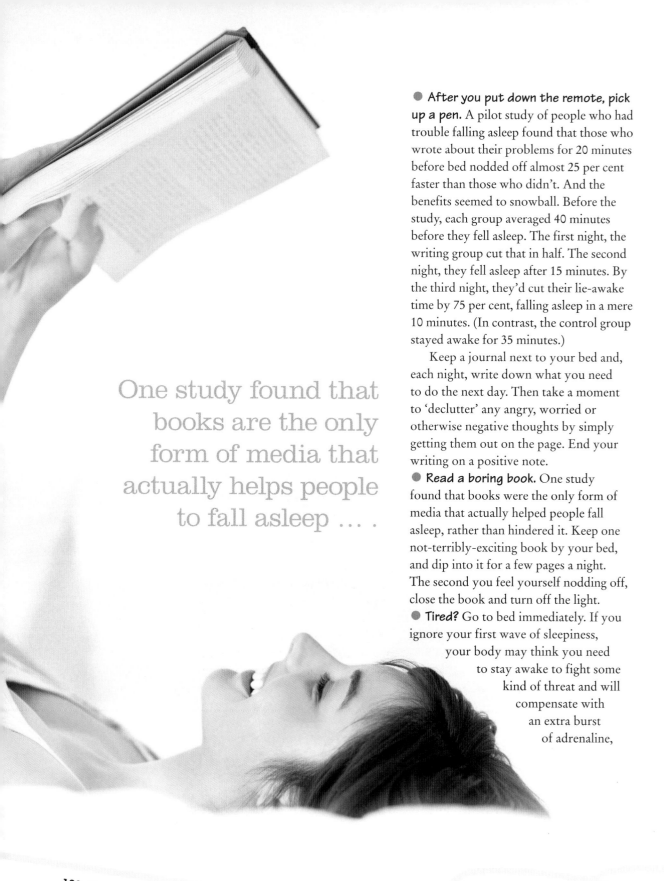

One study found that books are the only form of media that actually helps people to fall asleep … .

● **After you put down the remote, pick up a pen.** A pilot study of people who had trouble falling asleep found that those who wrote about their problems for 20 minutes before bed nodded off almost 25 per cent faster than those who didn't. And the benefits seemed to snowball. Before the study, each group averaged 40 minutes before they fell asleep. The first night, the writing group cut that in half. The second night, they fell asleep after 15 minutes. By the third night, they'd cut their lie-awake time by 75 per cent, falling asleep in a mere 10 minutes. (In contrast, the control group stayed awake for 35 minutes.)

Keep a journal next to your bed and, each night, write down what you need to do the next day. Then take a moment to 'declutter' any angry, worried or otherwise negative thoughts by simply getting them out on the page. End your writing on a positive note.

● **Read a boring book.** One study found that books were the only form of media that actually helped people fall asleep, rather than hindered it. Keep one not-terribly-exciting book by your bed, and dip into it for a few pages a night. The second you feel yourself nodding off, close the book and turn off the light.

● **Tired?** Go to bed immediately. If you ignore your first wave of sleepiness, your body may think you need to stay awake to fight some kind of threat and will compensate with an extra burst of adrenaline, giving you a second wind. That adrenaline might last several hours in your bloodstream and can interfere with subsequent attempts to fall asleep.

## WHEN SLEEP WON'T COME

● **Get out of bed.** Limit your non-sleeping time in bed. Try sticking to the 20 minute rule, which states that

pharmacist or GP to find out if insomnia is a common side effect. Culprits include antidepressants, decongestants and some asthma medicines and blood-pressure-lowering drugs.

● **Engage in pre-sleep relaxation therapy, aka sex.** Orgasm floods the system with endorphins, opiate-like chemicals released from the pituitary

## Tired? Go to bed immediately.

you can remain in bed only if you are asleep within 20 minutes, at any time of night. Any longer and you have to get up and leave the room to do something else, such as reading or knitting. (Don't watch TV.) Designate a comfortable warm spot where you can go for this quiet time. Put your lamp on a dimmer and have a portable CD player and headphones ready so you can listen to a meditation or relaxation CD. As soon as you feel ready to sleep again, head back to bed.

● **Play musical beds.** In order to break a cycle of insomnia, some people find it helps to sleep in another bed. If you've had several nights of poor sleep, make up the guest-room bed or the couch. If you've been awake for 20 minutes in your own bed, move there. Often the change of environment helps break the cycle of repetitive thoughts and anxiety.

● **Talk to your doctor.** As we get older, health conditions that cause pain or discomfort, such as arthritis, heartburn or chronic obstructive pulmonary disease (COPD), can interfere with sleep. Talk to your GP about how best to manage your condition and preserve health-promoting sleep at the same time. If you're taking a prescription drug, check with your

gland that reduce pain and increase feelings of wellbeing, and oxytocin, the bonding hormone that induces a sense of contented relaxation – perfect for sleep.

● **Lose a few pounds.** If your snoring keeps your partner awake, you may have obstructive sleep apnoea, a serious sleep disorder in which breathing is disrupted, causing you to wake repeatedly during the night. If you are regularly tired during the day and have been told that you snore, make an appointment with your doctor or with a sleep specialist (see below). He or she may suggest that you use a continuous positive air pressure (CPAP) device to keep your airways open at night. For some people, surgery will help, too. But for many, losing just 10 per cent of their weight can help reduce sleep apnoea.

● **Talk to the professionals.** If sleep problems are starting to interfere with your life, consider seeing a sleep specialist for an assessment. Your GP may be able to refer you to a sleep centre, or you can sometimes book an appointment yourself; treatment is often offered through the NHS as well as privately. At the centre, your sleeping issues will be addressed by one or more experts, who will try to determine the reasons for your problems.

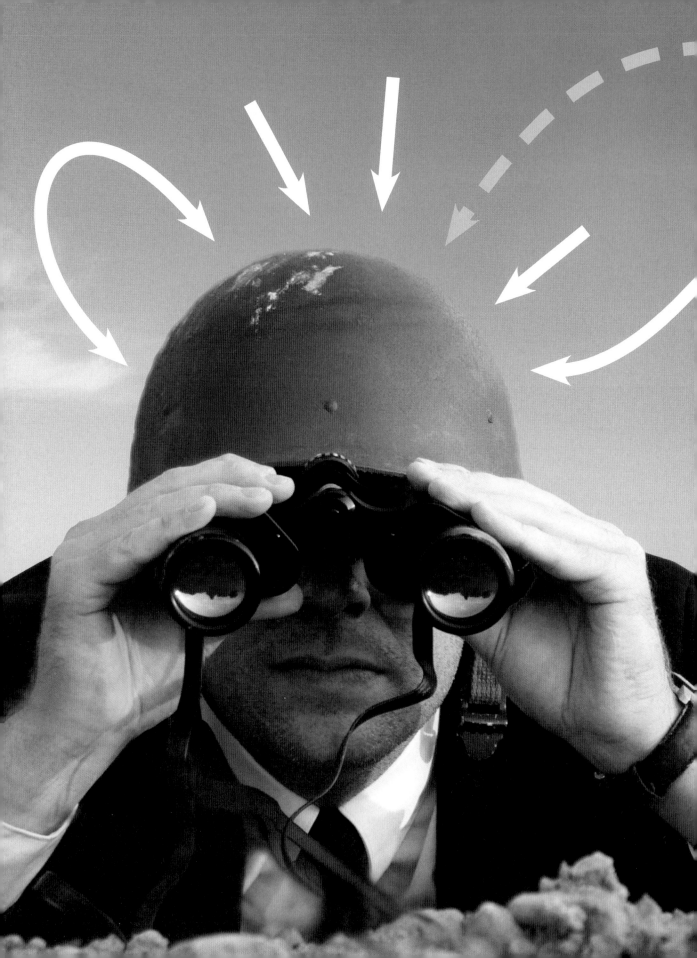

# FIVE BRAIN ENEMIES
## AND HOW TO BEAT THEM

part 3

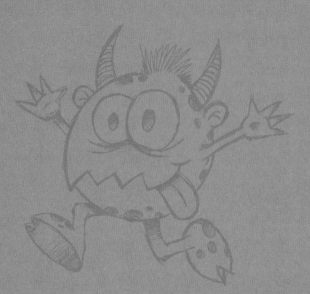

# ENEMY 1

## Stress & anxiety

**Redundancies and unemployment are rising. The economy's in decline, the planet's in jeopardy.** Add in family squabbles, health problems and, for some people, a never-ending to-do list and too little time in which to do it, and you start to understand why so many of us feel like a hamster on a non-stop exercise wheel.

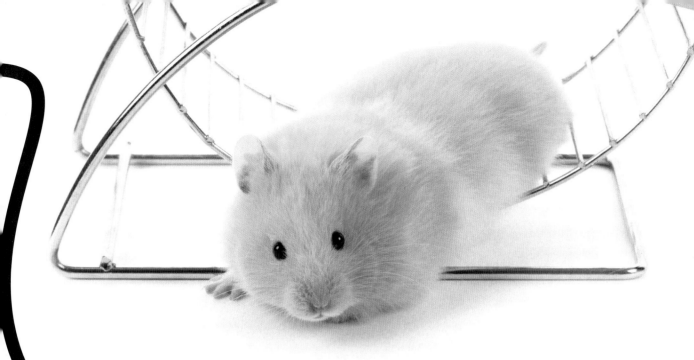

## Learn to cope with the hamster wheel of life.

**A**lthough it's just one of the many bodily organs affected by stress, the brain alone decides what is stressful and what is merely exciting. Some pressure is good for you – it keeps things interesting, challenges you to develop your skills and prepares you to deal with whatever life throws at you.

Short bursts of stress excite the neurons in your hippocampus and make you more alert. Especially during early adulthood, small increases in the stress hormone cortisol can increase the activity in your prefrontal cortex, enabling you to make memories and even helping you retrieve them.

The problem is that a number of the stressors in our lives are neither exciting nor short-lived; some simply make us anxious. Too many of us routinely worry and fret over broken lifestyles or ongoing issues that don't seem to get resolved, leaving us tense much of the time. The toxic effects of chronic pressure can contribute to harmful conditions such

as heart disease and diabetes, and also adversely affect cognitive function.

While small cortisol rises may improve the mental performance of young adults, in older adults, an excess of cortisol makes it more difficult to form new memories or to recall them later. The more cortisol in the blood, the less activity takes place in a part of the brain called the right middle frontal gyrus, an area that records memories of events. Ongoing stress can even shrink key sections of the brain.

One study found that the hippocampi of people who'd experienced five years of high cortisol levels were 14 per cent smaller when compared to those of more easygoing people of the same age. (Depression is also associated with a smaller hippocampus.) Once the hippocampus starts to shrink, it's less and less able to control stress, creating a vicious circle. Stress hormones can even alter the function of the hippocampus, changing the way it handles memories.

# STRESS: DISPOSE OF THE BAD, EMBRACE THE GOOD

If stress is so bad for us, why can't we just learn to relax? For some people, that's easier said than done.

The stress response is different for every brain and every body. Some people may look at a challenge and feel a burst of noradrenaline, the 'fight' hormone. They might seize the moment, meet the challenge and attack the situation head-on. Others might sense that circumstances are getting out of their control and, after the initial burst of noradrenaline, the 'flight/anxiety' hormone adrenaline will surge higher. These people might decide to flee or otherwise manage the anxiety, but not fight back (or tackle the challenge directly). A third group might undergo the same initial reaction, but instead of fighting or fleeing, they might give up,

seeing the entire situation as hopeless. Believing yourself ill-equipped to handle a task in this way triggers an extra release of cortisol from the adrenal glands.

## FINDING YOUR LEVEL

What we all need is a happy medium – enough challenge to make life interesting and mentally stimulating, but not so much that the brain drowns in neuron-killing cortisol. In other words, to be stressed but not stressed out. You may never be able to control the outside stresses that come your way completely (though taking a long, hard look at your lifestyle is a good start), but you can control how you respond to them.

One of the very best ways to improve your response to challenging situations is to convince yourself that you are equal to the task and that you have the resources you need to tackle the problem and succeed. That one single shift in attitude can make the difference between a thrilling, engaging life and a constant slog of never-ending worry – not to mention the difference between a healthy brain and a weak one. By shoring up your self-confidence as well as your coping mechanisms, you can go out and tackle the world and whatever it throws at you.

## DE-STRESS YOUR THOUGHTS

● **Imagine the worst-case scenario.** Sometimes, forcing yourself to think of the worst thing can be the best thing for an anxious brain. If you find yourself trapped in 'what-ifs', a common state of mind for people with chronic anxiety, try facing your fears head-on: 'If the stock market doesn't recover, I'll lose my savings and I'll be forced to live on the street.' When you say it out loud, doesn't

## BRAIN POWER

The brain creates our sense of time by dividing the flow of events into a sequence of frames. A normal brain detects on average about ten events per second. The brain's 'clock' mechanism is based on the regular rate at which certain brain cells fire. Damage to the area involved can make time appear to slow down or speed up.

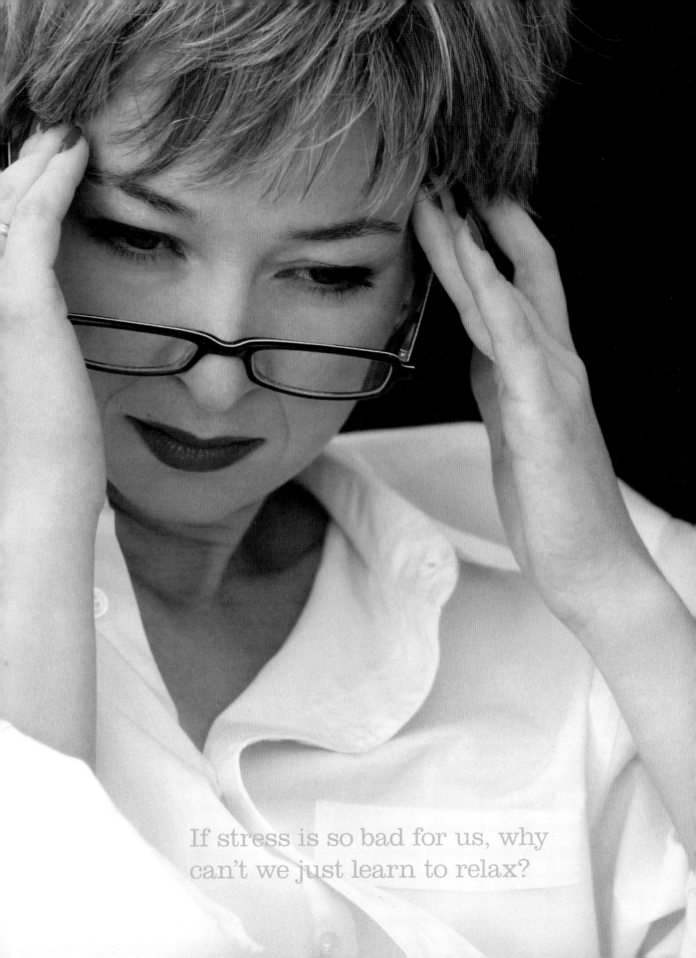

If stress is so bad for us, why can't we just learn to relax?

## IS IT JUST STRESS – OR CHRONIC ANXIETY?

If you've experienced excessive worry or tension regularly for more than six months you may have Generalised Anxiety Disorder (GAD). People with GAD often expect disaster to strike. They seem excessively concerned about health issues, money, family problems or difficulties at work. Even when they know they don't have reason to worry, people with GAD still fret about things for longer than others. They may experience physical symptoms, such as sweating, nausea, fatigue, headaches, muscle tension, twitching, light-headedness or a constant need to go to the bathroom.

If this sounds like you, take heart; you have many options. Just talking to a counsellor may help. The most effective treatment is often cognitive behavioural therapy, which teaches people new techniques to help them break negative thought patterns and react differently to everyday situations.

Exercise, plenty of sleep and meditation are also proven balms for the raw nerves of chronic anxiety.

it seem a little far-fetched? What's more likely to happen instead?

Imagining worst-case scenarios accomplishes two things: it helps you see how irrational some fears really are, and it lets you confront a more reasonable fear directly so that you can at least prepare a tentative plan for recovery.

● **Create a personal mantra.** If you're going through a stressful period or have a tendency to worry, a personal mantra can help you to refocus your mind on positive thoughts. To create yours, make a list of the three things that matter to you most. Then think of one word that represents each. Choose positive, powerful words that resonate deeply with

you. Let's say your top three priorities are a close family, good health and your work. Your mantra might be something like 'Love, strength, goals.' Whenever you're presented with a challenging situation, recite your mantra in your head. Speak the words to yourself as you walk down the street, go into a meeting or work in your garden, timing them with each step or arm movement. And value these areas equally so that if any part of any one is threatened you can call on the strength of the others.

● **Label the feeling.** One of the cornerstones of mindfulness meditation is learning to recognise stress and other emotions without giving in to them. Here's an example of how it works: you remember that your performance review at work is next week, and you're not sure what your boss is going to say. Your heart starts to pound or your mind starts spinning with possible scenarios. Rather than trying to talk yourself out of the stress or pretending that it's not there, examine it objectively and label your feelings. You might say 'nervous' or 'anxious', analysing the emotion as a scientist would. With practice, this technique has been shown to help people offset the cascade of negative emotions that comes from stress.

● **Create a 'worry' jotter.** Worriers need a place to deposit their negative thoughts. Keep a small notebook handy, and whenever you feel yourself starting to get anxious about something, open it and set down your feelings – write down everything that's concerning you, without thinking about how you're saying it or whether you've said it a thousand times before. Putting thoughts down on paper can help break a repetitive cycle of worry, which can deplete your capacity for performing other cognitive tasks.

One British study found that worriers performed worse on a cognitive test when they were thinking about a current problem, suggesting – unsurprisingly – that chronic fretters have less working memory capacity when they're preoccupied with a concern than when thinking about other topics. Just getting worries out of your head and down on paper can help.

● **Keep a 'happy' journal, too.** If your worry jotter is a strictly functional notebook, make this journal a beautiful, hardback book with good-quality paper – an object that you love to look at and feel in your hands. Write in this journal for 5 minutes a day, jotting down the top three things that made you happy that day. Make them detailed and specific.

Instead of writing 'I enjoyed seeing my family', write 'I'm so pleased my granddaughters came for dinner tonight. I love hearing about what they're doing. I'm so grateful they live nearby so that I can watch them grow up.' Over time, doing this routinely will help you start to notice all the good things each day as they happen.

● **Learn to focus and calm your thoughts.** To quieten down the chatter in your mind, simply close your eyes and focus on your breath, feeling it flow in and out of your nostrils. If thoughts pop up about shopping, your bills or the state of the economy, notice them, then redirect your attention to your breath. Keep doing this for 5 minutes. At first you might spend 20 seconds truly focused on your breath and 4 minutes and 40 seconds redirecting your thoughts

Write in a 'happy' journal for 5 minutes a day, jotting down the top three things that made you happy that day.

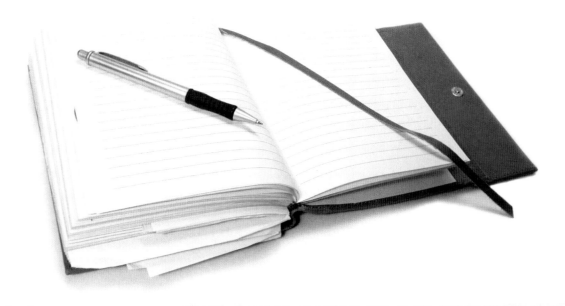

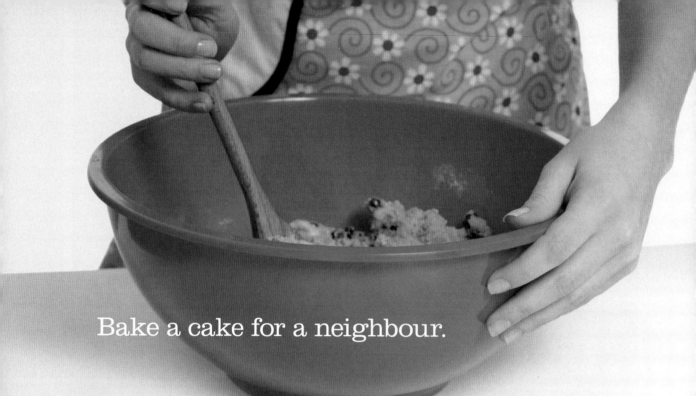

Bake a cake for a neighbour.

# 15 EFFECTIVE stress-busters

**1** Bake biscuits or a cake for a neighbour.

**2** Call a friend to let off steam, then have a mutual morale-boosting chat – but limit it to 10 minutes each so that you don't get too bogged down.

**3** Cancel one item on your schedule.

**4** Go to bed at 9pm tonight.

**5** Have sex (preferably with your partner!).

**6** Smile for no reason.

**7** Listen to your favourite album.

**8** Stroke your own or a friend's dog or cat.

**9** Cut out pictures from magazines of a travel destination you want to visit.

**10** Make funny shapes with your grandchildren's modelling clay or draw moustaches on photos in a magazine.

**11** Write a to-do list, then do the easiest thing on it.

**12** Walk to the nearest green space and spend 10 minutes looking at the flowers and greenery and smelling the air.

**13** Sit in a silent room or building, such as a church, or in a quiet garden or other outside space.

**14** Read the comic strip in your newspaper.

**15** Watch a funny video on YouTube (go to www.youtube.co.uk). Try searching for 'funny animals'.

away from your worries, but that ratio should improve with practice.

This little 5 minute exercise – which, by the way, is meditation, though you don't have to think of it that way – has been shown to lower heart rate, respiration, blood pressure, anxiety, pain, insomnia and the production of cortisol. It's a simple and effective method of stress reduction.

Want better focus? Meditation has been shown to activate frontal brain areas associated with attention; regular meditation can actually increase grey matter concentration in those brain regions involved in learning and memory processes.

● **Clear clutter.** Often, chronic stress and indecision go hand in hand. What's the connection with clutter? People who accumulate clutter tend to have trouble deciding what to do with their things ('I'll keep this catalogue/insurance form/ magazine article until I can find the time to deal with it'). In one study, compulsive hoarders and non-hoarders were asked to make decisions about whether to keep or discard an item. In the hoarders, MRI scans showed much more activity in brain areas that regulate decision making and attention, and control emotions. In other words, they had a much harder time deciding.

Take control of your clutter and you'll probably discover a greater sense of control over your life. Start with one small area. For example, make it an unbreakable rule to tidy and clean the kitchen worktop every single night, even if that means piling things on to another surface. Wipe it down with cleanser so that it really shines. Savour the sight of that clean surface to reinforce your

progress. Then add another rule: clear and clean the table or your computer desk. And another: clean out the sink. Continue until you can maintain several areas of your home without clutter.

Conquering clutter is a constant battle with no finishing line – you must continue to make those decisions, and not put them off, if you want to stay on top of things. Make it easier by getting rid of items you don't need. Pass them on to other people via freecycle (www. uk.freecycle.org) or a charity shop, or try putting them up for sale on eBay (www. ebay.co.uk) – freedom from clutter is its own reward, but a few extra pounds wouldn't hurt either.

## CARVE OUT TIME FOR 'R & R'

● **Have a break at lunchtime.** Make sure your midday break really is a break and get out of work mode. Don't sit at your desk with a sandwich, or chat with colleagues during your lunch hour. Leave

Make sure your midday break really is a break and get out of work mode.

the office – go for a walk round the block or take a packed lunch to the nearest park – or find a quiet space in which to relax and clear your mind of work issues. In one six month study at the University of Wuppertal in Germany, workers who engaged in just 20 minutes of progressive muscle relaxation over their lunch break experienced less emotional, mental, motivational and physical strain in the afternoons than those who spent their lunchtimes engaging in small talk.

● **'Punch out' even if you don't have a time card.** When you've finished work for the day, make sure you really stop. If you don't, your body (and brain) will never get a chance to recover.

Staying late at work, taking work home or being available by email or telephone during family hours may even be counterproductive. Make a deal with yourself to leave at a specific time every night. Doing so will force you to remain efficient and productive until the minute you leave. Don't take work home with you, and be sure to switch on your out-of-office email notification every Friday night. Not only will this help you to 'switch off', but people who try to reach you will appreciate knowing exactly when you'll be able to get back to them.

If you absolutely must stay connected, decide in advance on one designated time every day to check your voicemail and email; give yourself half an hour to scan through and respond to only the most critical items. Then disconnect for the rest of the day.

● **Take at least two holidays a year.** Sometimes, holidays are the only complete break from stress our bodies get. Yet nearly a quarter of British workers don't take all the paid holiday time to which they're entitled – even though 96 per cent of us know that holidays are important to our health and wellbeing. Those who shun holidays are at increased risk of heart disease and are 20 per cent more likely to die of any cause in a given year. Don't be one of them. Consider your holidays to be doctor's orders. Take one in your favourite haunt (even if it's a bed-and-breakfast nearby), the other one in a new place. The anticipation of visiting the old familiar place will help decrease stress, while the novelty of the new will stimulate new brain connections. When you do get away, make sure it's a proper break – a shocking 43 per cent of people say they think about work while on holiday, 12 per cent take work-related phone calls and 7 per cent even take their laptop with them to do some work while they're supposed to be 'getting away from it all'.

● **Watch a funny film.** Laughing is one of the best ways to reduce stress and boost your immunity. Studies show that the effects of laughter are similar to those of exercise on the cardiovascular and respiratory systems. Laughing reduces stress hormones and boosts the body's natural pleasure-boosting and pain-killing endorphin hormones, not just at the time but for hours afterwards. Watching funny films is a cheap, easy way to bring a little more laughter into your life – in fact, one study suggested that just looking forward to seeing a funny movie had a profound stress-relief effect, decreasing cortisol by 39 per cent, reducing adrenaline by 70 per cent and increasing levels of feel-good endorphins by 27 per cent.

Everyone's taste is different, but British favourites (according to a poll by the *Observer* newspaper) include

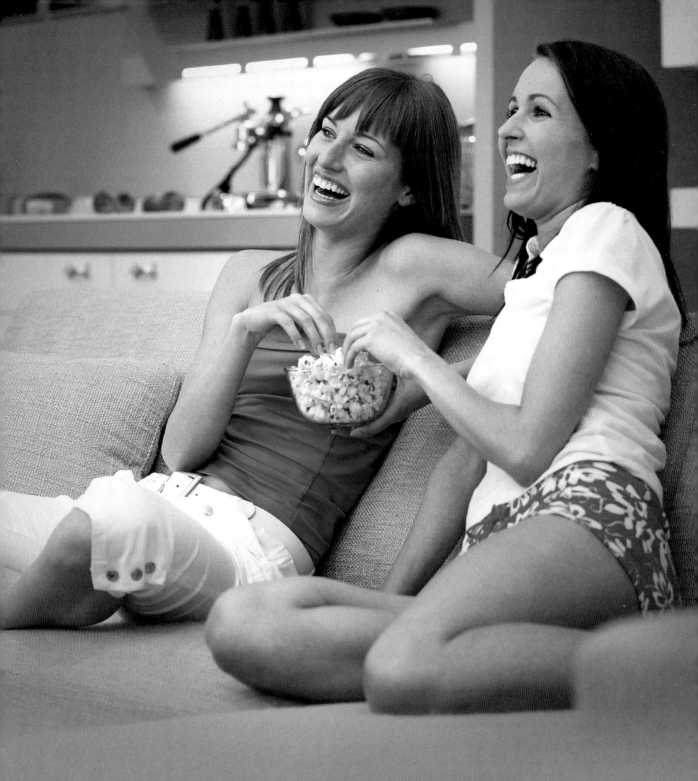

Watch a funny film.
Laughing is one of the best ways to
reduce stress and boost your immunity.

*Monty Python's Life of Brian, Airplane!, This is Spinal Tap, Some Like it Hot* and *Withnail and I*. Make a list of funny films you want to see and work your way through them all, or add them to your online film delivery service queue. You'll get a double benefit, first from looking forward to each film's arrival in the post, then from actually watching it.

### EASE THE PRESSURE IN YOUR SOCIAL CIRCLE

● **Stay away from competitive people.** If you find yourself around someone who makes you feel uncomfortable or with whom you have to compete, try to minimise your time with that person. Research shows that competition is one of the most potent stressors for any animal, human beings included.

Competitive people make you feel as if you should defend yourself or get another word in during conversations. In contrast, non-competitive friends love and accept you as you are; when you're with them, you'll never have the impulse to prove yourself. You'll walk away feeling appreciated, not insulted. Those friends can reduce cortisol and adrenaline and increase oxytocin and endorphins, all positive changes in your brain chemistry.

● **Hug someone you love.** It doesn't matter whether it's your partner, brother or sister, child or good friend – hugs are proven stress-relievers. One study found that the more hugs a woman got from her partner, the higher her levels of oxytocin (the 'cuddle hormone') and the lower her blood pressure and cortisol readings. Oxytocin helps bond people together. No wonder happier couples hug more often.

### DE-STRESS YOUR BODY

● **Get moving.** Perhaps the most effective stress-buster of all is physical activity. Regular exercise helps your body – your heart, your muscles, your nervous system – practise a positive response to pressure.

This is undoubtedly the most natural and healthy reaction: crises produce what is sometimes called the 'fight or flight' response – our bodies (like those of our ancient ancestors) prime themselves to fight or run away from a perceived foe. Sometimes, that's for the best – if, say, we were physically attacked or needed to jump out of the way of an oncoming vehicle.

More often, however, the source of stress is emotional. And the rising heart rate, increased blood sugar levels and raised levels of cortisol triggered by the stress response can severely strain the body's systems unless there is some physical release. Exercise or physical activity of any kind provides it and over time reduces levels of cortisol and other stress hormones, helping to increase our capacity to deal with emotional reactions and stressful situations.

If you're not particularly active, start with 10 minutes of walking, and be sure to do it every day – perhaps with a friend as that will help you both to keep it up until it becomes a habit. Then try to expand it by 5 minutes a week until you're walking for 25 minutes a day. Add in some sit-ups, modified push-ups and lunges on two or more days of the week. And if nothing else, at least make sure you walk as much as possible, take the stairs whenever you can and put some real energy into housework and gardening. Keeping active helps to combat stress and will keep your brain and body strong for years to come.

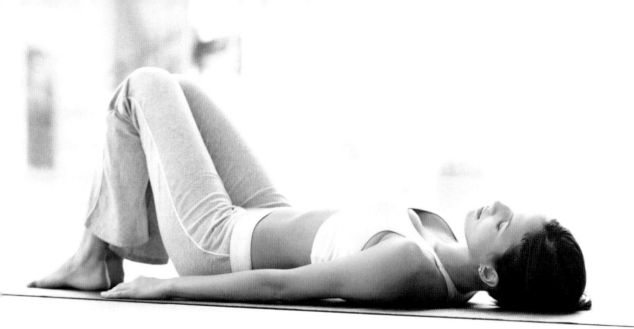

## Try a yoga class.

● **Do some deep breathing.** At least once a day, sit on a chair with your feet flat on the floor and take a slow, deep breath through your nose, expanding your belly (not your chest), then slowly release your breath through pursed lips. Repeat for several minutes. You'll get more oxygen to your blood – and to your brain – and melt away tension in your body.

● **Have a weekly massage.** Don't think of it as a reward – use it as a technique to build up your reserves. Numerous studies have found that having a massage can decrease anxiety, stress and pain. It releases encephalins, proteins that act like morphine in your brain, giving you a natural high, and increases dopamine and serotonin, neurotransmitters that enhance mood.

● **Try a yoga class.** In one German study, a group of women who considered themselves emotionally distressed signed up for a three-month yoga programme. The researchers split them into two groups; the first started the programme immediately, the others were told they were on the waiting list. During the three-month study period, the first group attended two 90 minute yoga classes each week.

After three months, when compared with the women on the waiting list, the women who did yoga demonstrated significant improvements in their perceived stress, anxiety, fatigue and depression. Those who'd previously suffered from headaches or back pain reported marked pain relief, and their cortisol levels plummeted.

The best way to learn yoga safely is from an instructor, not a video. Find a class for beginners, and bring a friend if you feel intimidated.

● **Supplement with fish oil.** As mentioned earlier, the omega-3 fats in oily fish help to keep your brain healthy (see page 65). According to a study from the Hôpital de la Cavale Blanche in Brest, France, fish oil may also help your body combat stress.

Researchers measured stress hormone levels in a small group of volunteers before and after they gave them an intense cognitive challenge. After taking fish oil for three weeks, the group was given a similar challenge and, this time, their stress hormone levels were significantly lower. The researchers believe the fish oil might influence the adrenal glands to produce fewer hormones in response to anxiety.

Study participants were taking more than 7g of fish oil a day, which is more than manufacturers typically recommend (usually 1g to 2g per day). Check first with your GP if you plan to try the higher dosage.

● **Steer yourself towards safer snacks.** Stress increases your appetite for fat and sugar. How do you beat your cravings? The truth is, if you're a stress-eater, you've probably spent much of your life reaching for food when times get tough – and such habits die hard. Your brain has grown accustomed to the satisfying dopamine and calming serotonin release that you get when you eat under stressful conditions.

If you must turn to food to help you cope with stress, crunch on carrots or celery, or have a bowl of low-fat yoghurt or cottage cheese. Avoid biscuits and sweets. You'll find that the fewer sugary, carbohydrate-loaded foods you eat, the less you'll crave them.

● **Cut out coffee.** Caffeine keeps cortisol and adrenaline at a raised level. If you're the stressed-out type, it's best to give up coffee altogether. If you can't or won't, keep to no more than two cups a day, no matter what, and drink them in the morning so that your body has plenty of time to metabolise the caffeine fully before bed. Or switch to decaf.

● **Quit smoking – with two friends.** Many smokers think that cigarettes help them to manage pressure, but surveys indicate that smokers are actually more stressed than non-smokers. Nicotine withdrawal can temporarily increase stress, but within a few weeks of quitting, once your body is used to being nicotine-free, the chances are your stress levels will decrease and continue to drop over time. By stopping, you'll also reduce your risk of cognitive decline and stroke.

Quitting with friends helps you all improve your chances of success. One recent study found that people tend to do best when whole clusters of friends and relatives stop smoking at the same time, usually in groups of three or more. It seems the group momentum encourages everyone.

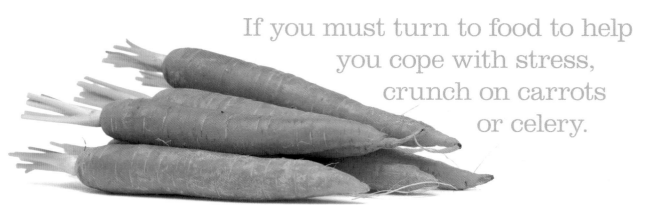

If you must turn to food to help you cope with stress, crunch on carrots or celery.

Cut out coffee altogether if you're the stressed-out type.

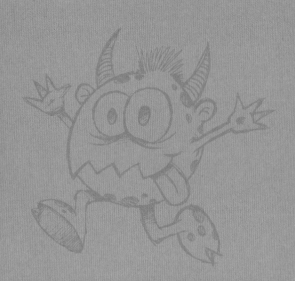

# ENEMY 2

## Depression

**Your mood and energy have been low, and you can't think straight. Coincidence? No.** Depression has real, measurable effects on memory and cognitive function. The good news: treating it can help bring back mental clarity, not to mention sunnier moods.

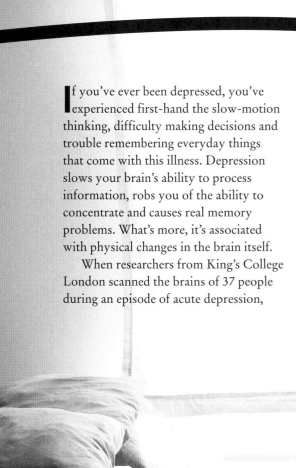

If you've ever been depressed, you've experienced first-hand the slow-motion thinking, difficulty making decisions and trouble remembering everyday things that come with this illness. Depression slows your brain's ability to process information, robs you of the ability to concentrate and causes real memory problems. What's more, it's associated with physical changes in the brain itself.

When researchers from King's College London scanned the brains of 37 people during an episode of acute depression, they found a reduced volume in the hippocampus – a brain area related to memory and learning – compared with non-depressed controls. Other studies suggest that depression disrupts the connections between the neurons which allow thought signals to zoom along from one cell to another.

The result? Difficulty forming and retrieving memories. Depression interferes with everything from finding your car keys to remembering words and names. One fascinating study has even discovered

Depression slows your brain's ability to process information, robs you of the ability to concentrate and causes real memory problems.

the bigger the memory problems can be, conclude the authors of a large study on people with depression. Depression also makes it difficult to take the steps proven to keep a brain sharp and active – such as exercising, learning new things, having new experiences and spending time with friends and family.

Instead, people tend to retreat and isolate themselves, a surefire recipe for dulled thinking all by itself. They may not look after themselves properly, leaving the door open for untreated medical problems that raise the risk of cognitive decline or even dementia, such as high blood pressure, diabetes and high cholesterol.

# FEELING GOOD AGAIN

When you are depressed, the most difficult task in the world can be finding the motivation to fight back. But your brain – and your heart and the rest of your body – depends on it. Help is out there.

Your best first step is to call your GP and make an appointment expressly to talk about your mood. Don't be embarrassed; depression is a medical condition like any other, and it needs to be treated. You may have to take the first step and raise the problem with your doctor, but once you do, it's his or her job to evaluate you and suggest the next step.

With treatment – whether it's an antidepressant or talking therapy – most cases of depression can be substantially relieved within 8 to 12 weeks. Without treatment, it could take months or even years, time that allows this illness to eat away at your brain, your life and your health.

that depression upsets your ability to remember where things are located. When British researchers used a virtual-reality game to test spatial memory in 49 people, they found that those who were depressed performed significantly worse than those who weren't. Volunteers were told to navigate through a virtual city in search of landmarks such as a cinema and a pool hall. Depressed people found a third fewer sites than non depressed participants.

## TREATMENT IS A LIFESAVER

If you suspect you or someone close to you is depressed, it's important to seek treatment as soon as possible. The longer the illness (and it is an illness) goes untreated, the greater the damage – and

● **Be persistent ... and patient.** You may have to try several antidepressants to find the one that's best for you. That's what happened in a landmark study of 3,700 people with depression. Seventy per cent eventually felt they had fully recovered, but only 37 per cent got relief from the first medication they tried. The rest tried up to four different therapies before finding the right one for them.

Plan to try a treatment for 8 to 12 weeks to see if it's working, stay in close contact with your doctor, and expect a big improvement. A successful treatment will allow you to feel like yourself again – perhaps even better – and will enable you to do all the things you used to do. Once you find the right treatment, stick with it. You may need your medication for 6 to 12 months, the usual length of a bout of depression, or longer if you've had depressive periods in the past.

● **Play with a dog for a few minutes every day.** When people who didn't own a pet played with a dog for a few minutes every day as part of a US study, their blood levels of the brain chemicals serotonin and oxytocin – both mood elevators – rose. You don't have to buy a dog to experience these feel-good effects – pet a neighbour's dog and offer to take it for walks, or volunteer at an animal shelter for some quality time with a furry friend.

● **Try cognitive behavioural therapy.** This practical, solutions-focused therapy is the most effective form of talking therapy and may help up to 75 per cent

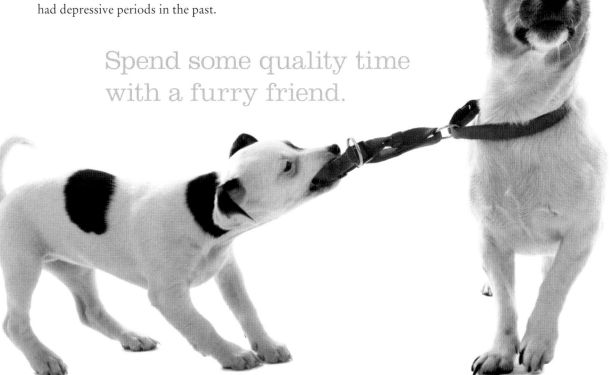

Spend some quality time with a furry friend.

*Continued on page 154*

# 12 SHORT PATHS to joy

Happiness can help you live longer, stay married longer, even earn a higher income, experts say. And while about 50 per cent of your outlook is encoded in your genes, you can teach yourself to feel more joy. Here's what works:

**1** **Keep a 'happy' journal.** Recognising all the good things in your life can boost your mood and your energy. And the more you do it, the more effective it is. Jotting down what you're grateful for five times a week worked better than three times a week, one study found. Or, every night as you fall asleep, think of five things that pleased you today.

**2** **Perform five acts of kindness this week.** Present flowers from your garden to a friend or help an elderly neighbour with his or her shopping. Altruistic acts are genuine mood-lifters.

**3** **Listen to the music that you love.** It triggers joy by unleashing feel-good brain chemicals called endorphins.

**4** **Cuddle … and more.** Physical affection and sex release endorphins, as well as the 'cuddle chemical' oxytocin, which strengthens your relationship with your partner.

**5** **Find a purpose.** Whether it's conventional religion, a sense of spirituality or feelings of closeness to nature, your family or your community, people with a strong sense of meaning in their lives tend to be happier.

**6** **Laugh out loud.** Watch a funny film, tell a joke or ask your friends and family to share some jokes and funny stories. A good giggle or guffaw raises levels of feel-good brain chemicals.

**7** **Adopt a happy posture.** Square your shoulders, stand up straight and, when you walk, take big, quick steps. That's the body language of a happy person – and studies show that acting as if you're happy can help you feel happier.

**8** **Do something new.** Then do something else new. Trying new things turbo charges positive emotions.

**9** **Set up clear work/home boundaries.** Turn off your mobile phone or BlackBerry and shut down your laptop when you get home. This can reduce stress in your house and also help you feel closer to your partner, children or grandchildren.

**10** **Appreciate what's 'good enough'.** You didn't lose as much weight as you'd hoped this week … but did you lose something? That's a victory, not a defeat. In large studies, people with more realistic expectations tend to be happier than those seeking perfection.

**11** **Unleash your inner Matisse.** Create a greeting card, decorate a cake, plant a herb garden, try a new craft. Creative endeavours allow us to enter a timeless, worry-free state called flow that's both absorbing and thrilling.

**12** **Imagine that you're already happy.** Shut your eyes and see yourself doing something that makes your heart sing. Experts say this 'thought experiment' boosts confidence and helps make happiness a habit.

Present flowers from your garden to a friend.

of people recover from depression. And studies show that it may also be a good way to protect your brain from future bouts of depression. Cognitive behavioural therapy usually comprises 8 to 16 sessions and is aimed at changing the thoughts and feelings that may lead to depression. One British study of 123 people with depression found that it cut the chance of a relapse in half. Ask your doctor for a referral to a psychologist specifically trained as a cognitive behavioural therapist.

● **Reach out to a friend.** Talking over what has happened in your day, in person or by phone or email, helps to emphasise the good points and process what's not so good so that you're not turning it over and over in your mind. In another UK study, when 86 depressed women were paired with volunteer friends, 65 per cent of the women felt better. In fact, regular social contact worked as effectively as antidepressant medication and psychotherapy. Frequent contact with a close friend can boost your self-confidence and encourage you to make other positive changes, such as taking up a new interest, going for long walks or starting an exercise programme, all of which will help to lift the depression.

● **Tackle the garden … or just get outdoors.** Too many of us spend our days in a man-made environment, shut away from the sun, the earth, green plants and the blue sky. Get back to nature – depending on where you live, it may be as simple as walking out of your front door.

● **Add a 10 minute walk two to three times a day.** Walking has been shown to lift mild to moderate depression –

Tackle the garden … or just get outdoors. Too many of us spend our days in a man-made environment.

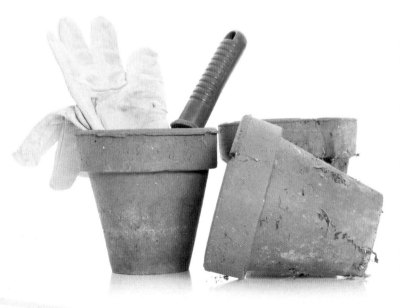

plus you get a dose of mood-boosting sunshine. One study of older adults found that ten weeks of regular exercise was 20 per cent more effective at reducing depression symptoms than medication. However, because depression may make you want to do anything but exercise, many doctors recommend combining the two treatments.

● **Let in more light.** Bright light therapy can ease seasonal affective disorder, a type of depression some people experience during the winter months when sunlight is in short supply. It may also ease other types of depression. The therapy involves sitting in front of a special light box for 20 minutes to an hour shortly after waking each morning. You can purchase a light box for home use from a variety of sources, many of them online, with prices starting at around £50.

● **Take omega-3 supplements.** There is some evidence that taking fish oil can help relieve mild to moderate depression. In one study at the University of Pavia in Italy, 46 depressed women aged between 66 and 95 took either omega-3 supplements or a placebo for eight weeks. Both depressive symptoms and quality of life improved in the treated group. See Brain booster 1: Diet, starting on page 62, for other ways in which these supplements can benefit your brain. To treat depression, a dose as high as 4g a day may be effective. However, to avoid any adverse reactions, you should discuss this first with your GP as this is more than the 1g to 2g per day that manufacturers typically recommend.

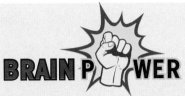

**BRAIN P WER**

Excitement enhances memory formation, while depression inhibits it. Laying down memories depends on physical processes that are influenced by certain chemical messengers in the brain, which ebb and flow according to mood. The higher our emotional state when a new experience occurs, the more likely we are to remember key details of that experience.

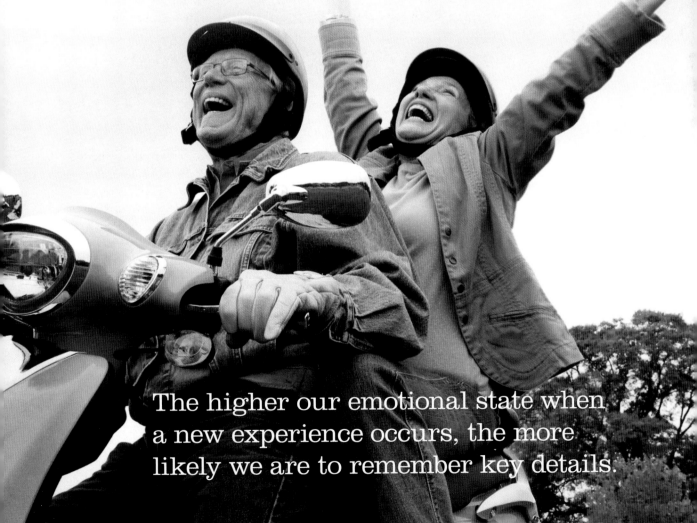

The higher our emotional state when a new experience occurs, the more likely we are to remember key details.

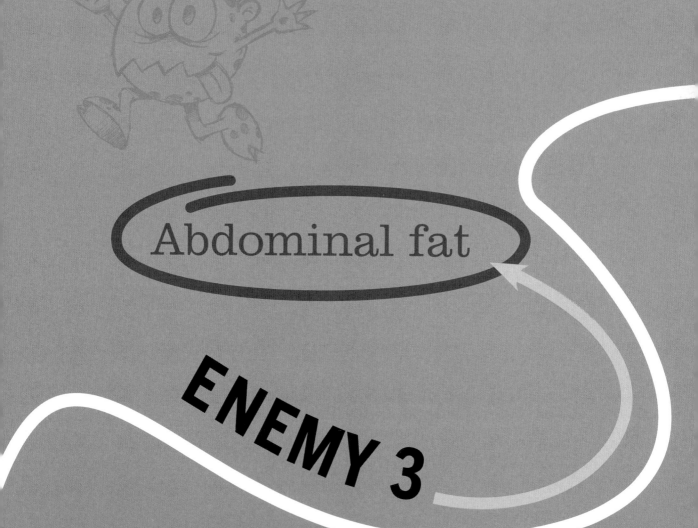

# Abdominal fat

## ENEMY 3

You've heard of 'gut instinct', a certain inkling that tells you when someone's being less than truthful or that points you towards the right path when you have to make a snap decision. In fact, your abdomen can affect your brain in far more damaging ways.

## If your waistline increases, over time you can expect your brainpower to decrease.

The trouble begins when fat accumulates around your belly, invading and surrounding your internal organs like butter melting into the surface of a crumpet. Doctors have known for years that this type of fat, also called visceral fat, increases the risk of heart disease, diabetes and even some types of cancer. Now they're beginning to recognise the dangerous role it plays when it comes to your brain. The bottom line: if your waistline increases, over time you can expect your brainpower to decrease.

Read on to find out whether an increasing middle is putting you at risk of cognitive decline, and discover simple strategies to send this hidden fat packing.

## BRAIN-SHRINKING BELLY FAT

The fat in your abdomen isn't like the flab that causes bottoms to jiggle or thighs to thunder. It's actually biologically active, secreting chemicals and hormones that affect your health, including your ability to remember where you parked the car or the name of your second cousin, not to mention balance your household accounts without tearing out your hair.

Even if no one could accuse you of having a beer belly, you may still have too much of this fat. (See Risky waistlines, page 159.) This is potentially worrying.

Here's why …

● **Too much abdominal fat is associated with poorer cognitive function.** In one study of 917 people who hadn't had a stroke and didn't have dementia, a higher waist circumference or waist-to-hip ratio (another measure of abdominal fat) was linked with lower scores on tests of intelligence and cognitive function. The association was reduced among more physically active participants.

● **It's linked with damage to brain connections.** Your brain cells communicate with each other via a superhighway of connections – think of them as information cables – called axons. Brain scans of people with wide waistlines show areas of damage to these cables. Such impairment is typically seen in people with dementia. But some experts think axon damage may drain memory and thinking power even in people who don't develop dementia.

● **It's related to lower brain volume.** People who are overweight or obese in middle age seem to be more likely to develop cognitive impairment or even dementia in later life. In an attempt to understand why, scientists took body measurements and performed brain scans on 733 people with an average age of 60. They found that measurements of total brain volume were lower among those who had a higher body mass index (BMI), waist circumference or waist-to-hip ratio, and more subcutaneous or belly fat. They observed that abdominal fat especially was linked with reduced brain volumes.

And a 2011 study of Swedish twins, suggested that middle-aged people who were overweight (with a BMI of between 25 and 30) or obese (BMI over 30) were 80 per cent more likely to develop dementia, vascular dementia or Alzheimer's disease than those with a healthy-range BMI (20 to 24.9).

● **It's part of metabolic syndrome.** Belly fat is an important component of metabolic syndrome, a cluster of risk factors that includes high blood pressure, abnormal blood lipids and raised blood sugar and insulin levels. Scientists don't always agree on which components make up the syndrome, or how many need to be present to diagnose the condition, but abdominal fat seems to be critical.

Metabolic syndrome often leads to diabetes and heart disease. Now it has also been linked with cloudy thinking. In one Dutch study, people with metabolic syndrome scored about 10 per cent lower on tests of mental processing speed and about 6 per cent lower on memory tests than those without it.

In fact, evidence of a link between metabolic syndrome and brain function is so strong that some experts now talk about 'metabolic-cognitive syndrome'. Some – though not all – studies suggest that people with metabolic syndrome in middle age are more likely to go on to develop cognitive decline in later life.

In the French 'Three-City Study', involving more than 7,000 people aged 65 or over at the start, those with at least three of five criteria for metabolic syndrome had a significantly increased risk of cognitive decline two or four years later. They were 22 per cent more likely to have lower overall mental function and 13 per cent more likely to have reduced visual working memory than people without metabolic syndrome.

People who are overweight in middle age are more likely to develop cognitive impairment or even dementia in later life.

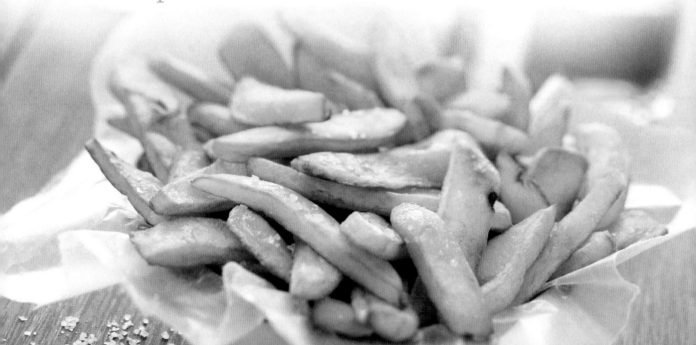

# Risky WAISTLINES

Check the numbers below to get a sense of the risk your waistline poses to your overall health.
To calculate your waist-to-hip ratio, measure your hips and your waist using a tape measure (see Are you at risk? below). Then divide your waist measurement by your hip measurement. A ratio of 1.0 or more in men, or 0.85 or more in women, indicates that you are carrying too much weight around your middle. This increases your risk of diseases linked to obesity such as Type 2 diabetes and heart disease.

| | HEALTHY WAIST RANGE | HIGH-RISK WAIST RANGE | VERY HIGH-RISK WAIST RANGE |
|---|---|---|---|
| Men | Less than 37in (94cm) | 37–40in (94–102cm) | More than 40in (102cm) |
| Women | Less than 32in (80cm) | 32–35in (80–88cm) | More than 35in (88cm) |

● **It's a factor in insulin resistance.** Belly fat churns out chemicals that make the body less sensitive to insulin, the hormone that lets blood sugar into cells, a condition known as insulin resistance. When glucose can't get into cells as easily, levels rise in the blood, prompting the body to send out more insulin in a bid to reduce blood glucose to normal levels. Insulin resistance can lead to diabetes, so it's sometimes referred to as 'pre-diabetes'.

Even if blood sugar levels aren't high enough to qualify as diabetes, raised levels can still be harmful. High insulin elevates triglycerides and other 'bad' fats, and interferes with kidney function, increasing blood pressure – so the vicious circle also worsens metabolic syndrome. And the combination of high blood glucose with high insulin is bad for your brain. Researchers suspect it's one reason that people with Type 2 diabetes score lower on memory tests than those without it.

● **It increases inflammation.** Inflammation is a tough concept to grasp, but think of it as your body's response to injuries of all sorts, even at the microscopic level. Abdominal fat increases inflammation, which appears to affect the brain. In one Finnish study, 97 women aged between 60 and 70 at the start had blood tests to measure low-level inflammation and were then followed for 12 years. Researchers found that memory (but not overall cognitive function or speed) was progressively worse the higher the level of inflammation to begin with.

## ARE YOU AT RISK?

To find out, measure your waist on bare skin. Use a soft, flexible measuring tape (the kind used for sewing). It may help to do this in front of a mirror. Feel for your hip bone on one side, then for the bone at the lower end of your ribcage on the same side. Take a measurement midway between – for most people this is about the level of your naval. Make sure the tape is straight, not twisted, and don't pull it too tight. Take your measurement at the end of a normal exhalation of breath (don't suck your tummy in).

What do the results mean? According to the NHS, health risks begin at more than 32in (80cm) for women and 37in (94cm) for men (see Risky waistlines, page 159). More than a third of adults now have too large a waist circumference, compared with less than a quarter 20 years ago. If both BMI and waist circumference are considered in assessing risks of health problems, 20 per cent of men are estimated to be at increased risk, 13 per cent at high risk and 21 per cent at very high risk. Equivalent figures for women are 14, 16 and 23 per cent.

### THINNER PEOPLE, TAKE HEED

Not overweight? Don't assume you can safely ignore the threat; there's a convincing body of evidence that even some relatively thin people have too much visceral fat hiding inside. When British researchers took MRI images of the torsos of more than 700 women and men, they made a sobering discovery: 45 per cent of the thin women and 65 per cent of the thin men had enough visceral fat to raise their risk of health problems. The scientists concluded that these TOFI (Thin on the Outside, Fat on the Inside) people were actually pre-overweight – they didn't exercise much and ate diets packed with high-fat, high-sugar foods.

## WHITTLE YOUR MIDDLE TO SAVE YOUR BRAIN

Everyone has some visceral fat, but if you're overweight, you might be carrying around 5lb to 10lb (2.2kg to 4.5kg) of it. The good news: it's easier to lose than the stubborn fat on your hips, thighs

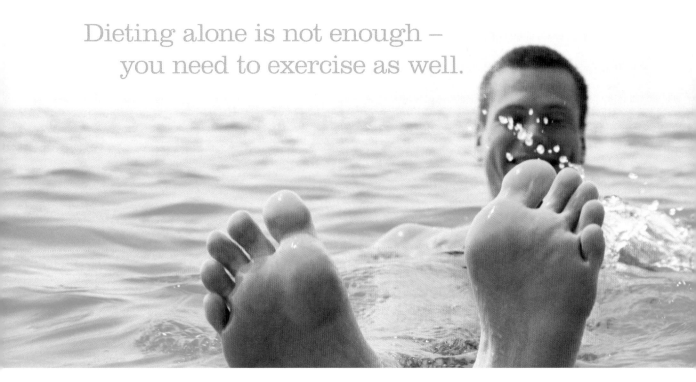

Dieting alone is not enough – you need to exercise as well.

and bottom, and a little effort yields big rewards. In one study, when 173 women walked briskly for just 50 minutes, three times a week, the average reduction in their waist measurements was 2in (5cm) – and they lost 13 per cent of their abdominal fat. You have many options:

● **Brisk walking, swimming or cycling.** Aerobic exercise – the kind that gets your muscles moving in a steady rhythm and your heart pumping – is your first line of defence against belly fat. In one study of overweight men, those who exercised for an hour three times a week at a moderately brisk pace (able to hold a conversation but not enough breath to sing Happy Birthday) lost a significant percentage of the visceral fat packed around their hearts, Japanese researchers report. (Visceral fat can occur anywhere in the torso, including the heart.)

Several studies suggest that weight-loss programmes which include physical activity are far more effective than diets alone for trimming this brain-dulling flab. In one study, 33 obese post-menopausal women with diabetes followed either a low-calorie diet or an exercise plan, or a combination of the two for 14 weeks. By the end, both the diet and the diet-plus-exercise groups had lost weight and had a reduction in total and subcutaneous (under the skin) abdominal fat.

In contrast, the exercise-only group had not lost any weight, but did have a lower body fat percentage and had reduced total, subcutaneous and visceral (internal) fat, despite the lack of overall weight loss. Visceral fat also reduced in the diet-plus-exercise group, but not in the group using dieting alone. Researchers concluded that dieting alone is not enough; exercise is needed as well

## BIGGER MIDDLE, SMALLER MEMORY

The link between abdominal fat and mental performance isn't just a theory; unfortunately, it may have practical consequences. French researchers gave word-recall tests to 2,223 women and men aged from 32 to 62 years, then repeated the test five years later. People with wide waistlines performed 35 per cent worse than those who were svelte.

in order to lose visceral fat If you choose not to exercise, you're allowing this fat to continue to grow. When 175 overweight, sedentary women and men volunteered for an exercise study, those who were given the most vigorous routines – equivalent to jogging 20 miles a week – reduced their belly fat levels by 7 to 20 per cent, while those in the no-exercise control group saw belly fat levels rise by 9 per cent to 17 per cent in eight months.

● **Add strength-training.** Sit-ups and crunches may make your tummy look tighter, but you can't spot-reduce deep ab fat. What does work: a whole-body strength-training routine (one that works all the muscles, including the legs, arms, abdominals and back). In one study of 164 overweight and obese women, those who strength-trained twice a week lost almost 4 per cent of their body fat and after two years were more successful at keeping off belly fat than those who didn't.

Strength-training increases your metabolism by building muscle mass, which means your body will burn more calories round-the-clock. More muscle also means you'll burn more fat and calories during aerobic exercise, supercharging your fat-fighting efforts.

● **Banish the 'bad' fats.** Ice cream, fatty meats, whole milk, cheese and cream are all full of saturated fat, which is particularly likely to raise your odds of developing too much visceral fat. By contrast sticking to a Mediterranean diet – which is low in saturated fat – is linked with less abdominal fat and a lower waist circumference, irrespective of an individual's BMI, according to a study of nearly half a million Europeans.

flakes, can help your brain not only by preventing blood-sugar rises, which are toxic to brain cells, but also by fighting visceral fat. People whose diets boost blood sugar the most tend to have more body fat, especially around the belly.

Researchers from Tufts University in Boston, USA, assessed dietary intake and body fat in 2,834 people taking part in the USA's Framingham Heart Study. They found that those with lower amounts of abdominal fat tended to eat more whole grains, but people with more abdominal fat ate more highly processed grains.

## Try peanut butter and banana sandwiches ...

● **Welcome the 'good' fats.** There's more and more research to suggest that eating more monounsaturated fats discourages the accumulation of belly fat and may even help you shed it more easily. When Spanish researchers studied the impact of three diets – one packed with monounsaturated fats, one with saturated fats and one with carbohydrates – they discovered that the 'good fat' diet helped slash abdominal fat. The others didn't.

To get more of these good fats, snack on a small handful of unsalted nuts instead of crisps, use olive oil in place of butter or other vegetable oils, have avocado slices on your sandwich rather than cheese, and opt for nut butters on your toast, in your sandwich and at snack time. Try peanut butter and banana sandwiches as a midafternoon pick-me-up.

● **Eat more fibre and fewer refined carbohydrates.** Eating whole-grain bread and whole-wheat pasta instead of white, highly processed products, and high-fibre cereal instead of rice-based cereals or corn

Whole fruit and vegetables are also excellent sources of fibre. A Harvard School of Public Health study of 486 women found that those who ate the most fruit and vegetables – not a huge quantity, equivalent to 1½ apples, a serving of cooked green beans and a handful of baby carrots a day – were 20 per cent less likely to have a dangerously large waist.

● **Put it all together.** People who exercised for 30 minutes at least five times a week, cut saturated fat, increased fibre and lost 7 per cent of their body weight (roughly 10lb/4.5kg if you weigh 10st/63kg) saw their visceral fat trimmed by a very significant 18 to 22 per cent.

● **Soothe stress.** High levels of the stress hormone cortisol prompt your body to store more abdominal fat – perhaps an ancient survival mechanism, intended to maintain fat in emergencies. But many of us feel under constant pressure, so cortisol sends fat into our torsos constantly. Fight back by de-stressing daily. (See Enemy 1: Stress & anxiety, starting on page 134.)

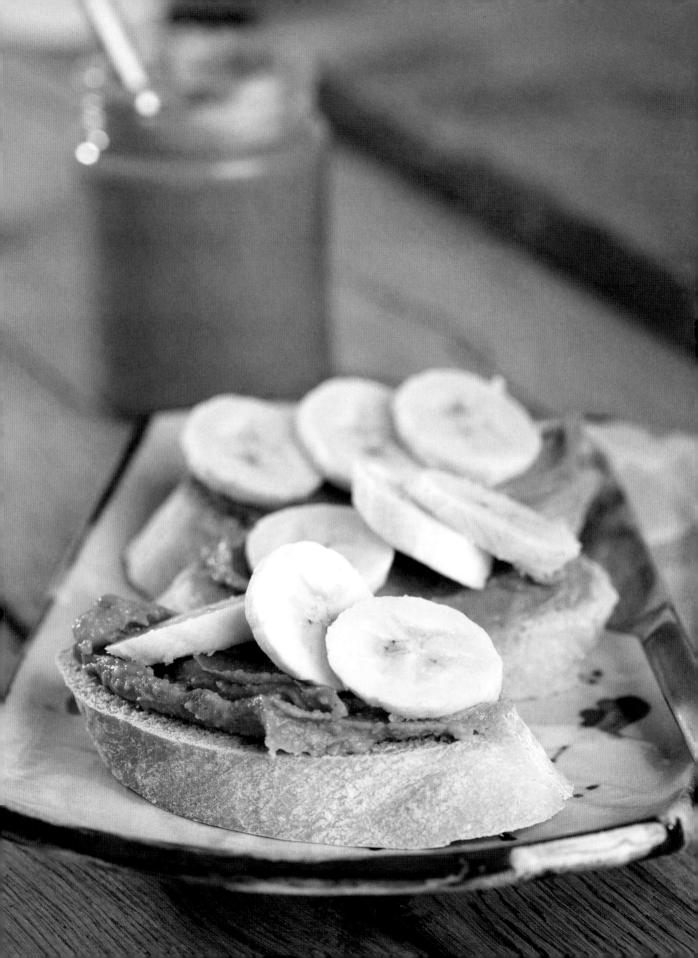

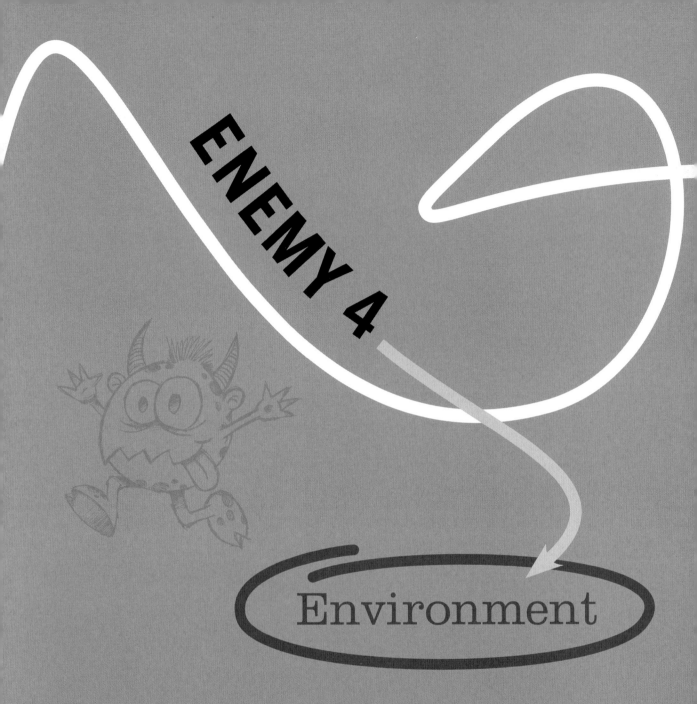

# ENEMY 4

## Environment

**When was the last time you walked through the woods, felt the wind in your hair or got mud on your shoes?** If it's been a while, your brain may be paying the price. Experts estimate that adults today spend at least 90 per cent of their time indoors, caught up in modern man-made environments that pose subtle threats to their mental clarity.

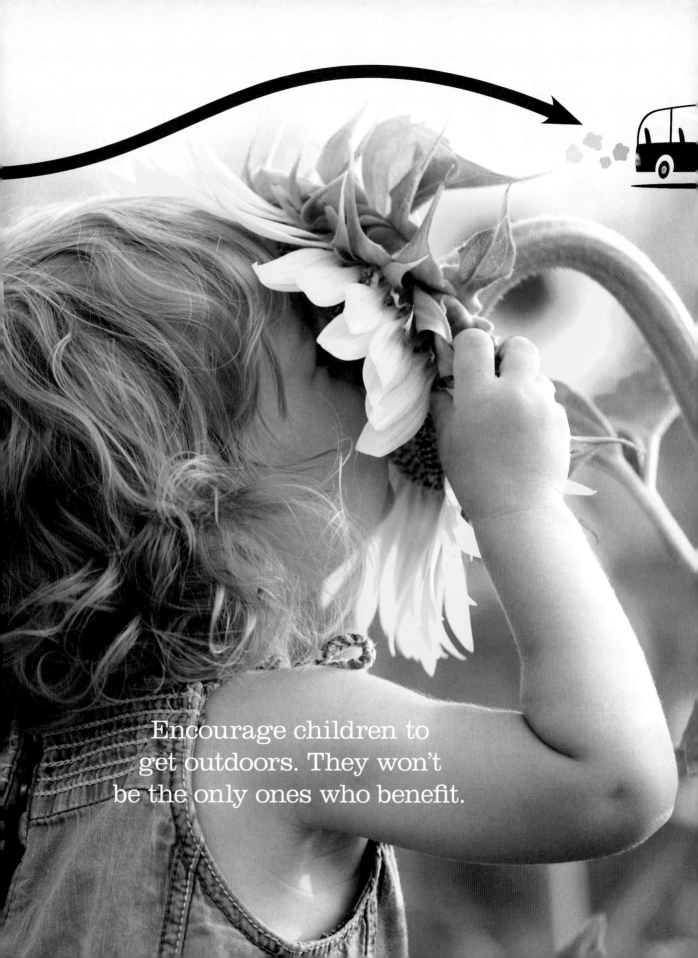

Encourage children to
get outdoors. They won't
be the only ones who benefit.

What's so bad about life indoors? For a start, there's the lack of alertness-boosting natural light, the shortage of fresh, oxygen-rich air and, if you live with a smoker, the exposure to brain-exhausting secondhand smoke. And let's face it, being in our offices and living rooms simply can't deliver the deeply restoring experience of the great outdoors.

In fact, spending time in natural surroundings can have such a positive mental effect that some doctors recommend outdoor time to patients who are so overwhelmed with stress that they can no longer think clearly.

Here, then, are five ways in which you can make your environment more brain-friendly, minimise real environmental hazards and protect your brain from some of the perils of modern-day life.

# EMBRACE NATURE

Adults and children alike report spending more time watching TV and playing with computers, mobile phones and video games than enjoying a walk round the block, an afternoon in the country or a back-garden barbecue. Even visits to parks and other scenic outdoor areas are declining. Experts call this growing disconnection from the outside world 'nature deficit disorder', and there's plenty of evidence that if you're not getting outside much, your brain is missing out.

Exposure to greenery has been shown in numerous studies to boost thinking skills, speed mental processing and reduce stress. Evidence suggests that even artificial plants may produce similar benefits.

Why do our brains seem to work better when the surrounding scene is natural? Some might argue that the answer lies in our prehistoric beginnings, when human beings lived and survived in the wild. It's not unreasonable to suggest that our bodies respond best to the natural environment in which – for the most part – human life evolved.

The trouble is, most of us spend little time in nature – 25 per cent less today than 20 years ago. These strategies can help you get back in touch.

● **Take a long walk in the park or countryside.** The University of Michigan in the USA boasts a large, well-maintained arboretum. To test the effects of nature on memory, university psychologists presented 38 students with a memory challenge – repeating a sequence of numbers backwards – before and after strolling through either the arboretum or the nearby town for 50 to 55 minutes. The nature group's scores on the 'after' test improved significantly; those of the urban walkers did not.

The great outdoors can also recharge your cognitive batteries. Spending just 2 hours a week outside helped 74 women who'd been newly diagnosed with breast cancer to overcome extreme mental fatigue – the kind that makes everyday decision making and activities (such as planning a meal, holding a conversation or balancing the monthly accounts) nearly impossible.

● **Fill your home with houseplants and your garden with greenery.** An environment that includes plants also appears to boost recall, reactions and creativity. In one Japanese study, men who could see plants during creative word-association tests scored higher than men who couldn't. In another study, having-plants in the test room was correlated with faster reaction times. In a third study, people taking the driving theory test achieved higher scores when there were green plants on the desk.

Plant greenery and flowers where you can see them from the windows you look out of most often, and open your curtains on the pretty view. No garden? Plant container pots on your patio or balcony. And fill your home and office with plants.

● **Invest in windowsill herbs.** Growing rosemary, for instance, is doubly beneficial; the herb is not only pretty but also its strong, resinous scent will perk up your brain every time you take a sniff. (Studies show that inhaling either rosemary or basil increases the brain's production of beta waves, which signal heightened awareness.) Rosemary, which grows well near sunny windows, is tasty with healthy grilled fish, meats (especially lamb) and vegetables.

● **Surround yourself with images of nature.** Simply hanging a photograph or painting of a beautiful natural scene in your home or office could help boost your memory. Psychologist Rita Berto

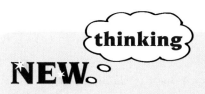

### NEW thinking

**Multi-tasking: bad for your brain?**
You may be able to walk and send texts or even read a magazine while watching your favourite TV programme. But 21st century-style multi-tasking feats may be too much for the brain.

'Despite having these incredibly complex and sophisticated brains, with 100 billion neurons processing information at rates of up to a thousand times a second, human beings have a crippling inability to do two tasks at once,' says neuroscientist Rene Marois, PhD, associate professor of psychology at Vanderbilt University in Tennessee, USA. In brain-scan studies, Dr Marois found that the brain region crucial for decision making seems able to process just one task at a time. Other research shows that asking your brain to switch between activities actually wastes time – and that doing one thing at a time may be more efficient.

Mental juggling may also impair your cognitive capacity. Brain-imaging studies show that when volunteers did two things at the same time, the brainpower available for each job dropped to less than half. A better plan: do one thing at a time when you have something mentally challenging to do.

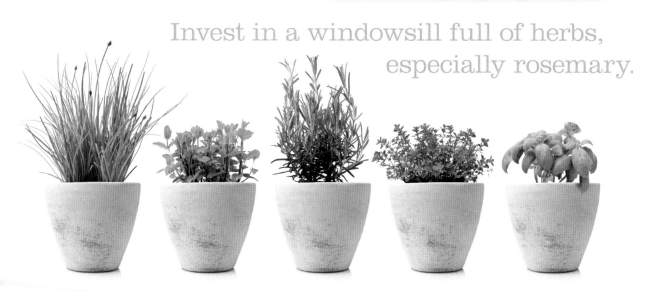

Invest in a windowsill full of herbs, especially rosemary.

from the University of Padua in Italy tested students' ability to complete a sustained attention task. Some were then shown photographs of natural scenes that other students had classed as relaxing, interesting and appealing, while others were shown photos such as ugly streetscapes or industrial scenes that had rated low on the same scale.

A third group was shown pictures of geometric patterns as a control situation (because it requires little effort to look at these). Then all of the students took the attention test again. The students who had viewed the natural photographs performed significantly better than they had on the first test, while there was no significant improvement for those who had looked at the 'ugly' photos or geometric shapes.

Eat outside …

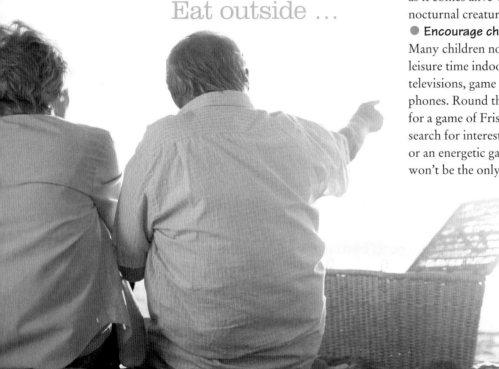

Other research has come to similar conclusions, and many scientists believe that natural scenes can have a 'restorative' effect on cognitive function. The findings suggest that having natural areas near your home or work, and enjoying them, is vital for tip-top thinking.

● **Move meals and parties outside.** Do you have a picnic table? You're ready to begin. Food eaten outdoors tastes extra good, and sitting in the garden or on a patio or balcony encourages you and your fellow diners to linger longer and enjoy each other's company, not to mention the fresh air.

● **Explore the world by moonlight.** Too busy for a daytime nature break? Night-time is good, too. Star-gaze, sign up for an after-hours walk at a local nature centre or simply sit outside listening to the sounds of your garden as it comes alive with all sorts of nocturnal creatures.

● **Encourage children to get outdoors.** Many children now spend much of their leisure time indoors, glued to computers, televisions, game consols and mobile phones. Round them up in the garden for a game of Frisbee, a treasure hunt, a search for interesting leaves or insects, or an energetic game of tag. The children won't be the only ones to benefit.

# THE BRAIN NEEDS PEACE AND QUIET

Deep within your inner ear, tiny 'hair cells' quiver, quake and shimmy along to the sounds in your world, from background music on the radio to your neighbour's noisy lawnmower to the quiet rustling of trees in the woods. These microscopic bristles convert sound waves into electrical signals that travel to your brain, delivering important information about what's happening round about you. But too much noise can overload your brain circuits, leading to that 'it's-so-loud-I-can't-think-straight' feeling.

In studies comparing schools situated near noisy airports, roads and railway lines with those in quiet areas, researchers have found links between noise pollution and problems with concentration, reading ability, memory and performance on tests. It seems highly likely that noisy environments have similar effects on adult learning, especially as older brains are more easily distracted by noise.

## NOISE IS A HEALTH HAZARD

Too much noise can also raise blood pressure – bad for the brain. When researchers checked the blood pressure levels of 140 adults living near London's Heathrow Airport and three other major European airports, they found that both the top and bottom numbers rose by 6 to 7 points whenever there was a 'noise event' – such as a plane flying overhead.

In another study at Imperial College London of nearly 5,000 people aged 45 to 70 living close to one of six major European airports, a 10 decibel increase in noise from night-time aircraft increased

## ARE YOU 'NOISE-SENSITIVE'?

If sounds affect you more profoundly than they do your friends, colleagues or family members, you may be among the estimated 1 in 13 people who are noise-sensitive. Experts aren't sure whether hyperacusis – the medical term for unusual intolerance of ordinary environmental sounds – is something you're born with or whether it's the result of early environmental exposures (it's also not clear whether growing up in quiet surroundings or amid noise increases the risk).

The effects are real. According to a survey at Uppsala University in Sweden, people with hyperacusis suffered difficulties in concentration and increased tension when noise levels were high. They also reported sensitivity to light and colours. If noise bothers you, seek quiet – your brain will thank you.

the risk of hypertension by 14 per cent. Average daily road traffic noise was even more hazardous, with men in the highest exposure group having a 54 per cent increased risk of high blood pressure. Over time, elevated blood pressure increases the risk of cognitive decline and age-related problems with mental processing, memory and reaction time.

## FINDING YOUR LEVEL

How much noise is too much? That depends on the situation, and on you. The loud music you enjoy as you dance at a party would make it difficult to concentrate if you were working. The traffic outside your window may be background sound by day, but could rob you of the deep, restorative sleep your brain needs at night for optimal performance tomorrow.

● **Turn off the TV and radio when you're trying to concentrate.** Subtle changes in brain activity, beginning in middle age, make it more and more difficult for our grey matter to tune out distractions and concentrate on the task at hand, whether it's reading, driving or writing a report at work. A study at the University of Otago in New Zealand tested groups of 32 older and younger people in a virtual-reality mock-up of a shopping precinct, complete with sounds and designed to simulate conditions of high or low distraction by varying the amount of visual stimulation and auditory noise. Each person was given two memory tasks to complete while walking down the street. As expected, the older people found it harder to remember than the younger group. Most striking was that in these conditions, more like those of real life than most laboratory memory tests, their difficulties were markedly accentuated when they were in a noisy environment.

● **Reduce night-time noise.** A snoring bedmate, the rush of traffic outside your bedroom window, a loud air-conditioner or noisy neighbours can all disturb your sleep and lead to diminished brainpower by reducing the amount of time you spend in phases of deep sleep, when memories are locked in place and the brain restores itself.

Earplugs can help, as can moving your sleeping quarters to the quietest part of the house. As for the snorer, ask him or her to roll over, experiment with a snoring aid or get an evaluation for sleep apnoea (a potentially serious condition) if the problem is extreme. A small Canadian study found that bedmates of snorers suffered hearing loss in the ear closest to the person making all the noise.

● **Buy a white noise machine or CD.** These generate a consistent, calming sound that covers other noises. They can help you fall asleep and stay asleep till morning. You can buy them easily online.

● **Invest in double glazing.** If you live in a noisy area, you can't necessarily pack up and move to a quieter place, but you can make sure your windows keep out as much sound as possible.

● **Boycott loud restaurants and events.** If you have to raise your voice to talk to your dining partner, the restaurant is too loud; take your business elsewhere.

● **Wear earplugs.** In one informal review, published in an online American magazine, reviewers found that cheap polyurethane earplugs were more effective, comfortable and easy to use than pricey customised silicon plugs or extra-fancy versions that deliver white noise directly into your ears. Keep a pair by your bed, in your bag or in your briefcase. In one Israeli study of factory workers, those who started wearing this type of earplug no longer experienced noise-related rises in the stress hormone cortisol, which in excess doses can be toxic to brain cells.

# IMPROVE YOUR AIR QUALITY

Fresh air doesn't just smell good, it supplies the oxygen your brain needs for snappy thinking and all-round alertness. But newer, energy-efficient buildings don't always provide enough of this vital brain fuel. Modern ventilation systems may not exchange indoor and outdoor air as frequently as older, 'leaky' buildings do. Plus, even if enough oxygen is coming

# Smoke-free ZONE

It's not just your heart and lungs that suffer if you smoke: the toxicity may affect your brain too. Research in patients with established Alzheimer's-type dementia has shown that heavy smoking, heavy drinking or the presence of the ApoE4 gene (see page 187) were associated with an earlier onset of disease by two to three years. In patients with all three risk factors, dementia was likely to have been diagnosed a staggering ten years earlier than in patients with none of these risks.

This implies that even if you are destined to develop the disease, avoiding smoke (as well as heavy alcohol consumption) could delay its onset. Secondhand smoke is also a significant danger, especially if you live with a smoker. In a study of almost 5,000 older non-smokers, published in the *British Medical Journal*, Cambridge University researchers found the group with the highest levels of cotinine (a marker for recent secondhand smoke exposure) had 44 per cent higher rates of cognitive impairment than those with the lowest levels.

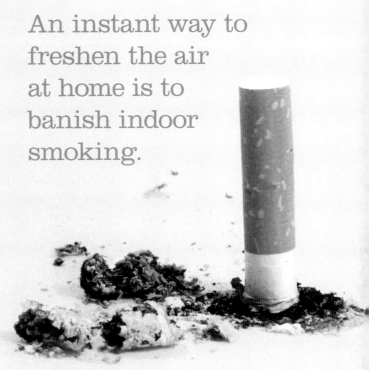

An instant way to freshen the air at home is to banish indoor smoking.

## EXTRA BRAIN BOOST?

When you quit smoking, using nicotine replacement therapies such as patches, gum, inhalators or lozenges may offer a surprising side benefit. While nicotine is toxic in higher doses, several studies suggest that, without all the additional harmful chemicals in tobacco smoke, a small amount can enhance cognitive function in the short term (using nicotine is not recommended, however, unless you are a smoker trying to quit).

In one study at Sussex University, young volunteers used either a nicotine or a placebo nasal spray. When they were given tests of prospective memory (remembering to do something) 15 minutes later, the results were significantly better in the nicotine group.

In another small study, researchers gave 11 patients with memory impairment a nicotine patch to wear for 16 hours a day. They determined that after four weeks the nicotine patch had improved the patients' reaction time and attention.

And Korean researchers who tested the effects of nicotine patches on 63 older men found their memory improved after receiving the nicotine.

in, the building's ventilation system may not circulate fresh air effectively.

Airtight rooms are low in oxygen and high in sleepiness-causing and fatigue-inducing carbon dioxide. Outside air contains about 350 parts per million of carbon dioxide; in some studies, levels in office buildings have risen to 1,000 parts per million or higher – enough to cause drowsiness and foggy thinking.

● **Open the window.** If you feel drowsy, get headaches or lack mental energy and you live or work in an energy-efficient building (many structures built after 1970 are classed as energy efficient), you may be breathing recirculated air that's not fully oxygenated. If possible, open a window or door to the outside – or go out for a walk at lunch, and have a 10 minute outside break in the afternoon.

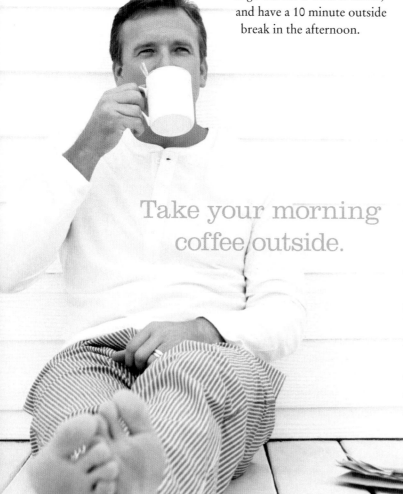

Take your morning coffee outside.

● **Combat dehydration.** If you spend a lot of time in an air-conditioned space, beware of dehydration, which causes drowsiness and lethargy and adversely affects concentration. Just 2 per cent of body weight lost in fluids can result in reduced physical and mental performance. Keep the temperature at about 19°C to 23°C, and try to maintain a comfortable level of humidity. Central heating can also cause the atmosphere to dry out. So if the air around you feels too dry, buy a humidifier or place bowls of water above radiators, or around the room. Plants and vases of fresh flowers will also contribute to the humidity, as well as breathing out oxygen.

## LET THE LIGHT SHINE IN

The best wake-up call for the human brain? Sunshine. When the dawn's early light strikes the human eye, it sends a signal to brain regions that control alertness, taking you from drowsy to bright-eyed and bushy-tailed, fast.

In a study from the Surrey Sleep Research Centre in Guildford, lights in a large British office building were fitted with experimental 'blue-white' bulbs for four weeks. The 94 participants reported increased alertness, concentration and work performance, along with reductions in irritability, blurred vision and evening fatigue. Researchers suspect that the blue-white light is effective because it mimics energising natural light.

Bright light may even slow down dementia. When Dutch scientists installed extremely bright lights in long-term care centres, people with dementia scored

5 per cent better on thinking tests and reported depression dropped by 19 per cent. The lights used in the study aren't available for home use – they were three times brighter than typical home lighting, on a par with television studio lighting – but it makes sense for people with or at risk of dementia to live in well-lit environments.

● **Pull back the curtains first thing in the morning – then get outside.** Your eyes and brain may be especially receptive to the energising effects of natural light first thing in the day, studies suggest. Take advantage of this window of opportunity by flooding your home with sunshine. Then get outside, either by taking a walk (good for the brain) or by lingering on your patio or in the garden with a cup of coffee (another brain-booster).

● **Enjoy a stimulating dose of natural light later in the day.** Half an hour of sunshine is all it takes to increase alertness. That's another good reason to devote part of your lunch hour to a stroll.

● **Turn on the lights.** During the morning and afternoon, make sure the area where you're spending your time is brightly lit. After dinner, dim the lights to signal that it's time to wind down.

# TACKLE CLUTTER

Some people thrive on chaos, but for most of us, a messy world creates stress and distraction. Piles of papers and stacks of stuff remind us of all the things we should be doing (such as opening our post, paying our bills) and simultaneously make it harder to get anything done.

The mess around you could even contribute to poor decision making and fuzzy thinking. Many studies of navigation screens in fighter jets show that too many details (known as visual clutter) interfere with a pilot's ability to find a target. And websites with too many extra features on one page prevent viewers from locating the information they're seeking.

Of course, clutter is in the eye of the beholder. Some studies suggest that a messy desk may actually be more conducive to creativity than a neat one. But if clear thinking and less stress is your goal, it's probably time for a clear-out.

● **Do a clean sweep.** Choose three surfaces you see as soon as you walk into a room and do a 5 minute 'keep or toss' blitz on each. If you can return objects to their rightful locations, do so. If not, designate a box for items to store later. Throw away everything you don't use or need.

● **Dig deeper with the A-B-C method.** When you have time, attack a room with this approach. Start with cupboards, to make room for other objects that need a home, then tackle the clutter. Place stray items into one of three piles: A for 'Always used'; B for 'Used only occasionally', such as for holidays or seasonally; and C for 'Not used for over a year'. Store A items in easy-to-reach spots in cupboards and drawers. Place B items on a special shelf or at the back of storage units. Dispose of C items (if they're valuable, make plans to sell or donate them – see page 141).

● **Buy some organisers.** You can't clear clutter if you don't have a place to store the items you want to keep. Investigate large stationery shops, with whole sections devoted to helping you organise your life. Buy a set of accordion-file folders for paperwork, some under-the-bed storage boxes for jumpers and other bulky clothing, a basket for current magazines, back-of-door shoe hangers and so on.

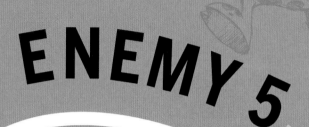

# ENEMY 5

## Medical causes

**Don't blame your advancing age for memory slips, cognitive slowdowns and attention deficits –** at least not until you've ruled out common, seemingly unrelated medical issues that can affect your brain. Rediscovering your own mental self may be as simple as getting a problem such as high blood pressure, high cholesterol or hearing loss under control.

# BLOOD PRESSURE CONTROL

Take a brittle, worn-out garden hose, turn the water on full force, and what happens? You get lots of little leaks, and maybe even a full-blown puncture. If you have high blood pressure, this messy scenario could unfold deep within your brain as fast-moving blood slams against the walls of fragile blood vessels. You could end up with tiny leaks that damage surrounding brain tissue (blood that escapes blood vessels is toxic to brain cells), plus a greater risk of a brain-altering, life-affecting stroke.

The bottom line: if you want to protect your brain, keep your blood pressure in the healthy range. In the large Tromsø study of over 5,000 subjects in Norway, high blood pressure at the start was associated with poorer performance on multiple memory and cognitive performance tests seven years later.

High blood pressure begins to threaten your memory and dull your thinking skills far earlier and at lower pressure levels than doctors ever realised in the past. Even slightly high pressure – levels considered normal or near-normal less than a decade ago – eroded memory, focus and verbal skills in one recent study.

If your levels are healthy now, you're not off the hook; high blood pressure becomes more common with age, affecting half of those over the age of 75. In the Newcastle 85+ study of more than 1,400 people aged 85 and above, nearly 60 per cent had hypertension. It's never too early – or too late – to take some pressure off.

● **Quit smoking.** The nicotine in tobacco constricts blood vessels and raises your blood pressure by 10 points or more for an hour after you smoke just one cigarette.

## AIM FOR THE RIGHT NUMBERS

Doctors in the UK base their treatment of high blood pressure on the British Hypertension Society's classification:

| Category | Systolic blood pressure (mmHg) | Diastolic blood pressure (mmHg) |
|---|---|---|
| Optimal blood pressure | <120 | <80 |
| Normal blood pressure | <130 | <85 |
| High-normal blood pressure | 130–139 | 85–89 |
| Grade 1 hypertension (mild) | 140–159 | 90–99 |
| Grade 2 hypertension (moderate) | 160–179 | 100–109 |
| Grade 3 hypertension (severe) | >/= 180 | >/= 110 |
| Isolated systolic hypertension (Grade 1) | 140–159 | <90 |
| Isolated systolic hypertension (Grade 2) | >/= 160 | <90 |

## BLOOD PRESSURE BLIPS YOU SHOULD NEVER IGNORE

● **Your blood pressure's 'high-normal':** if your BP is at the high end of normal (see page 175), you won't usually need treatment, but it's sensible to take lifestyle measures to reduce it. Some people at higher risk of complications may benefit from taking medication, though, including those who've had a heart attack, stroke or TIA (see page 181).

● **It's creeping up slowly:** in one study, women's blood pressure inched up by 8 to 10 points each decade, men's by 4 to 5 points, between the ages of 35 and 64 – enough to land you in the pre-hypertensive or hypertensive category.

● **It's high only in the GP's surgery:** don't ignore so-called white-coat hypertension – elevated readings that occur in the doctor's surgery only. In a study at Queen Elizabeth Hospital, Birmingham, people with white-coat hypertension scored significantly lower in memory tests than people with normal or even borderline high blood pressure.

If you want to protect your brain, keep your blood pressure in the healthy range.

● **Lose weight sooner rather than later.** Whittling 8lb to 10lb (3.5kg to 4.5kg) from your body weight can trim 4 to 5 points from the top number (systolic pressure) in your reading and 1 to 2 points from the bottom number (diastolic pressure). The best way to begin is to exercise for at least 30 minutes most days of the week. The sooner you start, the better: researchers suspect that, over time, chemicals churned out by body fat can make artery stiffness – which causes high blood pressure – hard to reverse.

● **Eat more fresh produce, whole grains and low-fat dairy products.** Calcium and other minerals in low-fat milk, yoghurt and other dairy products have pressure-lowering powers. So do the potassium, vitamins and antioxidants in many fruits and veggies (such as bananas, melons, spinach and sweet potatoes) and the fibre in whole grains and fresh fruit and veg.

● **Cut back on high-salt foods.** Cutting your salt intake by just 0.75g per day (that's about the amount in two slices of processed cheese) reduces systolic pressure by 2 to 4 points and diastolic pressure by 1 to 2 points. Cut out more salt, and blood pressure drops even lower.

The biggest sources of excess sodium (the main salt component) in our diets are processed foods such as canned soups, beans and vegetables, microwavable meals and side dishes, bottled salad dressings, salty snacks, hot dogs, sausages and cold meats, pickles and cheese.

● **Move – away from the screen.** In a major study of more than 14,000 people in Norfolk, television viewing was associated with higher blood pressure, and physical activity with lower pressure. In women who watched fewer than 2 hours of TV per day and who did more than 1 hour per week of vigorous exercise, diastolic blood pressure was on average 2.7mmHg lower than that of women who watched more than 4 hours of TV daily and did no vigorous activity. The equivalent figure for men was 3.6mmHg.

● **Take the blood pressure medicines you're prescribed – and make sure they're working.** Blood pressure medication can halve the risk of a stroke. But research shows that these medicines can't protect your brain if they're not lowering your blood pressure to healthy levels. That's important news for the six in every ten people who don't take their blood pressure medicines as directed, or who skip them entirely, and for the others who don't attend follow-up appointments to ensure that their medication and dosages are working.

## MINERALS THAT LOWER BLOOD PRESSURE

Potassium, calcium and magnesium all play a major role in keeping blood pressure low. Find them in these foods.

**Potassium:** Baked potato with skin, tomato sauce, butter-beans, orange juice, cooked spinach, butternut squash, bananas, raisins and prune juice.

**Calcium:** Low-fat yoghurt, low-fat milk, cooked spinach, green leafy vegetables and broccoli.

**Magnesium:** Whole grains, nuts, shellfish, cooked spinach and pumpkin seeds.

# KEEP YOUR CHOLESTEROL NUMBERS UNDER CONTROL

Could ordering the grilled salmon instead of the cheeseburger help you think faster? Could taking a stroll after dinner instead of watching a quiz show strengthen your memory? Could switching to porridge in the morning instead of a fast-food breakfast sharpen your mental clarity? The answer is yes, especially if your cholesterol levels are less than ideal.

Most of us know by now that unhealthy cholesterol levels – high LDL ('bad' cholesterol) and low HDL ('good' cholesterol) – are dangerous for the heart. But did you know that they're also dangerous for the brain? Remember that the brain is made up of a high proportion of fat. It's actually teeming with 'good' HDLs, which seem to protect against blood-vessel injury, brain plaques and inflammation. And as far as your brain is concerned, the more HDLs, the better. In one study of 3,673 people, all aged 61, those with low HDLs (below 1.1mmol/l) were 53 per cent more likely to have memory problems than those with high levels (over 1.6mmol/l). Those whose HDLs fell the furthest between the ages of 55 and 60 had the most trouble remembering words when tested.

Having high LDLs, the type of cholesterol that clogs the arteries, increases the risk of a stroke. Here's how to reduce LDLs and bolster HDLs.

● **Get tested.** If you're over 40 or have other risk factors for cardiovascular disease (such as a family historyw or diabetes), ask your GP for a cholesterol test. Your doctor uses your cholesterol level along with your age, sex, blood pressure and smoking status to determine your risk of developing cardiovascular disease – if it's more than 20 per cent over the next ten years, you may be offered treatment with a statin drug.

● **Eat for high HDLs and low LDLs.** This means serving yourself more fish, nuts, olive oil, oats, beans and fresh produce. When you eat meat, make sure it's lean. Go easy on cheese and butter, and buy skimmed or semi-skimmed milk plus low-fat yoghurt. This strategy cuts LDL-raising saturated fats and fills your plate with more of the good fats that protect HDL levels. It also gives you more soluble fibre, which whisks LDLs out of your body. Including walnuts or pecans may even nudge HDLs up a little.

● **Have a glass of wine or beer a day.** Studies suggest that drinking alcohol in moderation (no more than two units a day for women and up to three units for men) lowers LDL while raising HDL.

● **Achieve a healthier weight.** Gradually adjusting your diet and moving to a healthy weight could increase your HDL

## CHOLESTEROL – WHAT'S HEALTHY?

The UK government advises that in adults healthy levels are below 5mmol/l total and below 3mmol/l LDL cholesterol. The Joint British Societies' guidelines aim even lower, however, with 4mmol/l and 2mmol/l respectively, matching more stringent European guidelines.

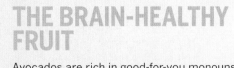

## THE BRAIN-HEALTHY FRUIT

Avocados are rich in good-for-you monounsaturated fat. In one study, adults who ate an avocado a day for a week reduced their total cholesterol by 17 per cent. Better still, their 'good' cholesterol levels rose while their 'bad' cholesterol levels fell. Add avocado slices instead of cheese or even butter to your sandwich and you'll get a double bonus: more brain-healthy good fat and less artery-clogging saturated fat. But eat them instead of, rather than in addition to other fats, as avocados are quite calorific.

Enjoy avocado slices instead of other, less healthy fats and you'll get a double bonus.

levels – every 6½lb (3kg) that you lose will make a measurable difference.

● **Walk briskly three times per week.** You can raise your HDLs by taking a fast stroll for half an hour three times a week. Adding three weekly strength-training sessions should improve them even more.

# PREVENT A STROKE

Suddenly, without warning, a blood clot closes off an artery. A fragile blood vessel bursts. Your leg, arm or face goes numb. You can't see straight, or speak, or walk. Your brain is under attack, and it may never be the same again. Moments after a stroke begins, brain cells die because they're deprived of oxygen-rich blood. A stroke occurring on the left side of the brain may cause paralysis on the right side of the body and affect speech, verbal short-term memory and understanding. A stroke on the right side of the brain may lead to visual memory problems and left side paralysis. Frontal damage can result in disorganised, compulsive or ultra-cautious behaviour and major personality changes. Strokes are also associated with an increased risk of dementia later on.

A stroke happens in no time at all. But some of the major health problems already outlined, which conspire to unleash a stroke, may be years in the making. These are the risk factors – all of which are treatable.

● **High blood pressure.** Your risk of a stroke begins to rise as soon as your blood pressure rises above 115/75, according to the landmark Framingham Heart Study. In fact, stroke risk doubles with every increase of 20 points in the top blood pressure number and/or 10 points in the bottom number. If you don't know your levels, write down the reading at your next GP visit so you can gauge whether it's going up or down. With your GP's help, make every effort to control it.

● **Off-beat heart rhythms.** Don't ignore atrial fibrillation – irregular heartbeats that can hurl clots into blood heading to your brain. Symptoms may include palpitations, chest pain or fainting. To avoid the risk of a stroke, seek early treatment.

● **High blood sugar and cholesterol levels.** Diabetes doubles or even triples your risk of a stroke; levels of 'bad' LDL cholesterol above 3.4mmol/l also raise the risk of strokes caused by blood clots

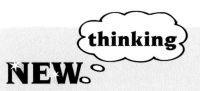

**NEW thinking**

**Silent stroke**

Experts are uncovering evidence of a type of stroke they've named a 'silent' stroke because it causes no symptoms at all. Like TIAs (see opposite), these can block tiny arteries in the brain, diminish brainpower, and increase the risk of a major stroke or more small strokes. As many as one in five adults over the age of 45 has had a silent stroke, yet most never realise it.

Does it matter if there are no symptoms? Yes – very much. In one study at Shimane Medical University in Japan, researchers scanned the brains of 933 people aged between 30 and 81 without any signs of neurological problems and found signs of a silent stroke in 10.6 per cent. On follow-up between one and seven years later, people whose brain scans had indicated a silent stroke were more than ten times more likely than the others to have had a full-blown stroke.

– notably of repeat strokes in someone who's already had at least one mini-stroke (see below). Controlling diabetes cuts stroke risk by 50 per cent; lowering LDLs can reduce it by up to 25 per cent.

● **Mini-strokes.** Days, weeks or months before having a major stroke, 30 to 40 per cent of people get a strange warning sign: a brief mini-stroke, called a transient ischaemic attack, or TIA. The symptoms are the same as those above, just shorter and less intense. They stop as swiftly as they start, but that doesn't mean the danger has passed. The risk of having a full-blown stroke in the next two days is 1 in 20; over the next three months, it's 1 in 10, unless you take action. Although the highest risk occurs early on, the danger persists in the long term. According to one study at the University of Glasgow of 795 patients who had had a TIA, after a follow-up of 14 years the percentage who'd succumbed to a stroke had reached 14 per cent.

What to do: call your doctor immediately and explain what has happened. He or she may want to put you on medication to prevent blood clots, lower your cholesterol and reduce your blood pressure. In a major study at Oxford University among 1,278 patients who had suffered a TIA or stroke, early treatment was associated with an 80 per cent reduction in the risk of a full-blown or recurrent stroke over the next 90 days, from 10.3 to 2.1 per cent.

If you think you've had a mini-stroke in the past, also let your doctor know. Having had one means you may have more in the future. Your doctor will decide whether you'd be likely to benefit from taking a blood thinner or blood pressure medicine.

# KNOW THE signs of a stroke – AND ACT FAST

Clot-busting drugs can stop and even reverse brain damage caused by the most common form of stroke – an ischaemic stroke due to a blood clot – but only if they're administered within 3 hours of the start of a stroke. Too many people hesitate before calling for help and miss this precious window of opportunity.

If you suspect a stroke, the Stroke Association's **'Act FAST'** guidance recommends an assessment of three specific symptoms of stroke:

**FACIAL WEAKNESS** – can the person smile? Has his or her mouth or eye drooped?

**ARM WEAKNESS** – can the person raise both arms?

**SPEECH PROBLEMS** – can the person speak clearly and understand what you say?

**TIME** to call 999.

Other symptoms may include weakness on one side of the body, including the leg as well as the arm; numbness, tingling or a feeling of heaviness on one side of the body; trouble seeing, such as blurred or double vision, dimness or a sensation that a blind has been pulled down over the eyes; unsteadiness, dizziness, clumsiness, fainting; trouble walking, or a sudden loss of strength in the legs; a sudden, severe headache.

**If you or anyone around you develops any one of these signs, dial 999 to call an ambulance immediately.**

Many people who have had a heart attack or stroke in the past are advised to take a low dose (75mg) of aspirin daily, to reduce the risk of blood clots and ward off another attack. However, preventive aspirin is not now generally recommended for people without existing cardiovascular disease. According to a major review published in *The Lancet* in 2009, looking at clinical trial data from 100,000 people, although aspirin reduces the risk of a heart attack among those at high risk, for people at low risk any such protection is outweighed by the increased risks of internal bleeding. (To minimise this risk, those prescribed aspirin are advised to take it after food.) Aspirin can also cause allergic reactions.

However, if your doctor does recommend aspirin, there may be positive side effects. One well-designed study of more than 6,000 women aged 65 or older tested the effect of long-term use of low-dose aspirin (100mg on alternate days) on cognitive decline over a period of almost ten years. The women were evaluated at 5.6 years after the start of the study, then re-evaluated two and four years later. Researchers found that women on aspirin therapy were 20 per cent less likely to develop substantial decline in something they call category fluency – tests used to assess semantic knowledge, retrieval ability and executive functioning, in which people are asked to produce words quickly in a specified category, such as makes of car. The people who seemed to benefit the most from taking aspirin were those who had high cholesterol or who were smokers.

If you have not been prescribed aspirin for a heart problem, discuss the pros and cons with your doctor before self-medicating. Be sure to tell your doctor about all of the other pills you take, including prescription and over-the-counter medicines and even vitamins and herbs. Some may increase the risk of dangerous bleeding when combined with aspirin.

# CONTROL YOUR BLOOD SUGAR

High blood sugar is a 'major ager' of the human brain that can result in problems such as memory lapses and fuzzy thinking. You don't even have to have diabetes to suffer the consequences. Long before high blood sugar causes diabetes, it can damage blood vessels that bring oxygen and nutrients to the brain, doubling the risk of vascular dementia (the type caused by insufficient blood flow to the brain). It can even shrink the hippocampus, an area that stores memories and facilitates learning. In one study, high blood sugar was associated with a fourfold increase in memory problems.

High blood sugar not only damages arteries, it also encourages the build-up of artery-clogging plaque. It seems to increase inflammation in the brain, too, and often goes hand in hand with insulin resistance, a condition in which cells stop responding to the hormone insulin. Insulin resistance in brain cells affects how the cells function, and not for the better.

Full-blown diabetes even seems to be linked with a higher chance of developing Alzheimer's disease. In a study at Uppsala University in Sweden, 1,125 men aged 71 years and free from dementia at the start were followed for an average of 12 years. Having diabetes was associated with a 63 per cent increased risk of developing dementia or cognitive impairment. The good news: taking diabetes medications may offer some protection (see page 184).

If you have diabetes or pre-diabetes (blood sugar of 5.5mmol/l to 7mmol/l on a fasting blood sugar test), or you've been told you're at risk of diabetes, work with your doctor to prevent high blood sugar.

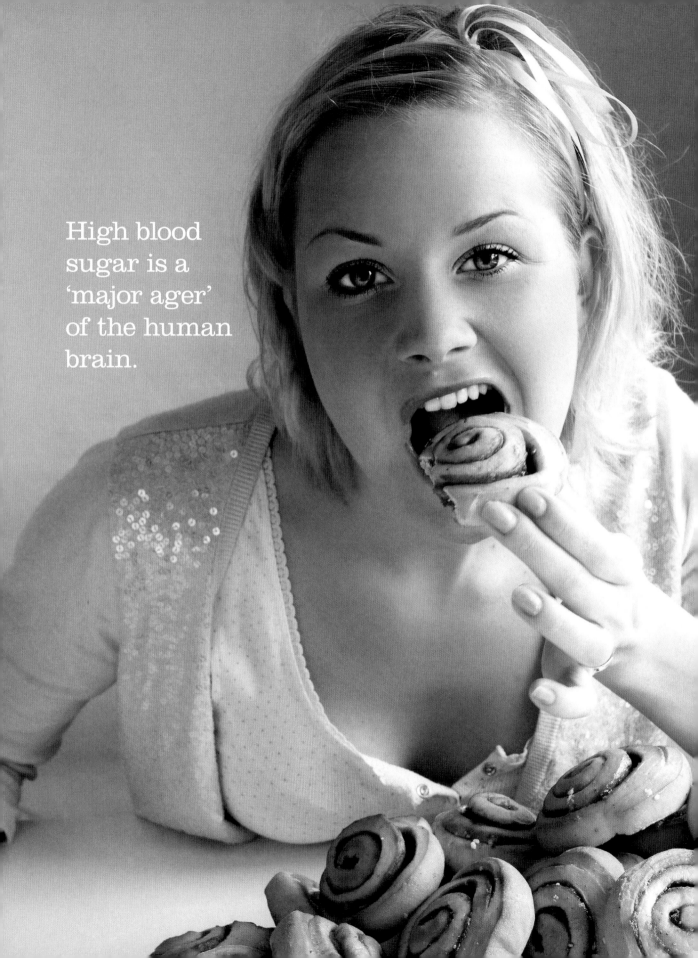

High blood sugar is a 'major ager' of the human brain.

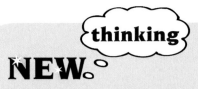

## NEW thinking

### Cellular link between diabetes and Alzheimer's disease?

Scientists investigating the links between Alzheimer's disease and insulin resistance in the brain have discovered in laboratory experiments that toxic proteins which accumulate in Alzheimer's disease lead to a dramatic loss of insulin receptors from the surface of affected brain cells.

That's a huge problem because, in the brain, the hormone insulin and its receptors not only help usher blood sugar into hungry brain cells, but also help nerve cells survive and form memories. Removing a neuron's ability to handle insulin, the scientists speculate, could cause nerve-cell damage similar to that of Alzheimer's disease.

Levels of brain insulin and of insulin receptors are already known to be lower than normal in people with the disease. Now, researchers hope that further studies will show whether diabetes drugs can protect neurons from this memory-robbing damage.

● **Check your blood sugar levels two ways.** If you have diabetes, it's important to perform daily blood sugar tests and keep track of the results as recommended by your doctor. But don't stop there. It's also wise to have regular blood tests to measure your glycated haemoglobin, or HbA1c, which is a valuable indicator of the long-term stability of your blood sugar over the previous 90 days. If you have Type 1 diabetes, you should be offered an HbA1c test between two and four times a year, or more frequently if your blood sugar control is poor. With Type 2 diabetes, HbA1c tests are recommended every two to six months.

● **Understand the blood pressure and cholesterol link.** About 70 per cent of people with diabetes also have high blood pressure and/or high cholesterol, yet surveys reveal that most worry only about their blood sugar. That's a mistake. Both high blood pressure and high cholesterol are even more dangerous to the brain when combined with high blood sugar. Put these risks on your radar – and take steps to control them.

● *Get the medicines you need.* If your blood sugar is creeping higher despite your best efforts, it may be time for diabetes medicines or insulin injections, or for a change in your medication regimen. Diabetes is a progressive health condition that often requires more intense treatment over time, even if you've done everything right. Don't shy away – your health and your brain are at stake. In one study of 145 people with Type 2 diabetes who were already taking one blood sugar-controlling drug, those who added a second drug for six months saw their blood sugar levels improve – and after six months, their scores on tests of working memory improved by 25 to 31 per cent.

## CATCH HEARING LOSS EARLY

Like tufts of grass waving in a breeze, tiny hair-like cells deep within your inner ear move in time to the sounds in your life. A child's winsome 'hello' might trigger a gentle shimmy, whereas the BANG! of fireworks could act more like gale-force winds, silencing a few of these sound-transmitting cells for ever. Lose enough of them, due to ageing, noise exposure or certain illnesses, and you have hearing problems that can be socially isolating – and bad for your brain.

Unless you've led your life well away from the influences of Western civilisation, the chances are that with age you will develop a little hearing loss. Between 24 and 40 per cent of adults over the age of 65 have difficulty hearing, as do up to half of people over the age of 75. In one study of people aged 50 to 94, researchers found that hearing loss was linked to loss of memory and cognitive skills. The reason: you may spend so much mental energy trying to work out what people are saying that your brain doesn't have a chance to focus on the information. On a practical level, hearing problems also simply mean more social isolation and less brain stimulation, both risk factors for age-related cognitive decline. How can you save your ears? These three steps are a good place to start.

● **See your doctor if you suspect you've lost some hearing.** If he or she suggests you try a hearing aid, be patient. The results are worth the effort it takes to get used to the device – and it could help you persevere with activities that can foster brain health.

Sometimes, the solution is even simpler. In one large study of people with hearing problems, researchers had to excuse one in ten study volunteers before the experiment even began – because their hearing problems improved significantly when doctors removed earwax.

● **Turn the music down.** If you use headphones or earbuds, your tunes are turned up too loud if others can hear what you're listening to.

● **Carry earplugs everywhere.** Wear them in places where you'll be exposed to any sound over 85 decibels, such as

## WHEN EVERYBODY'S MUMBLING: IS IT YOUR EARS?

You may have early signs of hearing loss – and should see your doctor – if you:

● Have trouble hearing the phone ring.

● Have difficulty following conversations when two or more people are talking.

● Turn up the TV volume so loud that others complain.

● Can't hear very well when there's background noise.

● Think everyone is mumbling.

near a lawnmower, at a rock concert, cinema or wedding with loud music – even in a loud health club. Don't rely on cotton-wool balls or bits of paper tissue in your ears; they'll screen out only about 7 decibels, while foam earplugs can block up to 32 decibels. Need more protection? Buy sound-deadening earmuffs.

Turn the music down.

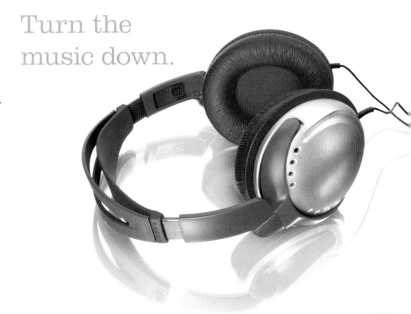

# DEMENTIA – MYTH AND REALITY

Many adults fear Alzheimer's disease and other dementias more than they fear heart disease (the number one killer), diabetes or cancer. We equate 'losing our minds' with losing our very selves. While there isn't yet a vaccine or cure for Alzheimer's, there is a vast amount of new knowledge about how to alleviate early symptoms and possibly delay the onset of disease.

Some people take every precaution and still develop dementia; others will do practically nothing and never get it. While the chance of getting Alzheimer's disease increases steadily with age, it is by no means an inevitable consequence of ageing. According to the Alzheimer's Society, about 1 in 50 people between the ages of 65 and 70 have some form of dementia, and this rises to about one in five people over the age of 80.

It's likely that the progressively increasing risk of dementia as you grow older is linked to diseases that become more common with age, such as hypertension, cardiovascular disease (heart attacks and strokes), age-related changes to neurons, DNA or cell structure and general weakening of the body's natural repair systems. The good news: with care, awareness and appropriate medical treatment, many of these factors are within your control.

And while age is the main risk factor for dementia, there are others. Women are slightly more likely to develop Alzheimer's disease than men, and not only because on average they live longer, although the reasons are ill-understood. On the other hand, men are more likely to get vascular dementia, probably related to their increased level of cardiovascular risk factors, such as heart disease and high blood pressure.

## SEEING, AND THINKING, STRAIGHT

There's a hidden connection between conditions that cause vision loss, such as age-related macular degeneration (AMD) and glaucoma, and dementia. When researchers followed 206 people with AMD for three years, they discovered that nearly 15 per cent showed signs of a decline in memory and other thinking skills, most likely because vision loss caused people to drop out of some of their activities. The lesson to be learned? Have regular eye tests to help preserve your vision, and do all that you can to keep participating in the activities you enjoy.

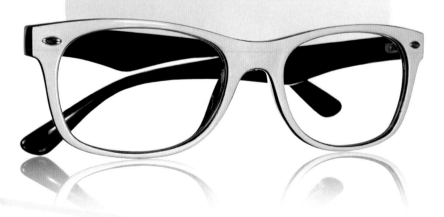

Have regular eye tests to help preserve your vision.

# IS IT depression, dementia OR BOTH?

For older people, depression can sometimes mimic dementia, and vice versa. This could make identifying and treating mood and memory problems tricky for you, your family and your doctor.

Although people with a history of depression before the age of 60 are four times more likely to develop Alzheimer's disease than those who have never been depressed, it's not clear if depression can trigger dementia ... or if treating depression lowers the risk of later-life dementia. Sometimes a diagnosis of Alzheimer's disease can trigger depression – as the person grieves deeply over the loss of memories, thinking skills and a big piece of his or her identity.

Some studies indicate that certain antidepressants can make daily life easier for Alzheimer's sufferers who are also depressed, even though these drugs won't improve their thinking problems (see also page 194) .

If you or your doctor suspect you may have Alzheimer's disease, it's important to get a referral to a specialist experienced in diagnosing the disease. An early diagnosis raises the chances that medication may be able to improve cognition and possibly slow the course of the disease.

Genes also play a prominent role, and sometimes dementia runs in families. One specific gene, called apolipoprotein E4 (ApoE4), is strongly associated with Alzheimer's disease – though not everyone who carries the gene will get the disease, and it can develop in people who do not carry the gene.

As well as cardiovascular diseases upping the risk of vascular dementia, there are some less common conditions that increase dementia risk. These include multiple sclerosis, Huntington's disease, Down's syndrome and AIDS/HIV. Severe or repeated head injuries also impart an increased risk of developing dementia.

## LIFESTYLE FACTORS

In addition to genes, gender and certain conditions, some of which are largely unalterable, lifestyle may play a role in the development of dementia. Most scientists now believe that someone's risk of developing dementia depends upon a combination of genetic and environmental factors.

Yet, even if you are most likely to develop it, there are steps you can take that can delay the onset of Alzheimer's disease, and which could certainly reduce your risk of vascular dementia, the type associated with disease affecting the brain blood vessels.

In one study that examined the effect of physical activity, the risk of dementia in people who exercised three times a week rose much more slowly than those who exercised less frequently. The active group's risk increased to 50 per cent only at the age of 92 – and by then, those who exercised infrequently had a 75 per cent risk. Exercise helps by lowering

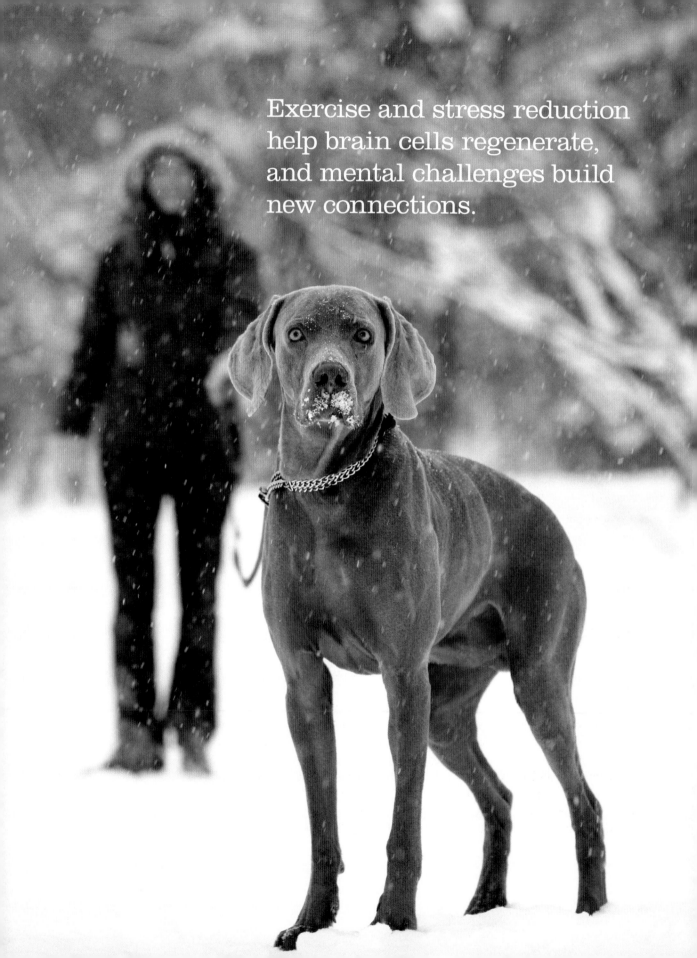

Exercise and stress reduction help brain cells regenerate, and mental challenges build new connections.

high blood pressure, protecting against diabetes, boosting blood circulation and encouraging the growth of new brain cells.

Studies that have looked at whether diet might influence the risk of developing Alzheimer's disease have produced conflicting results. But there is good evidence, as outlined earlier, that what you eat could have a big impact on your risk of cardiovascular disease, and thus of vascular dementia. In particular, there's evidence to suggest that eating a Mediterranean-style diet is associated with a reduced risk of dementia (see page 64). Experts think that this style of eating pampers the blood vessels and helps reduce inflammation, which may play a role in the development of brain diseases.

Ensuring that you keep your brain stimulated and engaged is also important, as is maintaining an active social network throughout your life. The evidence is pretty convincing that the combination of social, physical and mental activity, along with good control of medical conditions such as diabetes, high blood pressure and high cholesterol, gives you the best chance of preventing or delaying cognitive decline.

# TOP ANTI-DEMENTIA STRATEGIES

If you follow these tips, you'll be doing everything you can to avoid dementia later in life.

● **Keep blood vessels healthy.** Vascular dementia is the second most common form of dementia. It causes memory and thinking problems when blood vessels in

the brain can't deliver enough oxygenated blood to brain cells. This may happen when blood vessels are narrowed by atherosclerosis, contain leaks that damage surrounding brain tissue or have been damaged by a stroke.

Experts know more about preventing vascular dementia than they do about factors that could influence Alzheimer's disease at this point. You can take steps now to keep the blood vessels in your brain healthier, such as losing weight if you need to, exercising regularly and eating more fruit and vegetables to help keep your blood pressure low.

● **Maintain a cognitive reserve.** If having healthy blood vessels may help protect you from developing dementia, possessing a brain that's brimming with healthy nerve cells and connections between them could help to maintain functioning for longer if you do develop dementia. If you have a lot of cognitive reserve you can retain more of your abilities even in the face of the problems that dementia throws up.

How can you build and maintain cognitive reserve? By continually challenging your brain, looking after the health of your blood vessels, and keeping your brain healthy using the advice in this book so that it can grow new cells, as needed.

Exercise and stress reduction help brain cells regenerate, and mental challenges build new connections.

● **Don't smoke.** Smoking, as we've seen, is strongly associated with cardiovascular disease and thus with vascular dementia as well as age-related cognitive decline. In fact, according to Australian researchers who analysed 19 studies involving more than 26,000 smokers, former smokers and non-smokers, smoking is linked to a 40 to 80 per cent increased risk of all types of dementia or cognitive decline. If you smoke now, will quitting provide some protection? In this study, compared with current smokers, 70 per cent fewer former smokers developed dementia or cognitive decline.

● **Abstain from heavy drinking.** While moderate alcohol consumption (up to two units a day for women, three for men) may protect against dementia (one study found that it reduced the risk of vascular dementia by 71 per cent), overdoing it has the opposite effect. In fact, some experts suspect that one in ten cases of dementia results from brain-battering heavy drinking. Binge-drinking in middle age – downing a bottle of wine or five bottles of beer at a sitting – tripled the risk of dementia 25 years later, according to one Finnish study of 554 women and men.

● **Maintain healthy blood pressure.** High blood pressure increases the risk of dementia by 50 per cent, studies show. It damages the brain by causing small blood vessels to leak, triggering silent strokes and leading to major strokes. If you don't have high blood pressure, the strategies throughout this section, beginning on page 174, will help you prevent it.

If you already have high blood pressure, do whatever it takes to bring it down to healthy levels (optimal is below 120/80mmHg) and maintain it.

● **Keep a lid on blood sugar.** People with diabetes are significantly more likely to develop cognitive decline or dementia. But even if you don't officially have diabetes, high blood sugar levels may spell trouble. In a study at the Karolinska Institute in Stockholm, 1,173 people

aged 75 or above who had no dementia or diabetes at the outset were followed for nine years. Those whose blood sugar levels at the start indicated borderline levels verging on diabetes (called borderline diabetes, defined as a random blood glucose level of 7.8mmol/l to 11.0mmol/l) had a 67 per cent increased risk of any type of dementia and a 77 per cent risk of Alzheimer's disease. Further analysis suggested that the association was present only among people who did not carry the ApoE4 gene linked with Alzheimer's disease (see page 187).

Reduce the risk of high blood sugar by maintaining a healthy body weight, exercising regularly and eating well. Keep calories under control and ease off on simple carbohydrates such as white rice and white bread, along with all sugary foods and drinks. If you're at risk of diabetes, work with your doctor to be sure your blood sugar levels are checked often enough to spot problems early. If you have diabetes, make strict blood sugar control a priority. Research shows it really does protect the brain.

● **Stay in touch with friends.** Maintaining regular contact with three, four or more friends – in person, on the phone or even just via email – is one key way to protect your brain and your memories.

In one study of 2,200 women, those who remained sociable as they got older had a 26 per cent lower rate of dementia than those who didn't. Similar results have been shown in men. Socialising at home with your partner may not be enough, though. While researchers found that women with large social networks who made daily contact with friends had the lowest rates of dementia, being married didn't make a difference. Satisfaction with relationships and feeling supported in them may be the most important factors.

A study in Bordeaux, France, that followed over 2,000 older people for 15 years found that those who reported feeling satisfied with their relationships had 23 per cent lower rates of dementia than those who didn't. And participants who said that over their lifetime they had received more support than they gave were 53 per cent less likely to develop Alzheimer's disease than those who didn't feel that way, and 55 per cent less likely to develop any form of dementia. The researchers concluded that the quality, rather than quantity, of relationships may be crucial.

● **Exercise at least twice a week.** Walking, swimming, gardening, washing the car … whatever you do, make sure you do it at least twice a week (the minimum exercise frequency associated with a lower incidence of dementia in studies). 'Light' exercise (gardening or strolling) was associated with a 35 per cent lower risk of Alzheimer's disease and dementia

Stay in touch with friends; it's one key way to protect your brain and your memories.

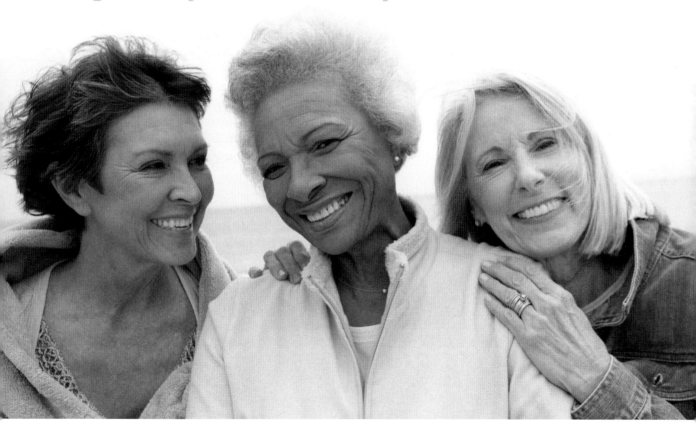

*Continued on page 195*

# Alzheimer's disease
## MEDICATIONS

Until we know exactly what causes Alzheimer's, we probably won't be able to develop drugs to cure it. In the meantime, the good news is that a handful of drugs have been approved for use in the NHS that will help to alleviate the symptoms of cognitive decline in up to half of those treated. According to a survey of 4,000 people by the Alzheimer's Society in the UK, those using cholinesterase inhibitors (see below) often experience improvements in motivation, anxiety and confidence, in addition to memory and thinking.

A hospital specialist must prescribe these drugs initially, but your GP may be able to provide repeat prescriptions. Your progress will be reviewed regularly and drug treatment will be continued if it is having a worthwhile effect on your symptoms.

### CHOLINESTERASE INHIBITORS

In your brain, chemicals called neurotransmitters are crucial to carrying messages from one brain cell to the next. People with Alzheimer's disease are often low on one of these chemicals, called acetylcholine, because the cells that produce it are damaged or destroyed. The following drugs (also known as cholinesterase inhibitors) help preserve acetylcholine by inhibiting an enzyme called acetylcholinesterase, which breaks it down. They don't cure Alzheimer's, but, in some people, they can help slow the course of the disease (according to the Alzheimer's Society, between 40 and 60 per cent of people with the disease benefit from these drugs).

**Donepezil (Aricept).** This is the drug most often used. While it may be prescribed to ease symptoms of mild to moderate dementia in Alzheimer's disease, several international studies have found that it may also help to protect higher function of patients with mild cognitive impairment as well as vascular dementia.

**Galantamine (Reminyl).** The newest drug in this class, galantamine boosts acetylcholine and also helps the brain use it more effectively. It may be used to treat mild to moderately severe Alzheimer's disease, and is available in both liquid and tablet form.

**Rivastigmine (Exelon).** Rivastigmine may be prescribed for people with mild to moderately severe Alzheimer's disease, and is also licensed for dementia associated with Parkinson's disease. It is available as capsules, liquid or patches.

### NMDA ANTAGONISTS

It is possible to have too much of a good thing. In normal quantities, the neurotransmitter glutamate activates neurons. But too much glutamate can be toxic to the brain and may cause some of the neuron degeneration that occurs with Alzheimer's disease. NMDA antagonists work by blocking the receptors on cells that normally receive glutamate, thereby reducing the 'static' between cells and allowing them to 'talk' to each other more effectively. They have been used in Germany since the 1980s for any kind of dementia, and also for depression.

**Memantine (Ebixa).** Memantine is available as tablets or oral drops and may be used to treat moderate Alzheimer's disease in people who cannot take cholinesterase inhibitors for some reason. It may also be prescribed for people with severe Alzheimer's disease.

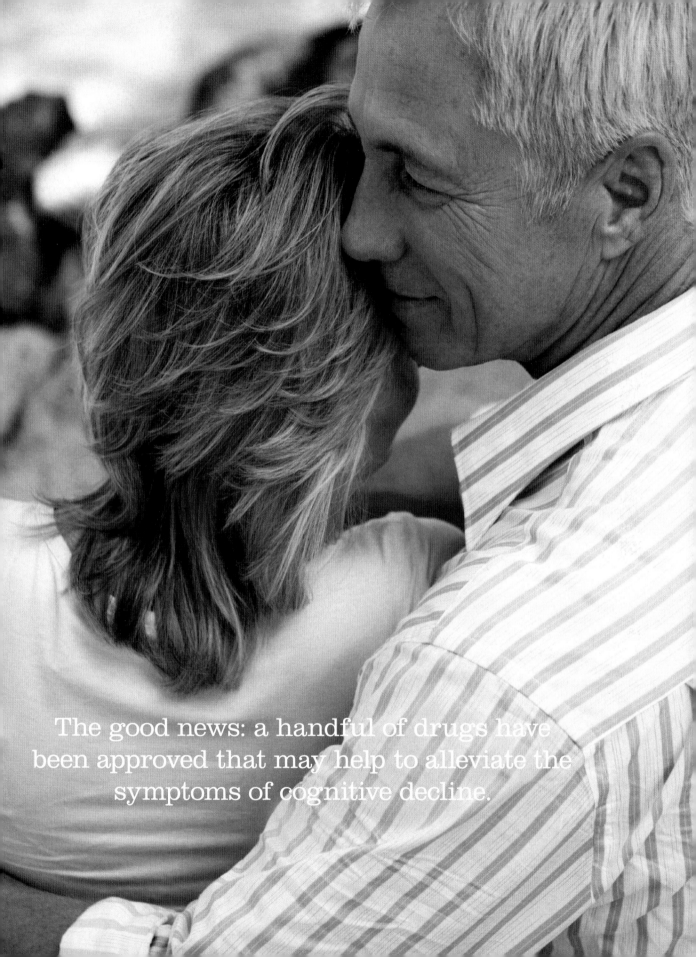

The good news: a handful of drugs have been approved that may help to alleviate the symptoms of cognitive decline.

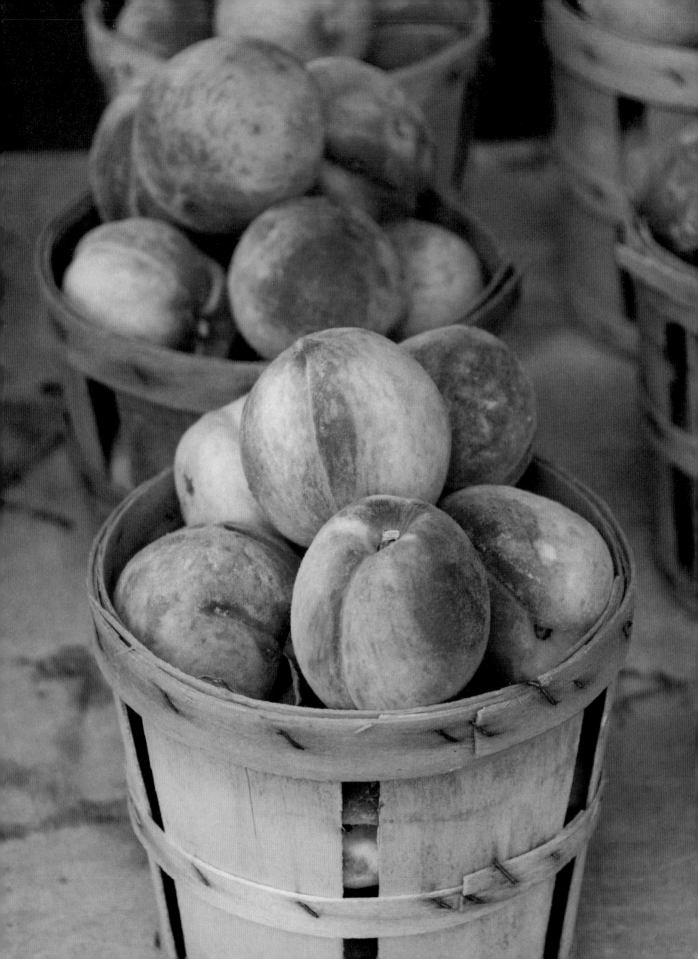

in one recent Swedish study of 3,334 sets of twins. Regular, moderate exercise was associated with 50 per cent less risk.

Even among older or inactive people, or those carrying the ApoE4 gene, exercise is linked with a lower risk of Alzheimer's disease. In one study of 2,263 men aged 71 or older, inactive volunteers who started an exercise programme had only half the risk of dementia compared with those who did not. In another study, without cognitive impairment followed for an average 4.5 years showed that those with the highest adherence to a Mediterranean diet were 28 per cent less likely to develop mild cognitive impairment (MCI) compared with those with the lowest adherence. Among 482 people who had MCI at the start, progression to Alzheimer's disease was reduced by up to 48 per cent in those eating a Mediterranean diet.

## Eat Mediterranean style – it's associated with a lower incidence of cognitive decline and dementia.

people who exercised just twice a week were half as likely to have dementia 21 years later as those who were inactive, even if they had inherited the ApoE4 gene for late-life Alzheimer's (see page 187).

Exercise helps the brain use blood sugar more efficiently, avoiding gluts and shortages that may harm some brain regions. It also boosts blood circulation, protects brain cells from injury and helps fuel new cell growth in areas we use for complex thought.

● **Eat Mediterranean-style.** As explained earlier (see page 64), the combination of foods in a Mediterranean-style diet – fruits, vegetables, whole grains, fish, nuts and olive oil – is associated with a lower incidence of cognitive decline and dementia.

In one study of 1,880 older people, those whose diets most closely adhered to a Mediterranean pattern had a 40 per cent lower rate of Alzheimer's disease during an average five-year follow-up compared with people whose diets were the least similar. A further study of 1,393 people

● **Wear a helmet if you cycle or ski.** Experts are divided over whether mild head injuries (such as the time you slipped on the ice and banged your head hard) increase the risk of dementia. But they're certain that moderate and severe head injuries do. So wear protection whether you're bungee-jumping, cycling around the block or skiing down the slopes.

● **Challenge your brain every day.** 'Use it or lose it' is an apt phrase when it comes to brainpower. Many studies have shown that people with a higher level of education or a mentally stimulating lifestyle have a lower risk of cognitive decline and dementia.

If your brain is continually active and engaged in new or stimulating tasks, you build a cognitive reserve that may help to compensate for early symptoms of dementia. And you'll have a much more interesting life to boot. Here's the perfect opportunity to take the challenge and hone your cognitive skills – try the next section: 'Your Brain Fitness Programme'.

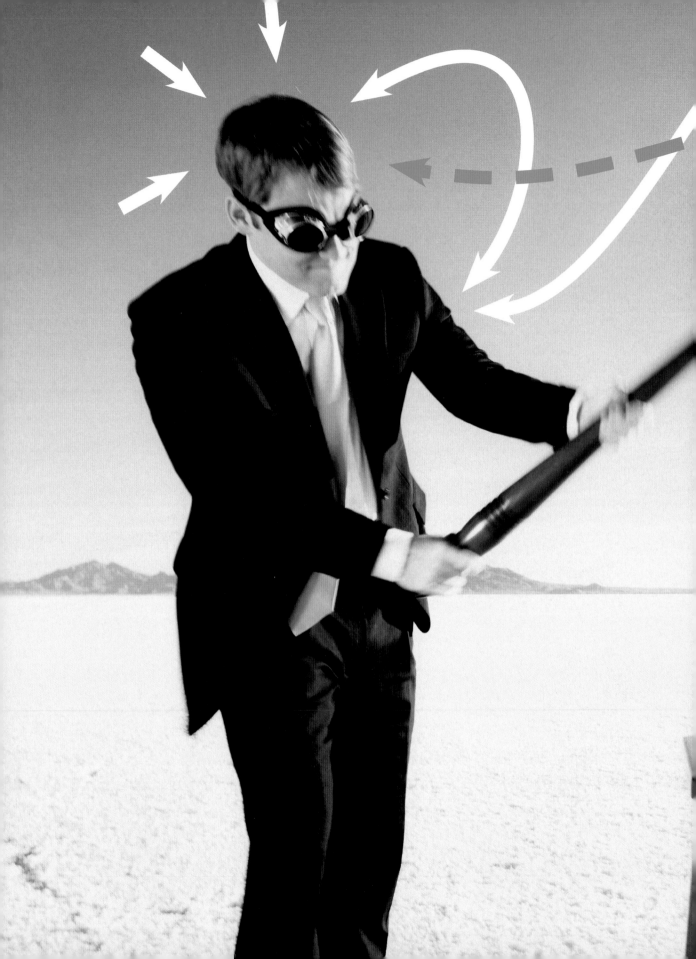

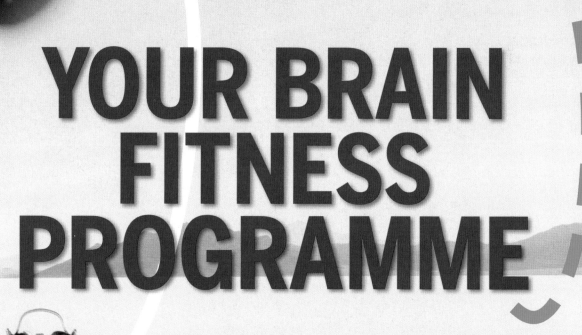

# YOUR BRAIN FITNESS PROGRAMME

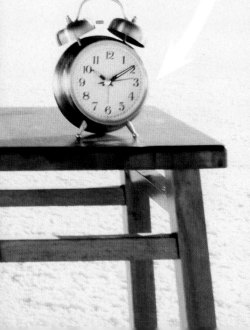

part 4

# INCREASE YOUR BRAIN POWER

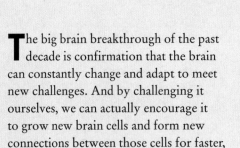

## in minutes a day

The big brain breakthrough of the past decade is confirmation that the brain can constantly change and adapt to meet new challenges. And by challenging it ourselves, we can actually encourage it to grow new brain cells and form new connections between those cells for faster, more efficient, more effective thinking.

In retrospect, it seems odd that scientists should find this surprising. Every other part of the body changes, including the bones, which seem rock solid but are constantly breaking themselves down and building themselves back up. The more you tax your bones with weight-bearing exercise, the stronger they are forced to grow. Likewise, the more you challenge your brain, the stronger it will become.

That's why this book includes a brain fitness programme. The exercises and strategies are designed to improve your performance in six main areas of cognitive function (see box, right). Try to do these and similar exercises and strategies for at least 20 minutes a day. You should feel more alert and 'with it' almost instantly once you give your brain a jolt of stimulation.

### THE EVIDENCE

In 2003, the prestigious US *New England Journal of Medicine* printed an article with the title 'Use it or lose it', discussing the potential benefits of staying mentally active. It appeared after a 5 year study by researchers at the Albert Einstein College of Medicine of Yeshiva University in New York suggested that leisure activities

– including reading, playing board games, playing a musical instrument and dancing – might reduce the risk of developing dementia by more than half.

That seemed an amazing benefit for such enjoyable activities. To date there is not sufficient evidence to confirm that this is always the case, as genes also seem to play a role in whether or not people develop dementia in later life. But what is becoming increasingly evident is that keeping the brain active throughout life can help to compensate for the natural cognitive decline that occurs with age.

## TRAINING HONES SKILLS

In 2006, the *Journal of the American Medical Association* published results of the study known as ACTIVE – Advanced Cognitive Training for Independent and Vital Elderly. People over the age of 65 were taught how to improve memory, reasoning and processing speed, then were evaluated immediately and five years later. After 10 short sessions, people who received the training not only did better in those areas than those who were not trained but also maintained their superior skills when they were retested five years

later. This shows that practising a skill can bring improvement at any time of life.

It may be, of course, that the shining examples of acute minds at an advanced age belong to people who have always enjoyed keeping their brains active. But this and other observational research does suggest that, with the right sort of stimulation – such as the tricks and strategies you'll find here – it is possible to combat some age-related problems, such as slower processing of new information and a slightly smaller capacity for storing short-term memories.

## BEFORE YOU BEGIN

Look back at your scores in the quiz on pages 8-9 to help you to determine a personal brain-boosting strategy. From your answers and the 'Where should I start?' panel below, you can work out which of the six areas of cognitive function you should focus on the most.

These exercises should be the beginning of your brain training, not the end. Your advanced studies need to take place out in the world. Opportunities to expand your brain power are all around you; you just need to reach out and take them.

## Where should I start?

In the quiz you took on pages 8-9, the questions addressed six areas of cognitive function. The more True answers you had in a particular category, the more help you need in that area. For easy reference, the following puzzles are colour-coded to address the same six areas – so you can choose which skills to practise first.

- ATTENTION AND FOCUS
- MEMORY
- PROCESSING SPEED
- VERBAL SKILLS
- NUMBER SKILLS
- REASONING SKILLS

# IMPROVE YOUR ATTENTION
## and focus

When was the last time you really lost yourself in a good book or became so enthralled with a project that hours flew by like minutes? It happens all the time in childhood but, as you get older, it can become much harder to focus intensely.

No one knows exactly why age tends to affect our ability to concentrate but one popular theory is that younger people have some sort of system that keeps irrelevant and extraneous information from interfering with attention.

Think of this system as mulch in a garden to keep down the weeds. A teenager has 'mulch' so thick that he or she can do maths homework with music blaring and occasionally stop to answer a text message. With age, though, the 'mulch' thins, allowing more and more distractions to creep in. When too many get through, they can affect how well we learn and remember, as well as how we perform certain tasks. Let's say you're driving along and spot some rubbish at the side of the road, which makes you wonder whether you took the refuse bag out of the kitchen, which reminds you that you need to pick up onions for dinner, which leads to thoughts of crying and eyes and your appointment with the optician next week. All of a sudden, your focus switches back to the road and you see that you've driven miles without realising it, and perhaps even missed your turning.

## ATTENTION, PLEASE!

No one can pay attention to everything. Information blasts into your senses constantly. Every colour, object, sound, taste, odour or physical sensation is taken into the brain and processed. But most of these inputs are ignored, as they should be. It would be exhausting to be hypervigilant at every moment; there's no real need to remember what kind of bird just flew by your window. Instead, you choose what to pay attention to, like the email you were reading when the bird flew by. It's that information that you hold in your short-term memory.

As you get older, you tend to have less working memory (as short-term memory is also called). Unless you pay close attention, the information just doesn't stick as well as it used to. That's one reason why an older person might have trouble moving back and forth between one task and another. Let's say you're trying to read alternately from two chapters in a book. When you switch chapters, you may lose your place in the first chapter and struggle to reorient yourself, while a younger person with greater working memory would have less difficulty.

## MORE ENERGY REQUIRED

Focus is closely linked to attention. If you think of attention as turning on a light in a dark room, focus is turning a laser beam on a specific object in the room. Focus is that intense level of attention that makes you feel as though you are burning memories into your brain. You lose some of that ability as you age, too. The small details simply vanish. If you read a passage in a book, you might remember the gist of it, but a younger person will be more likely to be able to recall exact sentences.

You don't lose your ability to focus entirely; it's just that it takes more energy and interest. What you gain is the ability to absorb a broader view of the world – a sum of the parts. Younger people tend to see the parts, but might miss how they fit into the bigger picture. The tips and exercises in this chapter are designed to help you improve both your attention and focus, so you can make it through *War and Peace* if you choose to, or at least a long newspaper feature. And the challenge of a new laptop, mobile phone or MP3 player should seem less daunting once you've finished here.

# HAVE A GO

These exercises challenge your attention and focus, training your brain to concentrate. Regardless of how well you do or how quickly you complete each exercise, you win as you are practising a skill that will help you to absorb and recall information.

## Read & remember ...

**For this exercise, you'll need a pencil.**

Below, you'll find a series of short articles. Read them carefully, trying to remember as much detail as possible. Then, without looking back at the article, answer the questions on the next page. You'll probably notice that it's easier to retain details when reading about topics with which you're already somewhat familiar. The same is true in real life.

### ● Read 1

Many people who enjoy solving crosswords have wondered how crosswords are made. Those who have tried to create a puzzle of their own, perhaps for a friend's birthday, were probably surprised at how difficult it was. No doubt they discovered that solving crosswords and making them up are two very different talents, each requiring its own set of skills. Yes, there is some overlap. You'll need a good vocabulary and a wide-ranging base of general knowledge to do both successfully. But the skill similarities pretty much end there.

Consider this analogy from the world of music. Playing the piano is very different from composing a symphony. There are, of course, people noted for excelling at both composition and performance – George Gershwin, Franz Liszt and Sergei Rachmaninov come to mind.

It's safe to say that solving crosswords is much easier than making them. And there's a special art involved in creating cryptic crosswords, which are very popular in Britain but, interestingly, much less common in the United States. Cryptic crosswords involve wordplay and solving a clue usually requires a degree of lateral thinking. Part of the clue is a straight definition but the rest includes coded language that a cryptic crossword enthusiast learns to unravel, for instance, 'about' may mean turning the letters of a word around.

And if you've ever wondered whether compilers of either type of crossword create the clues or the word diagram first, here's a hint: Try to make your own 3-by-3 crossword by writing the clues first; you'll quickly see the answer for yourself.

*Now answer questions on page 204*

## ● Read 2

The Euro is the official currency of most of the member nations of the European Union. The nations that use the Euro exclusively form what's known as the Eurozone. Euro coins and banknotes entered circulation on January 1, 2002, as the national currency of 11 countries: Austria, Belgium, Finland, France, Germany, Ireland, Italy, Luxembourg, the Netherlands, Portugal and Spain. The Euro is managed and administered by the Frankfurt-based European Central Bank. The inspiration for the distinctive € symbol was the Greek letter Epsilon, a reference to the cradle of European civilisation.

The Euro is divided into 100 cents. Euro coins come in eight different denominations, ranging from 1 cent to 2 Euros, although by Finnish law, cash transactions are rounded to the nearest 5 cents, so that 1 cent and 2 cent coins aren't needed. There are seven Euro banknote denominations, from 5 to 500 (€5, €10, €20, €50, €100, €200, and €500). Each denomination has its own size and colour, in part to help visually impaired people to recognise them.

*Now answer questions on page 204*

## ● Read 3

Have you ever watched a cartoon or children's programme where someone's cooked a soufflé and a tiny poke or a sudden loud noise makes it collapse?

Soufflés lend themselves to that sort of mockery because they're full of air. And 'soufflé', the past particle of the French verb 'souffler' (to blow) can sometimes mean 'blown up' or 'exploded'. Whether prepared as a savoury main dish or a sweet dessert, every soufflé is made from two basic components: a base of custard or a flavoured cream sauce, and egg whites beaten into a soft meringue. The base provides the flavour, while the egg whites provide the lift. Soufflés are traditionally served in flat-bottomed, round porcelain containers called ramekins.

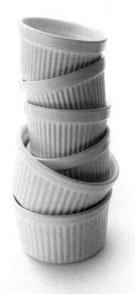

If prepared correctly, your soufflé will be puffed up and fluffy when you take it out of the oven. But be sure to serve it quickly – soufflés generally fall within 5 to 10 minutes.

*Now answer questions on page 204*

# Read & remember **QUESTIONS**

## Read 1 Questions

**1** Who is the first composer mentioned?

**2** What type of crosswords are much more popular in Britain than America?

**3** The two skills required both to solve and make general crosswords are a wide-ranging base of general knowledge and what else?

**4** What might the word 'about' suggest in a cryptic crossword?

**5** As implied by the passage, do crossword-writers create the clues or the word diagram first?

## Read 2 Questions

**1** What is the term for the group of European nations that uses the Euro?

**2** In what year did the Euro enter circulation?

**3** How many countries adopted it at the start?

**4** How many different Euro banknote denominations are there?

**5** What nation doesn't use the two smallest Euro coin denominations?

## Read 3 Questions

**1** What can 'soufflé' also mean in French?

**2** What ingredient provides the lift in a soufflé?

**3** What are soufflé containers called?

**4** What form do the egg whites take when beaten?

**5** How soon after being taken out of the oven will soufflés generally fall?

*Check your answers by rereading the articles.*

# Smart EVERYDAY STRATEGIES

All of us get distracted and lose our focus now and then. If it happens to you a lot, get in the habit of using these strategies to help compensate.

## ✳ Take notes

Writing forces you to pay attention and also helps move the information from short-term memory into long-term memory. And, of course, it provides a solid record if you need it later on.

## ✳ Carry a pocket-size recorder

For years, patient advocates have been advising people to take a small cassette or digital recorder when they see a doctor. When people are nervous or under stress, they may not accurately or fully remember what was said in an office visit. The same strategy can help in everyday life. If you carry a recorder, you can use a voice-activation feature to capture important conversations or even personal memos to yourself. You can then review the recording any time you want to.

## ✳ Invest in a pair of noise-reducing headphones

Unlike earplugs, these gadgets reduce or eliminate ambient sound while slightly muffling distinct sounds. For example, if you wear them in the office, you'll eliminate the hum of machinery and background chatter, while being able to hear someone speaking to you or the sound of a telephone ringing.

## ✳ Control sensory distractions

Take charge of the controllable distractions around you by turning off the music, television, and radio. If you are cold, put on a sweater. If you are hungry, eat. If the air feels stagnant, open a window. The more comfortable you are, the better you'll be able to focus.

## ✳ Find a quiet corner

If you don't have total noise control, take yourself to another location. Libraries are often quiet, or at least quieter than a busy home.

## ✳ Boost concentration with caffeine

Researchers from the University of Arizona in Tucson discovered that people over the age 65 who felt that their attention was highest in the morning (as opposed to 'night owls' who concentrate best late at night) could improve their focus by drinking 350ml regular coffee. Decaffeinated coffee didn't work. And this trick only works if you are already a coffee-drinker. If not, the side effects of caffeine – that jittery buzz – will only disrupt your attention.

# Name that shape ...

**For this exercise, you'll need a pencil and a watch or clock with a second hand.**

Below, you'll see a grid containing geometric shapes with the names of the shapes underneath. Your goal is to make sure that the shapes and names match, so that each shape has a correct name in the corresponding position on the grid. If you spot a mistake, circle the incorrect word and continue on.

For example:

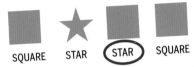

SQUARE    STAR    STAR    SQUARE

**Third word ('star') should be circled.**

These exercises will be scored for accuracy. But time is also important, so work as quickly as possible. When you have completed each one, write down the amount of time you needed to finish in the space provided at the bottom. Score the exercise before moving on to the next one. When you are ready, set the timer and begin.

## Shape card 1

| | | | | | | | | |
|---|---|---|---|---|---|---|---|---|
| SQUARE | SQUARE | STAR | STAR | SQUARE | SQUARE | SQUARE | SQUARE | SQUARE |
| STAR | SQUARE | STAR | SQUARE | STAR | STAR | SQUARE | STAR | STAR |
| STAR | SQUARE | STAR | STAR | SQUARE | SQUARE | SQUARE | SQUARE | SQUARE |
| STAR | STAR | STAR | SQUARE | SQUARE | STAR | SQUARE | SQUARE | STAR |

TIME............    ITEMS CIRCLED INCORRECTLY............    MISSED MISTAKES............

*Answers on page 265*

## Shape card 2

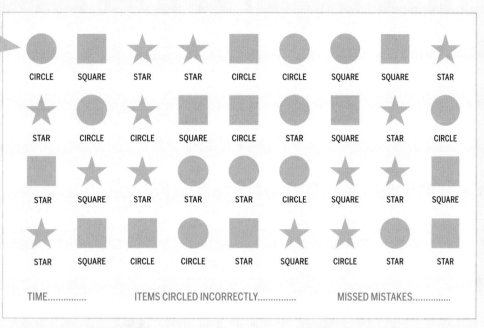

| | | | | | | | | |
|---|---|---|---|---|---|---|---|---|
| CIRCLE | SQUARE | STAR | STAR | CIRCLE | CIRCLE | SQUARE | SQUARE | STAR |
| STAR | CIRCLE | CIRCLE | SQUARE | CIRCLE | STAR | SQUARE | STAR | CIRCLE |
| STAR | SQUARE | STAR | STAR | STAR | CIRCLE | SQUARE | STAR | SQUARE |
| STAR | SQUARE | CIRCLE | CIRCLE | STAR | SQUARE | CIRCLE | STAR | STAR |

TIME...............     ITEMS CIRCLED INCORRECTLY...............     MISSED MISTAKES...............

*Answers on page 265*

## Shape card 3

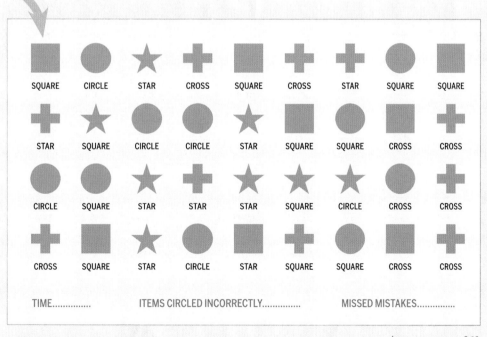

| | | | | | | | | |
|---|---|---|---|---|---|---|---|---|
| SQUARE | CIRCLE | STAR | CROSS | SQUARE | CROSS | STAR | SQUARE | SQUARE |
| STAR | SQUARE | CIRCLE | CIRCLE | STAR | SQUARE | SQUARE | CROSS | CROSS |
| CIRCLE | SQUARE | STAR | STAR | STAR | SQUARE | CIRCLE | CROSS | CROSS |
| CROSS | SQUARE | STAR | CIRCLE | STAR | SQUARE | SQUARE | CROSS | CROSS |

TIME...............     ITEMS CIRCLED INCORRECTLY...............     MISSED MISTAKES...............

*Answers on page 265*

## Shape card 4

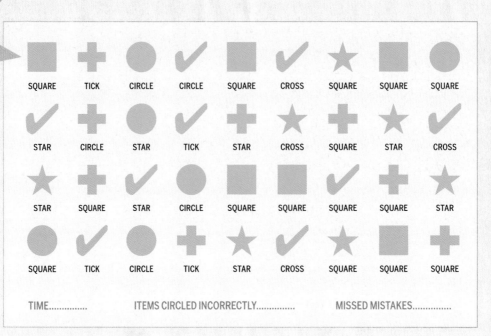

| | | | | | | | | |
|---|---|---|---|---|---|---|---|---|
| SQUARE | TICK | CIRCLE | CIRCLE | SQUARE | CROSS | SQUARE | SQUARE | SQUARE |
| STAR | CIRCLE | STAR | TICK | STAR | CROSS | SQUARE | STAR | CROSS |
| STAR | SQUARE | STAR | CIRCLE | SQUARE | SQUARE | SQUARE | SQUARE | STAR |
| SQUARE | TICK | CIRCLE | TICK | STAR | CROSS | SQUARE | SQUARE | SQUARE |

TIME............. ITEMS CIRCLED INCORRECTLY............. MISSED MISTAKES.............

*Answers on page 265*

## Shape card 5

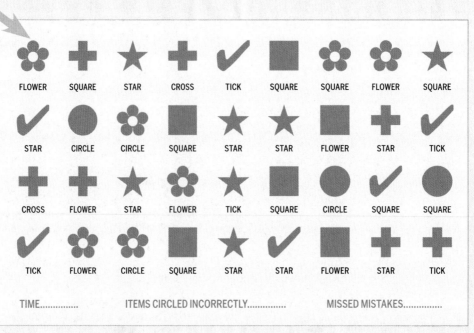

| | | | | | | | | |
|---|---|---|---|---|---|---|---|---|
| FLOWER | SQUARE | STAR | CROSS | TICK | SQUARE | SQUARE | FLOWER | SQUARE |
| STAR | CIRCLE | CIRCLE | SQUARE | STAR | STAR | FLOWER | STAR | TICK |
| CROSS | FLOWER | STAR | FLOWER | TICK | SQUARE | CIRCLE | SQUARE | SQUARE |
| TICK | FLOWER | CIRCLE | SQUARE | STAR | STAR | FLOWER | STAR | TICK |

TIME............. ITEMS CIRCLED INCORRECTLY............. MISSED MISTAKES.............

*Answers on page 265*

# Odd one out ...

**For this exercise, you'll need a pencil.**

Below, you'll see what looks like a number of identical items. Only one item in the group is different from the others. Find and circle that item. This is not a timed exercise.

● Odd one out  1

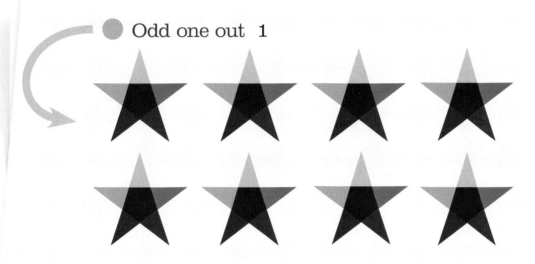

*Answer on page 265*

● Odd one out  2

*Answer on page 265*

## Odd one out 3

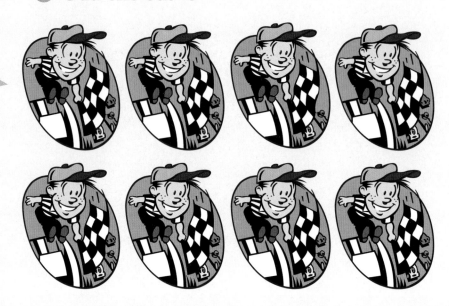

## Odd one out 4

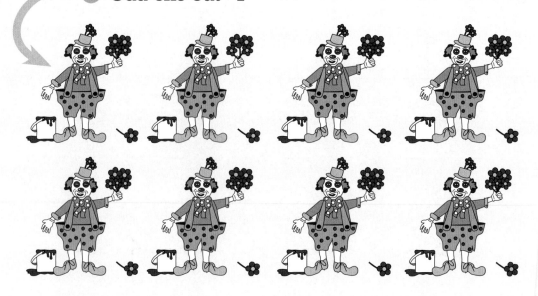

## Odd one out 5

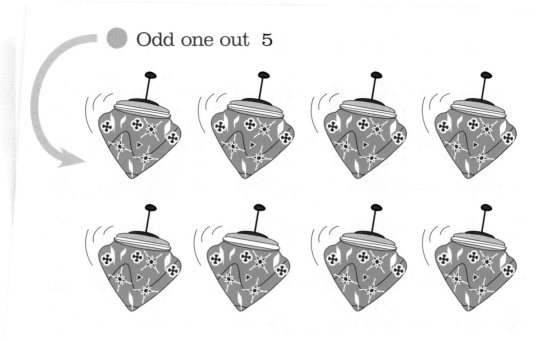

## Odd one out 6

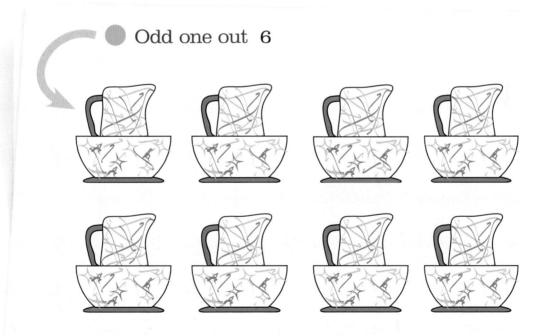

*Answers on page 265*

# Spot the difference ...

**For this exercise, you'll need a pencil.**

The picture pairs here are nearly identical, but not quite. Find the specified number of differences and circle them. This is not a timed exercise.

 Picture 1

There are three differences. Can you see them?

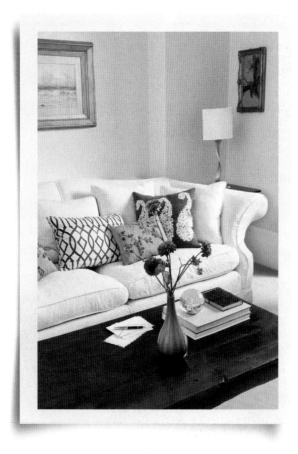

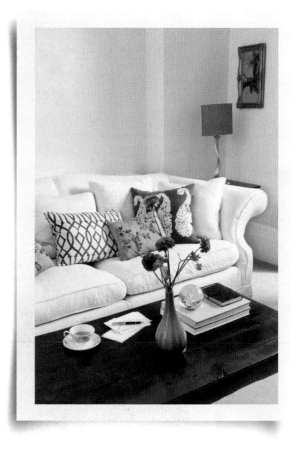

*Answers on page 266*

## Picture 2

Can you identify the four differences?

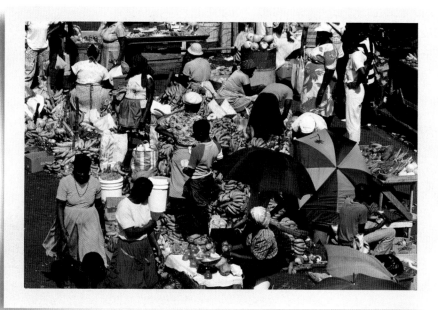

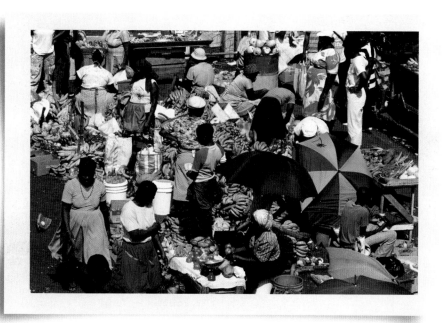

*Answers on page 266*

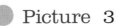 # Picture 3

There are five differences. Can you see them?

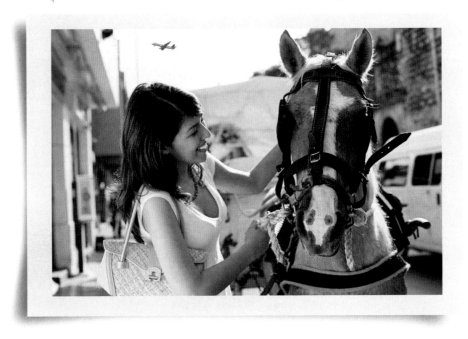

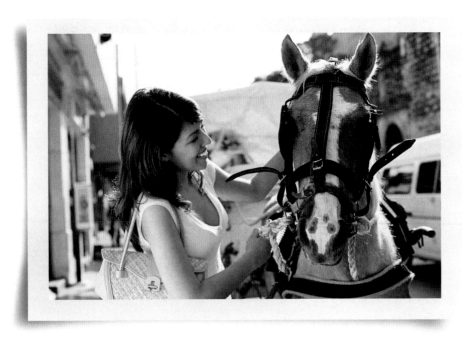

*Answers on page 266*

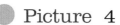
Can you spot the six differences?

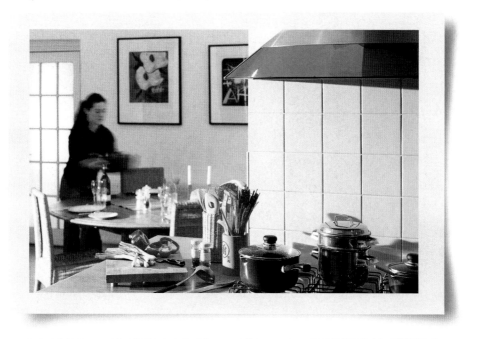

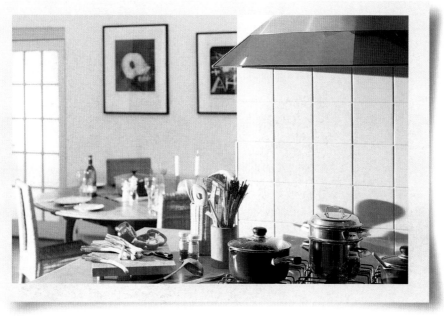

*Answers on page 266*

# Improve your MEMORY

**When people talk about their memory getting worse, they usually mean** those aspects of memory that allow them to function in the world – remembering appointments, the location of car keys, items on a to-do list, work deadlines, even basic facts.

**W**e can run into real trouble when our memory lets us down, especially when it comes to 'remembering' future events. Imagine if you forgot to pay your house insurance premium. That slip could cost thousands of pounds if the house were flooded or caught fire. Luckily, most memory slips are less serious.

## KEEPING TRACK

Keys, sunglasses, mobile phone, car in a multi-storey car park – if you haven't 'lost' one of these items in the past month, then you're doing well in the memory department. Misplacing objects is normal at any age, especially when you're under stress. You lose track of items because the brain is so darned efficient. When you perform routine tasks, your body goes on automatic pilot. Let's say that every day, you come home and drop the keys in the same general location. But if something interrupts you – perhaps the phone is ringing as you open the door – then your brain is preoccupied with the new task. Your automatic pilot disengages, you drop the keys somewhere new, and later you have to search to find them.

## RECALLING THE PAST

The ability to retrieve memories of past events declines with age. Recognition remains strong, but recall weakens. This is a fine but important distinction. Recall is the ability to pull up a memory simply by thinking about it. Recognition is the ability to remember once prompted with a cue. For example, if you were asked to name all the places to which you have ever travelled, your list would probably be incomplete. But if you were asked if you had ever been to Egypt, you could answer definitively yes or no.

If you want to remember on your own, you need to provide your own cues. That's one reason people buy souvenirs – to remind them of the details of a trip. For everyday purposes, we can use our imaginations instead.

## 'REMEMBERING' THE FUTURE

The most annoying of all memory problems involves prospective memory – the need to recall things that have yet to happen, such as an appointment or an anniversary. When this type of memory fails, we may forget to take medication, call at the supermarket for milk, or return a DVD on time. Experts who specialise in this aspect of memory call this 'remembering to remember'.

As far as the brain is concerned, this is much more difficult to pull off than other types of remembering, thanks to the gap in time between intending to do something and actually doing it.

Though everyone has prospective memory failures, some research has shown that these types of slips tend to become more common as we get older. One recent UK study of nearly 320,000 people, aged between 8 and 50 years, suggests that 'remembering to remember' starts to decline in early adulthood and throughout life. However, age is not the only determining factor. Stress, lack of sleep and the side effects of medication have all been shown to influence the forgetfulness factor.

## SMART EVERYDAY STRATEGIES

No one's memory is perfect. Yours doesn't have to be either. But it's easy enough not to lose your car keys or forget another appointment simply by using some commonsense strategies. Save your brain power for other things.

Establish routines. Boring as it seems, it really is easier to find things if you always put them in the same place. Put up a hook somewhere to hang your car keys and create a special folder for unpaid bills, for instance. Find repositories for all the things you tend to misplace.

If you have to put an item in an unfamiliar place, say what you are doing out loud, as in, 'I am putting my sunglasses on the table by the door'. All sensory channels create their own neural links to the information. By letting your ears register the information, you increase your chances of remembering it later.

## MEMORY CUES

Make full use of Post-it notes. Keep a pad of them in every room and stick a reminder where you are likely to see it. Concerned that you might forget to call a friend? Put a note on the phone and another in a spot that you are likely to notice during the day, such as on the television or on your computer keyboard.

Let technology remember for you. Mobile phones, Blackberries and other electronic devices have calendars you can set to remind you of what you need to do during the day. Some types of software have a 'notes' function you can program to remind you of what you need to do during the day.

Once you have learnt how to use these systems, you'll wonder how you ever got along without them. And yes, almost anyone can learn to use them. Researchers have taught people with significant memory problems – those with brain injuries and mild to moderate Alzheimer's disease – to use such devices successfully. Just make sure you keep a back-up, such as a wall calendar, day planner, or external hard drive.

Use checklists. People make lists for a reason: they work. Tick off each to-do item as you complete it. The more you have, the more likely you are to refer to it again and again, each time reinforcing your memory of the tasks there.

Plant a visual reminder. If you need to remember to take an umbrella, hang it on the door handle. Visual reminders can even help you to accomplish goals. For example, if you decide you want to begin a healthy diet tomorrow, put the porridge oats on the worktop the night before.

You can also use imaginary cues when planting a visual clue is impossible. If you go to a museum and have to check in a bag or briefcase, how can you remember to collect it? By using your imagination. Robert Logie, professor of human cognitive neuroscience at Edinburgh University suggests this: when you first realise that you will need to use prospective memory, look for physical landmarks to trigger it.

It could be a distinctive door or a statue or other permanent fixture. Then, imagine your item and the landmark together. In the museum example, you can imagine a briefcase blocking the doorway. In studies, these imaginary cues proved to be as effective as external cues. Imaginary cues work best when you are in an unfamiliar location or situation and therefore less likely to go on autopilot.

## DON'T PROCRASTINATE

Do it now, not later. Although this won't work in all situations, the best way to remember to do something is to do it while you're thinking about it. Instead of telling yourself to remember to make a phone call or pay a bill, why not do it immediately? Too often it's procrastination that makes us forget.

# HAVE A GO

These exercises challenge your recall of old memories as well as your retention of new information.

## You must remember this...

**For this exercise, you'll need a timer.**

Set the timer for 5 minutes. Read one of the questions, then close your eyes and remember all the details you can. Try to think on all sensory fronts: sight, sound, smell, taste and touch. Don't rush the process; take the full 5 minutes. After the timer goes off, open your eyes. Did you remember more than you thought you would?

- How did you celebrate your 13th birthday?
- How did you get to school in your last year at primary school?
- What do you remember about your best friend's wedding?
- What do you remember about your most recent holiday?
- Where and with whom was your first kiss?
- What was the best birthday present you ever got?
- What do you remember most about your grandparents?
- How did you spend summers as a child?
- Which dance steps or music groups were popular when you were in secondary school?
- What do you remember about the first job you ever held?
- What books have you read in the past year?
- What films have you seen in the past year?
- How did you and your friends spend your time after school when you were 10?
- What was your first pet?
- What was your most intimidating moment?
- When did you get your first bicycle?
- What was your favourite book as a child?
- Who was your favourite primary-school teacher?
- What did the first house you lived in look like?
- Who was your first love?

# Picture recall …

**For this exercise, you'll need a pencil and a timer.**

Set the timer for 2 minutes and study the picture below. After 2 minutes, turn the page. There you'll find a picture that is identical to this one except for a few details. Repeat for the other two pictures on page 221.

● Observe 1

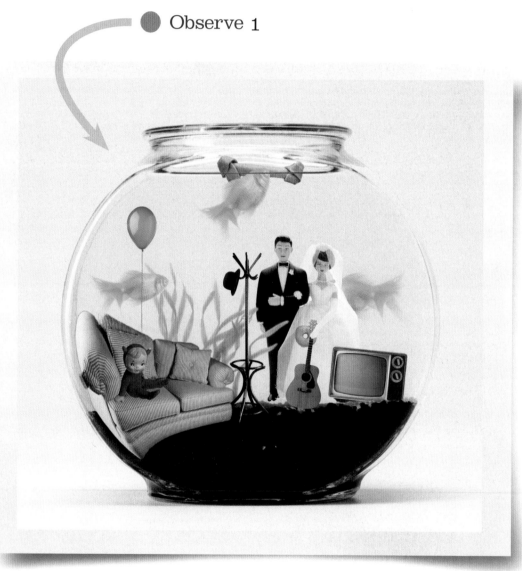

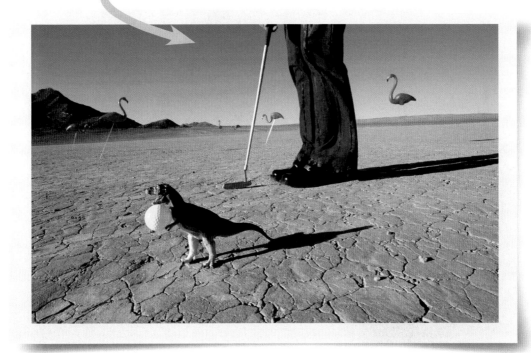

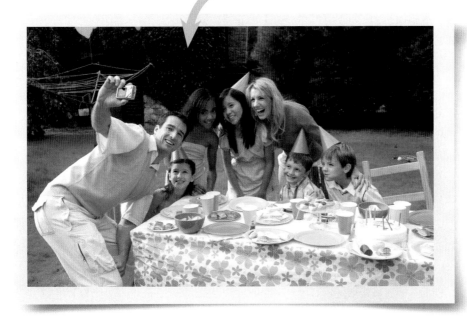

# Recall 1

Without looking back, circle the details that have changed. How many can you identify?

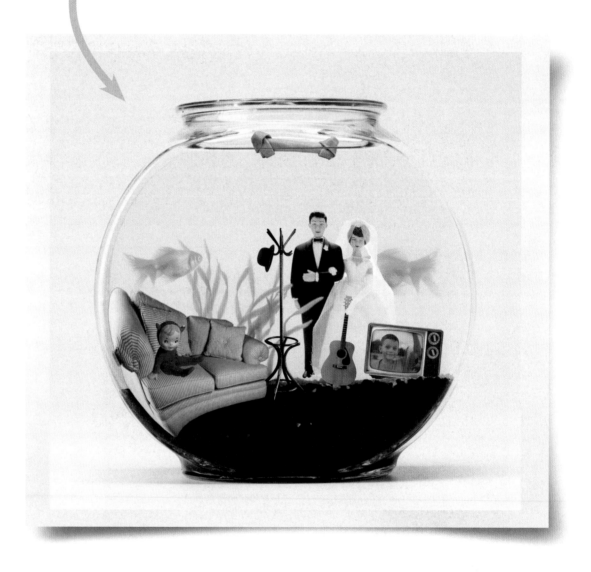

*Answers on page 267*

## Recall 2

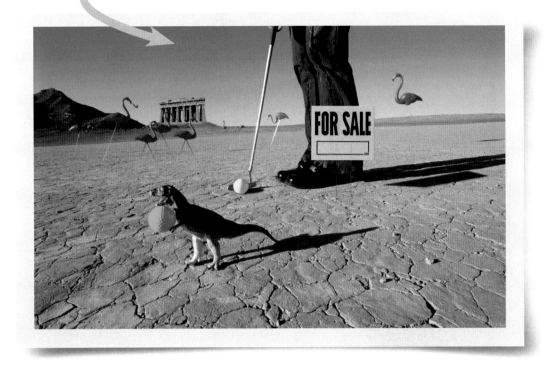

## Recall 3

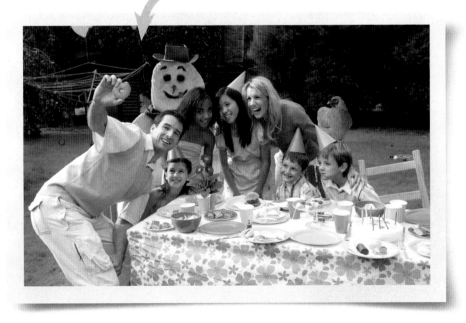

*Answers on page 267*

# Concentration ...

**For this exercise, you'll need a pencil and a timer.**

Set the timer for 1 minute and study the grid below. After a minute, turn the page. There you'll find a blank grid and two rows of objects. Match the objects to their proper locations on the grid. Repeat the exercise with all the following grids.

## ● Concentration 1

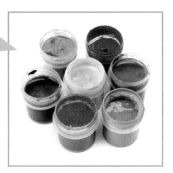 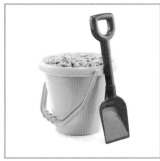 (row 1)

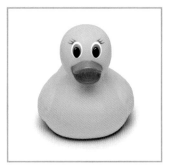 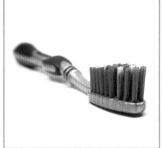 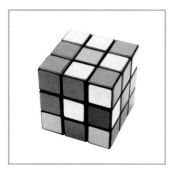 (row 2)

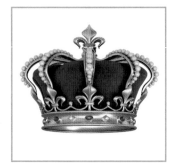 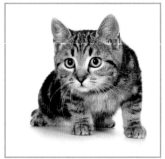 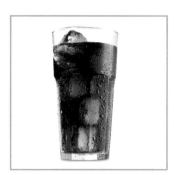 (row 3)

## Concentration 2

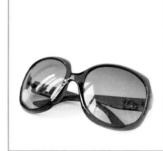
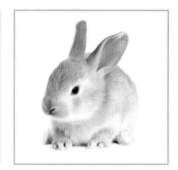

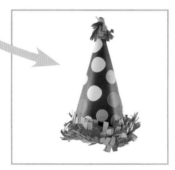
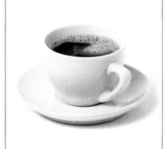
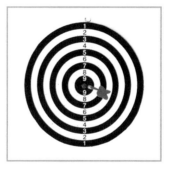

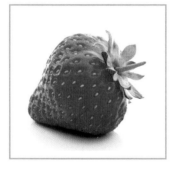
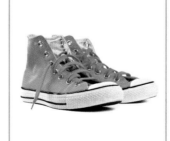
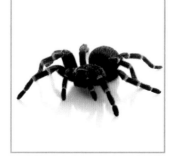

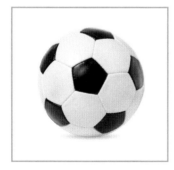

# Recall 1

Each picture is labelled with a letter. Try to recall where each picture was located on the grid, then write the letter associated with the picture in the proper place on the grid. Do the same for 'Recall 2' (opposite).

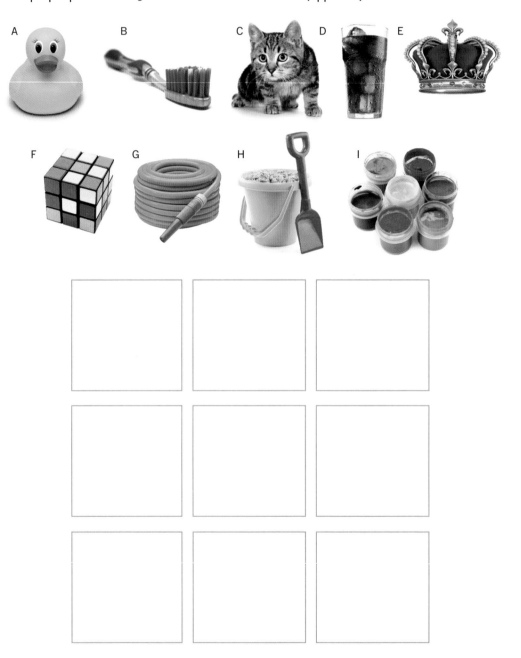

A    B    C    D    E

F    G    H    I

*To check your answers, turn back to page 224*

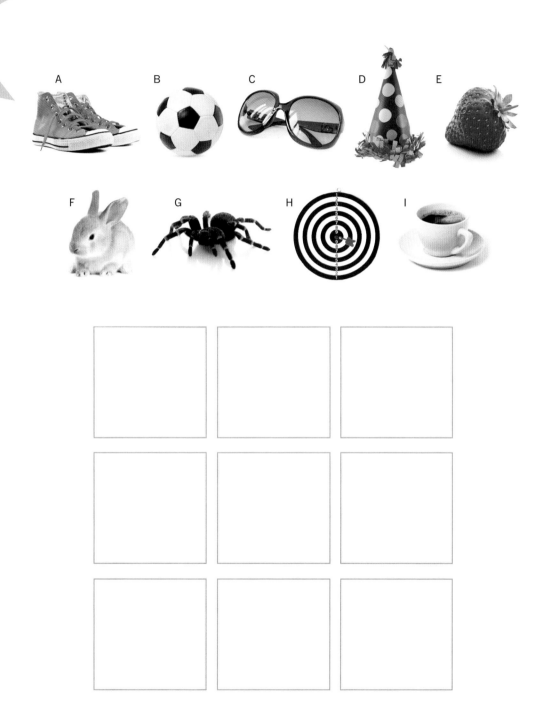

# Recall 2

A B C D E

F G H I

*To check your answers, turn back to page 225*

# Concentration 3

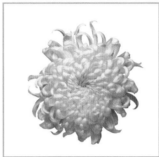 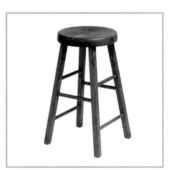

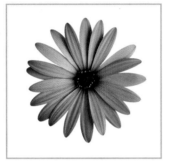 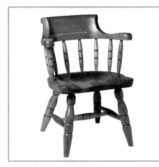 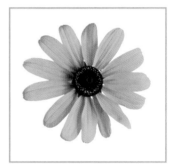

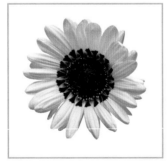 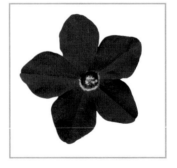 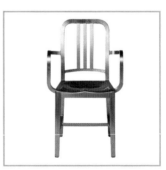

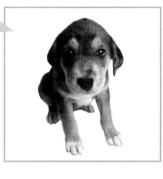 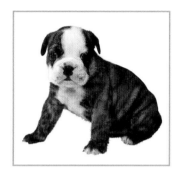 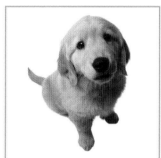

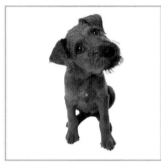 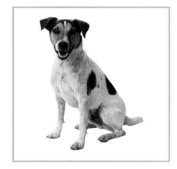 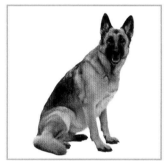

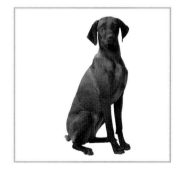 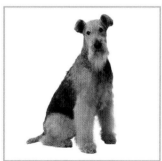 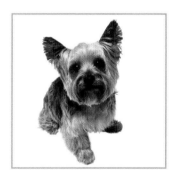

# Recall 3

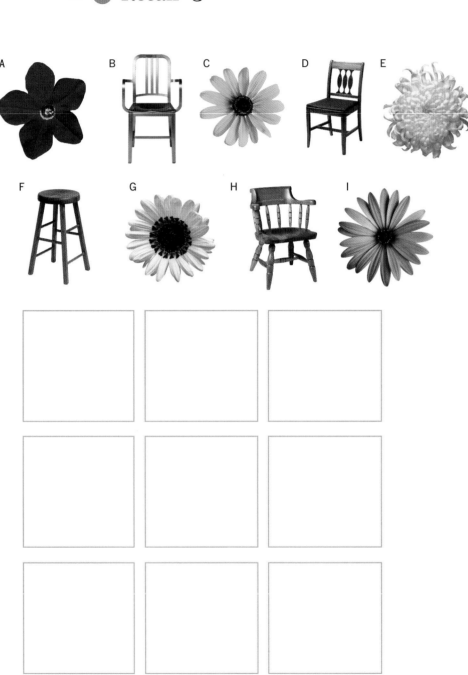

*To check your answers, turn back to page 228*

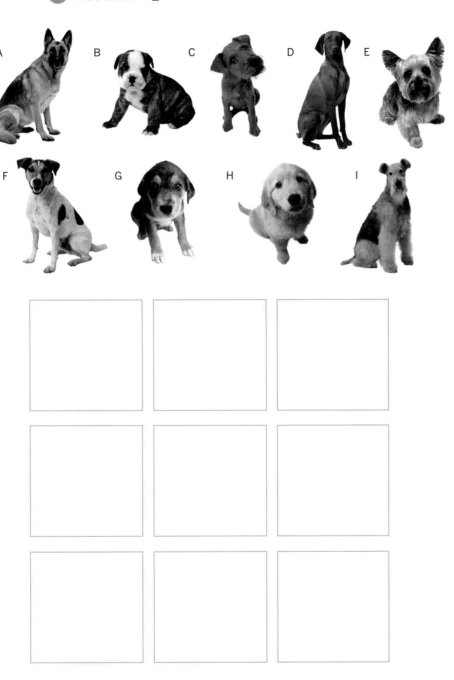

Recall 4

A  B  C  D  E

F  G  H  I

*To check your answers, turn back to page 229*

# Scents and sensibility ...

**For this exercise, you'll need a pencil and a timer.**

Certain scents have the amazing ability to transport you back to a particular time, place, or moment in your life. The olfactory bulb, the area of the brain that perceives smells, is part of the brain's limbic system, which plays a major role in long-term memory, especially emotional memories.

 Scent memories  1

Set the timer for 5 minutes. Look at the list below and choose one of the scents. If you happen to have access to the scent, take a good sniff. Then, sit down without any distractions and imagine the smell as best you can. Let your mind recall every detail of the memories it evokes. Don't rush the process; take the full 5 minutes. Later, come back and do this exercise with other scents from the list.

| | |
|---|---|
| cinnamon | old books |
| warm apple pie | wood smoke |
| hot chocolate | hay |
| freshly sharpened lead pencil | tobacco |
| fresh pine (or a pine-scented candle) | surgical spirit |
| roses | aftershave |
| cigars | nutmeg |
| wet dog | shoe polish |
| floral perfume | baking bread |
| baby powder | burning leaves |
| freshly mown grass | ripe Camembert |
| damp earth after a rainstorm | strawberry lip gloss |
| manure | lake water |
| homemade chicken soup | chlorine |
| mulled wine | |

## ● Scent memories 2

Think of a scent that has special meaning for you. Maybe it's the perfume your mother wore on special occasions, a former boyfriend's aftershave, bread baking in your grandmother's kitchen, a lilac tree from your childhood garden, a leather chair from your father's study, the smell of wood and sawdust from your uncle's workshop, or sausages frying over a campfire. The possibilities are endless. For each scent you think of, write down the memory you associate with it.

SCENT ...........................................................................................................

MEMORY .......................................................................................................

...........................................................................................................

...........................................................................................................

...........................................................................................................

SCENT ...........................................................................................................

MEMORY .......................................................................................................

...........................................................................................................

...........................................................................................................

...........................................................................................................

SCENT ...........................................................................................................

MEMORY .......................................................................................................

...........................................................................................................

...........................................................................................................

...........................................................................................................

SCENT ...........................................................................................................

MEMORY .......................................................................................................

...........................................................................................................

...........................................................................................................

...........................................................................................................

# Improve your PROCESSING SPEED

Have you watched a young child in action lately? They don't walk; they run. They don't sit; they fidget. As we get older, our bodies slow down. The same goes for our brains. We can learn and remember almost as well as we used to, but it might take our brains a bit longer.

The brain tends to operate more slowly with age because we naturally produce fewer neurotransmitters, the all-important brain chemicals that carry information across the gaps between brain cells. We also lose some of our white matter, the fatty substance that insulates the brain's high-speed information 'cables' (bundles of nerve fibres, really) that enable faster transmission of electrical signals from one part of the brain to another.

Lagging speed can affect our ability to understand a fast-moving scene in a movie, count change at the supermarket check-out, balance our accounts, or react to a car swerving in front of us on the highway. It can even affect how 'fast' the brain hears. Sounds that enter the ear take an extra moment or two to be registered and translated in the brain. Many older people are sent for hearing tests by family members who are later confused when the tests show normal hearing. The delay between hearing and responding is often interpreted as a hearing problem, when it is actually just a natural, if frustrating, slowdown in the brain.

That is also the reason why new memories do not form as quickly or as completely as they once did. But if we can't quite attain the thinking speed of our youth, there is no need for the mental equivalent of shuffling. Like a sprinter training for the Olympics, we can train our brains to go faster.

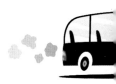

# Smart EVERYDAY STRATEGIES

While you're using the exercises in this book to help increase your processing speed, also consider these strategies.

## ❈ Be deliberate and calm

As with all mental processes, speed suffers when you are stressed. If you find yourself feeling pressured by your own or others' expectations, take a deep breath, relax and remind yourself that you deserve to take as much time as you need.

## ❈ Practise

Everything you do, you can do faster with practice. The general reaction to doing poorly at tasks is to give up trying, but if speed is your problem, avoidance of the task will only make it worse. Work at small projects by practising them again and again, the way you would practise if you were learning to play a musical instrument, and soon your brain will find the 'notes' in no time.

## ❈ Check out computer games

The same computer games your children and grandchildren play can help improve your ability to see, process and react to fast-moving objects. You can also train your brain using video games designed specifically to improve cognitive abilities, including processing speed (see 'Can playing computer games make you smarter?" on page 236). These can be played on a home computer or video game system. These may not necessarily speed up other mental processes, but there is some satisfaction in keeping up (if you can) with the digital skills of the young.

# CAN PLAYING computer games MAKE YOU CLEVERER?

**W**ith so many baby boomers living in fear of brain deterioration, it's no wonder that computer games designed to improve brain fitness are on the market. There's Nintendo's Brain Age, Posit Science's Brain Fitness, and CogniFit's MindFit, to name a few, plus web-based programmes such as www.lumosity.com or UK sites such as www.braintrainingpuzzle.co.uk/. Do they work? The answer is yes and no – depending on your goals, how hard you are willing to work (or, in this case, play), and which software you use.

Imagine a teenager who wants to improve his overall athletic ability. What should he do? He could run on a track to improve his speed and endurance, but that won't help his basketball skills. He could spend weeks perfecting his dribbling technique, but that won't help his ability to score a basket. And none of that training will help his golf game.

## VARIETY IS KEY

It's the same with brain training. Cognitive abilities come in many distinct types. The best programmes work on several types, including processing speed, visual acuity, listening, concentration and focus, reasoning, spatial orientation and memory. These encourage general brain improvement, as opposed to what might be called the Sudoku effect – if you do Sudoku puzzles day and night, you can become fast at filling squares with numbers, but won't get any better at counting change at the supermarket.

Detractors say there is no proof that any of the games really help improve mental function and that the business is overwhelming the science. But practising certain skills is undoubtedly beneficial. For instance, Posit Science tested its eight-week programme on older adults (aged 60 to 97) and claims that memory improved significantly, even months later. Larger studies are underway at most of the serious brain fitness companies to determine if and how these games might prevent or delay age-related memory problems or even dementia.

Bottom line: the games may help and can't hurt anything but your wallet. Many people enjoy them, but, you don't have to buy computer games to keep your mind active.

'Everything you do helps in one way or another,' says memory expert Robert Logie, professor of human cognitive neuroscience at Edinburgh University. 'Playing an instrument, joining a choir or a special interest club, taking an evening class or learning a language are stimulating and also offer social benefits.'

Buy games for fun, he adds, but don't neglect the rest of the world; there are plenty of fascinating non-digital ways to challenge your mind.

If our reaction time slows, the world can pass us by. We become frustrated, and it's not difficult to feel that others are annoyed with us as well. These exercises were designed to improve the brain's processing speed. Do them every day, at least once a day.

# HAVE A GO

## Speed sorting ... Repeat three times a day, if possible.

For this exercise, you'll need a pen, paper, a watch or clock with a second hand and a pack of playing cards.

### Speed sort 1

● **PREPARE** Shuffle the deck well and place it face down in front of you.

● **BEGIN** Note the time when you begin. Pick up the deck and sort the cards into four piles by suit. Do this as quickly as you can. When you finish sorting, look at the clock and note the time.

● **FINISH** Write down how long it took you to complete the exercise – and try to beat your time next time. Then, for your own information, look through the piles to see how accurate you were.

TIME...............

NUMBER OF MISTAKES...............

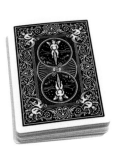
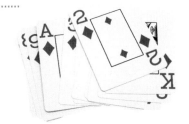
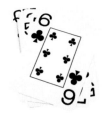
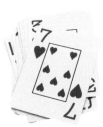
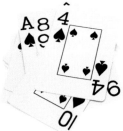

## Speed sort 2

**ONE STEP HARDER**

Note the time you begin. Quickly separate the deck into piles by suit, then take each pile and order the cards by number, with aces low and picture cards in this order: Jacks, Queens, Kings. Do not record your time until both phases of the exercise are complete.

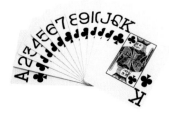
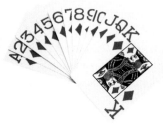
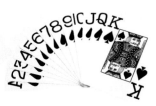
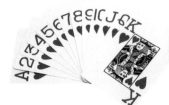

TIME.............. NUMBER OF MISTAKES..............

## Speed sort 3

**TWO STEPS HARDER**

Note the time you begin. Separate the deck into six piles – aces in one pile, picture cards in a second pile and four piles of numbered cards by suit. Do not record your time until all phases of the exercise are complete.

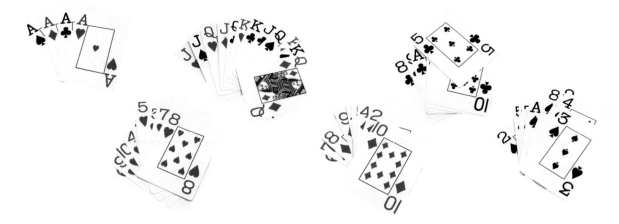

TIME.............. NUMBER OF MISTAKES..............

# Letter search ...

For this exercise, you'll need a pencil, paper and a watch or clock with a second hand.

● Letter search 1

In the grid below, find all appearances of the letter R, both capital and lower-case, any colour. When you are ready, set the stopwatch or note the time. Circle every letter R. Then go back and count how many appear in capital and how many in lower-case. Finally, count how many Rs appear in red. Note how long it took you, and see if you can beat your time in subsequent exercises.

| K | a | N | M | r | r | N | c | N | m | n | k | A | r | X | c | X | m | x | r | N | a |
|---|---|---|---|---|---|---|---|---|---|---|---|---|---|---|---|---|---|---|---|---|---|
| k | R | n | n | r | k | r | X | B | k | k | M | z | N | r | n | k | r | X | N | Z | N |
| a | x | m | Z | r | R | r | K | Z | N | X | k | R | X | n | k | k | n | R | a | k | X |
| x | r | x | n | Z | k | m | X | R | r | Z | c | m | x | Z | r | Z | m | X | Z | r | R |
| m | Z | c | Z | N | a | Z | n | Z | R | m | N | r | R | M | z | A | Z | m | c | k | R |
| R | m | z | n | X | r | Z | m | N | K | z | x | N | a | z | R | z | M | r | z | X | r |
| X | z | N | k | m | M | c | z | Z | r | c | X | R | N | n | z | K | R | a | K | k | n |
| c | m | z | R | z | k | c | M | N | Z | x | m | z | B | a | x | X | M | R | X | m | m |
| x | X | N | z | m | r | R | x | A | X | n | z | m | Z | X | N | z | M | n | X | a | X |
| n | X | A | k | r | n | m | x | R | a | X | R | R | r | m | c | R | n | B | a | k | z |
| k | x | z | M | Z | k | N | z | m | R | N | X | a | k | r | R | x | r | k | X | r | X |
| B | Z | r | X | r | K | a | Z | B | z | R | z | N | A | k | M | X | X | c | R | n | A |
| r | X | n | x | a | R | M | k | k | Z | x | r | X | k | a | c | K | x | R | n | R | z |
| c | x | z | N | R | x | c | M | m | R | n | z | B | M | x | R | z | n | R | z | x | M |
| N | R | r | R | z | r | R | n | Z | R | n | m | R | A | a | X | X | r | m | R | n | Z |
| R | z | R | z | N | z | B | x | R | R | r | Z | x | R | n | X | a | z | m | R | x | n |

Time...............    Number of capital Rs...............

Number of Rs in lower case...............    Number of Rs in red...............    *Answers on page 268*

# Letter search 2

In the grid below, find all appearances of the letter N, both capital and lower-case, any colour. When you are ready, set the stopwatch or note the time. Circle every letter N. Then go back and count how many appear in capital and how many in lower-case. Finally, count how many Ns appear in blue. Note how long it took you.

| K | a | N | M | r | r | N | c | N | m | n | k | A | r | X | c | X | m | x | r | N | a |
|---|---|---|---|---|---|---|---|---|---|---|---|---|---|---|---|---|---|---|---|---|---|
| k | R | n | n | r | k | r | X | B | k | k | M | z | N | r | n | k | r | X | N | Z | N |
| a | x | m | Z | r | R | r | K | Z | N | X | k | R | X | n | k | k | n | R | a | k | X |
| x | r | x | n | Z | k | m | X | R | r | Z | c | m | x | Z | r | Z | m | X | Z | r | R |
| m | Z | c | Z | N | a | Z | n | Z | R | m | N | r | R | M | z | A | Z | m | c | k | R |
| R | m | z | n | X | r | Z | m | N | K | z | x | N | a | z | R | z | M | r | z | X | r |
| X | z | N | k | m | M | c | z | Z | r | c | X | R | N | n | z | K | R | A | K | k | n |
| c | m | z | R | z | k | c | M | N | Z | x | m | z | B | a | x | X | M | R | X | m | m |
| x | X | N | z | m | r | R | x | A | X | n | z | m | Z | X | N | z | M | n | X | a | X |
| n | X | A | k | r | n | m | x | R | a | X | R | R | r | m | c | R | n | B | a | k | z |
| k | x | z | M | Z | k | N | z | m | R | N | X | a | k | r | R | x | r | k | X | r | X |
| B | Z | r | X | r | K | a | Z | B | z | R | z | N | A | k | M | x | X | c | R | n | A |
| r | X | n | x | a | R | M | k | k | Z | x | r | X | k | a | c | K | x | R | n | R | z |
| c | x | z | N | R | x | c | M | m | R | n | z | B | M | x | R | z | n | R | z | x | M |
| N | R | r | R | z | r | R | n | Z | R | n | m | R | A | a | X | X | r | m | R | n | Z |
| R | z | R | Z | N | z | B | x | R | R | r | Z | x | R | n | X | a | z | m | R | x | n |
| c | x | z | N | R | x | c | M | m | R | n | z | B | M | x | R | z | n | R | z | x | M |
| n | x | z | M | Z | k | N | z | m | R | N | X | a | k | r | R | x | r | k | X | r | X |
| R | m | z | n | X | r | Z | m | N | K | z | x | N | a | z | R | z | M | r | z | X | r |

Time...............          Number of capital Ns...............

Number of Ns in lower case...............          Number of Ns in blue...............          *Answers on page 268*

# Letter search 3

In the grid below, find all appearances of the letter K, both capital and lower-case, any colour. When you are ready, set the stopwatch or note the time. Circle every letter K. Then go back and count how many appear in capital and how many in lower-case. Finally, count how many Ks appear in green. Note how long it took you.

| K | a | N | M | r | r | N | c | N | m | n | k | A | r | X | c | X | m | x | r | N | a |
| k | R | n | n | r | k | r | X | B | k | k | M | z | N | r | n | k | r | X | N | Z | N |
| a | x | m | Z | r | R | r | K | Z | N | X | k | R | X | n | k | k | n | R | a | k | X |
| x | r | x | n | Z | k | m | X | R | r | Z | c | m | x | Z | r | Z | m | X | Z | r | R |
| m | Z | c | Z | N | a | Z | n | Z | R | m | N | r | R | M | z | A | Z | m | c | k | R |
| R | m | z | n | X | r | Z | m | N | K | z | x | N | a | z | R | z | M | r | z | X | r |
| X | z | N | k | m | M | c | z | Z | r | c | X | R | N | n | z | K | R | a | K | k | n |
| c | m | z | R | z | k | c | M | N | Z | x | m | z | B | a | x | X | M | R | X | m | m |
| x | X | N | z | m | r | R | x | A | X | n | z | m | Z | X | N | z | M | n | X | a | X |
| n | X | A | k | r | n | m | x | R | a | X | R | R | r | m | c | R | n | B | a | k | z |
| k | x | z | M | Z | k | N | z | m | R | N | X | a | k | r | R | x | r | k | X | r | X |
| B | Z | r | X | r | K | a | Z | B | z | R | z | N | A | k | M | x | X | c | R | n | A |
| r | X | n | x | a | R | M | k | k | Z | x | r | X | k | a | c | K | x | R | n | R | z |
| c | x | z | N | R | x | c | M | m | R | n | z | B | M | x | R | z | n | R | z | x | M |
| N | R | r | R | z | r | R | n | Z | R | n | m | R | A | a | X | X | r | m | R | n | Z |
| R | z | R | z | N | z | B | x | R | R | r | Z | x | R | n | X | a | z | m | R | x | n |
| k | R | n | n | r | k | r | X | B | k | k | M | z | N | r | n | k | r | X | N | Z | N |
| B | Z | r | X | k | K | a | Z | B | z | K | z | N | A | k | M | x | X | c | R | n | A |
| q | X | N | z | m | r | R | x | A | X | n | z | w | Z | X | K | z | p | n | X | a | Z |

Time...............          Number of capital Ks...............

Number of Ks in lower case...............          Number of Ks in green...............          *Answers on page 268*

The ability to communicate with others is perhaps the single most valuable skill a person can have because it gives voice to the self. In prisons, solitary confinement – separating an individual from nearly all human contact – has been known to unhinge people from their psychological moorings and drive them crazy.

# Improve your
# VERBAL SKILLS

Most of us will never experience solitary confinement, of course, but even small reductions in our ability to communicate and express ourselves can be distressing. When we are speaking and suddenly forget a word or a name, for instance, we feel as if our brains are betraying us.

The tip-of-the-tongue phenomenon, in which the word or fact we want feels close by but just out of reach, is universal. The information is right there, encoded in nerve cell pathways in our brains; we just can't always access it when we want to, especially as we get older.

You don't have to feel backed into a verbal corner. The research clearly shows that people who practise mental tricks to help them remember – known as mnemonic strategies – have an easier time recalling words, names and facts than people who wing it and hope for the best. You can improve simply by applying one of the techniques outlined here. Psychologists used to think that there was a single best mnemonic, but new theories suggest that any mnemonic technique is helpful. Read through them and try the one that fits your personal thinking style, or use more than one to meet different needs.

# Smart EVERYDAY STRATEGIES

While you're working on your word skills with the exercises in this chapter, also learn and practise the following strategies, which will help to ensure that you can access the words you need, when you need them.

## ❋ Make up a story

For lists of words you want to remember short-term, such as a grocery list or a to-do list, experts recommend making up a story that links the words. The story should be as visual as possible (otherwise you're just creating words to remember other words) and as silly or ridiculous as you can imagine.

For example, let's say you have three words to remember – lamp, strawberries, car. You could imagine turning on a lamp outdoors and finding strawberries growing inside the car and overflowing out the windows. The more imaginative or elaborate your mental pictures, the better your chances of remembering the items.

## ❋ Group words together

For long lists of words that don't have to be memorised in order, group similar words together. You decide which categories to use. If you have a grocery list, you can group the items by location in the store, by food group, by size, by price or by where you will store the items when you get home.

## ❋ Listen for the name

When you meet someone for the first time and want to remember his or her name, the first step is to listen! Most people are so focused on making a good impression that they forget to pay attention to the person they are meeting.

Focus on hearing the person's name. Immediately repeat the name ('Nice to meet you, Frank'), and use it again when addressing the person in conversation. This is often a problem in British culture, where it can seem a little odd and rather impolite to keep repeating a person's name in this way. Yet, this is a shame because saying it only once or not at all almost guarantees that the name will be forgotten.

## ❋ Let a name tell a story

When you hear the name, think about how the name sounds and what images it evokes. For example, if you meet Marina Taylor, you can easily visualise a marina full of boats and a tailor sitting on the dock mending sails. You can take the exercise a step further to help you recall this person, and their name, in the future. If Marina is a redhead, let every boat in the marina be painted red. It will be almost impossible to forget her name after such an elaborate visual image.

Not all names can be so easily translated into images. In those cases, use whatever associations come to mind. For example, if you meet Ted Sutton, who is balding, you might remember that you have a cousin or another friend named Ted who is also balding. And that your cousin was married to a woman who used to live in the south London borough of Sutton. So you can imagine your bald cousin Ted sitting in the middle of a south London street.

## ❋ Sound out difficult names

The first time you meet Wojciech Cieszko, you will probably have a tough time coming up with a story that fits his name. In such a case, ask him to repeat his name slowly. As he does, sound it out in your head and imagine writing the phonetic spelling out on a slip of paper. Now, mentally staple the paper to a mental snapshot of the person.

# HAVE A GO

Of all the memory problems people struggle with, weakened verbal skills may annoy us most because we have to use them every day. The exercises below will help to keep those skills up to scratch – and may prevent further erosion. But first, an exercise to test one of the 'everyday strategies' outlined on page 243.

**For this exercise you'll need a pencil and a blank sheet of paper**

## ● Memory jogger

Here's a list of words. Look at it for a minute, then turn over the book and write down as many as you can remember:

| |
|---|
| **oranges** |
| **currants** |
| **yoghurt** |
| **bread** |
| **cheese** |
| **breakfast cereal** |
| **ham** |
| **chicken** |
| **marmalade** |
| **deodorant** |
| **pet food** |
| **light bulbs** |

Now look at this new list:

| |
|---|
| **butter** |
| **bacon** |
| **flour** |
| **jam** |
| **apples** |
| **biscuits** |
| **orange juice** |
| **toothpaste** |
| **kitchen roll** |
| **foil** |
| **detergent** |
| **ice cream** |

This time, make up a story involving all the items, in any order. For instance, you might want to think of items on the list as cartoon characters in a children's story. Imagine a block of butter as Mrs Butter who sets off for some adventures that involve the strong smelling Mr Bacon who has just been covered in Flour by local prankster Jam Pot. This also makes the process of making up stories quite fun. Or you might prefer to generate something more logical, perhaps weaving the items into an account of everyday living, starring you. The mental images you conjure up as you compose your story will help the memory process.

Try making up your own story, using the list of words, then turn the book over and write down as many as you can remember. How did you do?

## Irregular words

**For this exercise, you'll need a pencil.**

Below are groups of words. Within each group, one of the words does not fit in the same category as the others or differs in another specific way. Circle the irregular word.

1 broccoli, carrots, spinach, peas
2 brick, bubble, football, globe
3 eagle, sparrow, ostrich, blackbird
4 tennis, ping-pong, rugby, volleyball
5 antagonise, anger, inspire, infuriate
6 Braille, Morse code, dominoes, zebras
7 duck, badger, camel, hog
8 tree, ball, watch, sock
9 plant, car, money, cash
10 television, radio, play, film

## Link-up

**For this exercise, you'll need a pencil.**

Below is a series of analogies. It's up to you to fill in the blanks. We've helped by providing the correct number of spaces needed.

1 DOWNPOUR is to RAIN as BLIZZARD is to: ___ ___ ___ ___
2 POUND is to PENNY as CENTURY is to: ___ ___ ___ ___
3 RECIPES is to COOKBOOK as MAPS is to: ___ ___ ___ ___ ___
4 CRICKET is to BAT as TENNIS is to: ___ ___ ___ ___ ___ ___
5 BLUE is to SAPPHIRE as RED is to: ___ ___ ___ ___
6 LION is to ROAR as BEE is to: ___ ___ ___ ___
7 HEN is to COCKEREL as FILLY is to: ___ ___ ___ ___
8 MOON is to CRATER as PAVEMENT is to: ___ ___ ___ ___ ___ ___
9 SPIDER is to CRAWL as SNAKE is to: ___ ___ ___ ___ ___ ___
10 BOILED SWEET is to SUGAR as TYRE is to: ___ ___ ___ ___ ___ ___

*Answers on page 268*

# Circle-grams

Try to find the word formed by the letters.
Hint: The trick is figuring out where to start.

### 1

U A Q L Y I T

### 2

L I A Z E E R

### 3

R E V S E E D

### 4

T P S I I A N

### 5

H E C E S S E

### 6

A E T H R T E

### 7

U L F H E O P

### 8

M I O N S O U

### 9

O M D E B N A

*Answers on page 268*

## Opposites attract 1

Match each word with its antonym by writing its number next to each letter.

| | | | |
|---|---|---|---|
| 1 | elated | ......... A | ally |
| 2 | inspired | ......... B | support |
| 3 | lazy | ......... C | beneficial |
| 4 | obscure | ......... D | affirm |
| 5 | adversary | ......... E | dejected |
| 6 | pernicious | ......... F | industrious |
| 7 | oppose | ......... G | mean-spirited |
| 8 | deny | ......... H | ignore |
| 9 | address | ......... I | evident |
| 10 | affable | ......... J | unmotivated |

## Opposites attract 2

| | | | |
|---|---|---|---|
| 1 | futile | ......... A | yield |
| 2 | penitent | ......... B | disparaging |
| 3 | courage | ......... C | ungainly |
| 4 | agreeable | ......... D | unpleasant |
| 5 | defy | ......... E | remorseless |
| 6 | incessant | ......... F | loquacious |
| 7 | taciturn | ......... G | useful |
| 8 | careless | ......... H | cowardice |
| 9 | elegant | ......... I | thoughtful |
| 10 | fawning | ......... J | intermittent |

## Matching pairs 1

Match each word to its synonym by writing a number next to each letter.

| | | | |
|---|---|---|---|
| 1 | settle | ......... A | resist |
| 2 | entreat | ......... B | compromise |
| 3 | acquiesce | ......... C | grave |
| 4 | disregard | ......... D | coarse |
| 5 | peevish | ......... E | wander |
| 6 | vulgar | ......... F | enlarge |
| 7 | roam | ......... G | petulant |
| 8 | oppose | ......... H | implore |
| 9 | amplify | ......... I | ignore |
| 10 | solemn | ......... J | comply |

## Matching pairs 2

| | | | |
|---|---|---|---|
| 1 | egotism | ......... A | covert |
| 2 | grateful | ......... B | rugged |
| 3 | approach | ......... C | fixed |
| 4 | rough | ......... D | overstate |
| 5 | immobile | ......... E | assiduous |
| 6 | imitate | ......... F | self-conceit |
| 7 | secret | ......... G | vanquished |
| 8 | exaggerate | ......... H | advance |
| 9 | persistent | ......... I | mirror |
| 10 | conquered | ......... J | appreciative |

*Answers on page 268*

In 2006, a 60 year-old Japanese man set a new world record by reciting pi, that never-ending mathematical number (taught in school as 3.14159), to 100,000 decimal places – from memory in 16 hours. So why do many of us have so much trouble remembering a simple phone number?

# Improve your
# NUMBER SKILLS

Recalling random sequences of numbers was first devised by a school teacher called Joseph Jacobs in 1887 to measure the mental ability of children in his class, and was used in a similar way by French psychologist Alfred Binet in the early 1900s.

We know that most people can hold between five and nine digits in their working, or short-term, memory. That's why landline phone numbers have seven digits (although there is often an area code to remember as well). People used to commit frequently used phone numbers to long-term memory simply by dialing them over and over again but today automatic and speed-dialling has made many of us more mentally lazy. And few bother to remember

11-digit mobile phone numbers other than their own. So, making the effort to recall other numbers from one day to the next requires strategies.

'Chunking', for instance, breaks down the numbers into groups that are easier to recall. Other techniques involve finding a way to relate to the numbers and link them to other pieces of information so they become meaningful (and therefore memorable), instead of random.

Research shows that using number strategies can improve memory skills tremendously, and scientists have worked hard to find the best technique.

However, research from the Karolinska Institute in Stockholm, Sweden, suggests that there is no single best memory strategy. So experiment and find out what works for you. Once you've done that your memory for numbers will improve significantly.

# Smart **EVERYDAY STRATEGIES**

There are several classic ways to remember numbers beyond the two listed here, but some are very complicated. One involves substituting words for numbers, which takes a great deal of practice. The two below are simple and can be used straight away.

## ✳ 'Chunk' them

Chunking larger numbers into small groups makes them easier to remember.  Try this yourself – look at the following series of numbers for about 5 seconds, then look away and try to write them down in the correct order.

**3-7-2-6-9-5-1-8**

Now try this again with a different set of numbers. You might find it helpful to say the numbers out loud then say them over to yourself until you can write them down. Look at the numbers for 5 seconds, then look away and try to write them down from memory.

**4-6-2   5-3-7   9-8-1**

This second time should have been easier, even although there were more numbers (9 instead of 8). Grouping or 'chunking' numbers can help to increase your digit span, and you will probably find that rehearsing or repeating numbers aloud or in your head also helps. This is the reason that telephone numbers are often written out in groups of threes or fours, rather than as a single long string.

## ✳ Give them meaning

Many mathematicians are particularly good at remembering numbers because they manage to find meaning in them. For instance, show a maths wizard the number 4824 and he might immediately think, four-digit number with the first two digits doubling the second two. If you don't happen to be gifted in this manner, find a different way to relate to the number. For example, a history buff might relate all numbers to significant dates, a librarian may place numbers in the context of the Dewey Decimal System, and a football fan may associate them with a favourite player's numbers or game scores. You can also relate them to the ages and birthdates of family members, or any other numbers you know that come quickly to mind.

If you don't work with numbers in your job, then you probably don't get enough of a chance to become comfortable with them. This is a relatively easy memory category, one that it is perfectly possible to improve. But it is also the one area that can evoke strong responses in some people. If you had bad experiences with maths when you were in school, you may still be suffering from number phobia. Don't worry, you're not going to be tested – these exercises will simply help you to manage the numbers in your life.

# HAVE A GO

## PIN codes ...

These days, most of us have far too many PINs (personal identification numbers) to remember. Take a look at each of the four PINs below, and try to make an association with the number to help you remember it. To increase the difficulty level, move on to the puzzle, 'Words & numbers' on page 253, before you go to page 252 to see if you can write in the PIN numbers you memorised.

**For example: 7613**

A person familiar with the song 'Seventy-six trombones' from *The Music Man* might think of that song for the first two digits. Someone with a 13 year-old child might use the child's age to remember the second two.

● PIN code 1
**Richard's ATM PIN: 4923**

● PIN code 2
**Edward's email PIN: 403214**

● PIN code 3
**Michelle's online banking PIN: 120489**

● PIN code 4
**Eric's online travel site PIN: 52547**

# Caller ID ...

Who's calling? Look at the names and phone numbers below. Try to remember which phone numbers are whose. Then turn to page 252 and see how well you do.

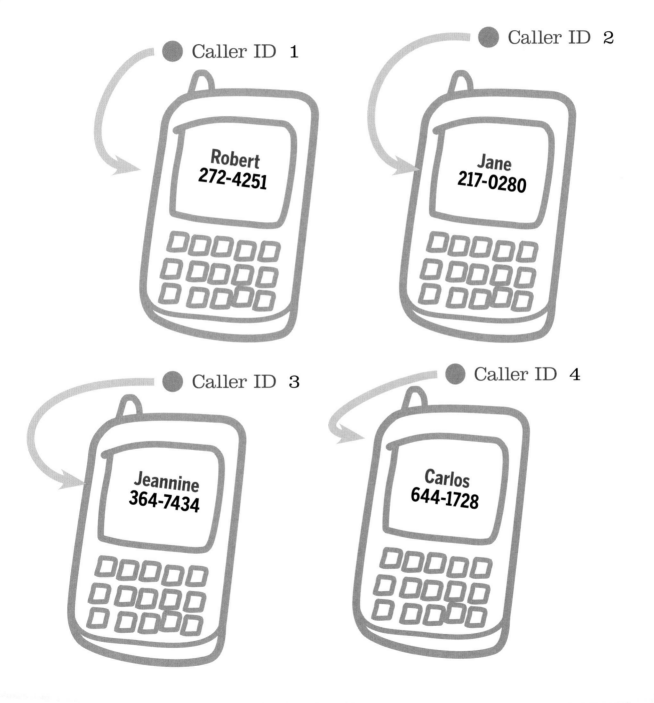

Caller ID 1

**Robert**
**272-4251**

Caller ID 2

**Jane**
**217-0280**

Caller ID 3

**Jeannine**
**364-7434**

Caller ID 4

**Carlos**
**644-1728**

# PIN codes ...

Write down the numbers you remember, then turn back to page 250 to see how you did.

**PIN code 1**
Richard's ATM PIN: ..................................

**PIN code 2**
Edward's email PIN: ..................................

**PIN code 3**
Michelle's online banking PIN: ..................................

**PIN code 4**
Eric's online travel site PIN: ..................................

Write down the numbers you remember, then turn back to page 251 to see how you did.

**Caller ID 1**
272-4251
A Jane
B Carlos
C Robert
D Jeannine

**Caller ID 2**
217-0280
A Jane
B Carlos
C Robert
D Jeannine

**Caller ID 3**
364-7434
A Jane
B Carlos
C Robert
D Jeannine

**Caller ID 4**
644-1728
A Jane
B Carlos
C Robert
D Jeannine

# Words & numbers ...

These exercises will help you to
solve everyday problems involving numbers.

## ● Words & numbers 1

Dan is a full-time university student who has a part-time job. His
girlfriend lives hundreds of miles away. On a particular day, his
classes end at 4pm, after which he immediately drives to his job,
arrives at 4. 15pm, and works for 3 ½ hours, plus a 45 minute
break for dinner. After work, he drives straight home, immediately
starts studying and continues studying for 2 hours and 10 minutes,
and then telephones his girlfriend at 11pm. How long did it take
Dan to drive home from work?

## ● Words & numbers 2

Dorothy loves entering contests by post. A few years
ago, she bought five books of twelve 39p stamps and
used 15 of them before the first-class rate went up to
41p per letter. If she already has seven 1p stamps and
eight 2p stamps, how much does she have to spend on
additional postage so she can use her remaining 39p
stamps to post her contest entries?

*Answers on page 268*

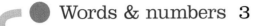

# Words & numbers ...

### ● Words & numbers 3

Jacqueline has 15 coins in her purse, all pennies, 20p and 5p pieces. If the total value of her coins is £1.03, how many each of 20p, 5p pieces and pennies does she have?

### ● Words & numbers 4

A certain airline has a weight limit of 12kg for a piece of carry-on baggage. Marc's empty suitcase weighs 1kg, and he has these items that he'd like to put in it for his flight:

Jar of snacks: 0.5kg
Travel iron: 1.5kg
Crossword dictionary: 1kg
Gift for his mother: 4kg
Laptop computer: 5kg

Which of these items should he take, if he'd like to take as much (by weight) as possible?

*Answers on page 268*

# Sums without symbols ...

Place arithmetic symbols **+, -, ÷, ×, =** (plus, minus, multiplication or division) between the numbers in each group below to get the result asked for.

For example:

**2, 3, 4, 5** to get **19**

Answer:

**2 x 3 x 4 – 5 = 19**

● Sum 1

**8, 6, 4, 11** to get **4**

● Sum 2

**10, 3, 8, 2** to get **30**

● Sum 3

**9, 2, 8, 4, 10** to get **50**

● Sum 4

**15, 5, 11, 6, 5** to get **100**

● Sum 5

**5, 4, 2, 4, 6** to get **6**

● Sum 6

**12, 2, 8, 4, 3, 4** to get **0**

*Answers on page 268*

# Improve your
# REASONING SKILLS

**Whether we realise it or not, we use reasoning skills every day. Reasoning actually involves various sets of skills,** such as categorising information (that animal looks feline, so it must be a cat), evaluating logic (if that man has only one arm, he wasn't the one who carried the heavy timber into the garage), extrapolation (estimating an outcome from the available evidence) and good old problem solving.

From the time we are old enough to think, our brains start looking for patterns in the seemingly random events of life. We also amass information we can draw on later. Every fact we learn and every problem we solve improves our ability to reason. In that way – experience by experience, decision by decision – we make sense of the world.

The evidence isn't clear about whether we lose the power to think logically and solve difficult problems as we get older, but research shows that everyone – young and old alike – can benefit from training and practice.

If you are not accustomed to doing brain gymnastics, then you may find this section particularly difficult. But remember that challenging your brain is the way to make it more capable. Think of these exercises as interesting puzzles to be solved. If you get tired or frustrated, stop and come back to them another day.

# HAVE A GO

## Logical or not?

This exercise requires you to pay attention to the story and follow the logic from sentence to sentence. First, read the paragraph and decide if all sentences are logical given the rest of the text. If not, underline the sentence or sentences that don't make sense.

### Puzzle 1

Betty and Bill were having Diane and Dave over that Wednesday evening to hear about their recent holidays, so Bill put a £20 note in his pocket and strolled over to Bestco's, the local grocery store, to pick up a few things that they needed. But Bestco's was closed when he got there – Bill had forgotten that Bestco's closes early on weekends. So Bill had to walk right across town, to the Mammoth Market, to get what he needed. He bought three varieties of cheese, crisps and a bottle of wine. He paid the total cost of £19.75 with his credit card, put everything in the boot of his car and went straight home. As soon as he got home, Diane called to postpone dinner until the following week.

*Answers on page 268*

# Logical or not?

## Puzzle 2

The semi-annual St. Patrick's Day celebration in Ballyhoo is eagerly awaited by one and all. It doesn't matter if you're from Iceland or not, everyone joins in the festivities. The fun starts early in the morning, with the traditional green-egg breakfast (thanks to some food colouring) served in the town square. The parade starts at 10am and lasts for about 2 hours. There is the marching band, of course, with all the flutes, tubas, cellos and trumpets, and elaborately constructed floats on which men in kilts play accordions. The non-musical marchers include representatives from the local schools, civic associations, and the police and fire departments, with the mayor in his green limousine at the very end. Then, everyone rushes to McSweeney's restaurant for the traditional corned beef and cabbage lunch.

## Puzzle 3

Since I've retired, I've become a pretty active user of the internet and get a lot of my news online, but I still like getting the newspaper every weekday morning (I'm much too busy on weekends to sit down with the paper). So my 'newspaper week' starts every Monday morning. The paper arrives like clockwork at 6am, which suits me fine since I'm an early riser. So, with my Monday morning cup of coffee in hand, I read the newspaper from page 1 to the back cover, including the sports news, local and international news, stock-market listings, comic strips and, of course, the daily crossword. After a quick breakfast, I kiss my wife good-bye and take the bus to the office.

*Answers on page 268*

## Puzzle 4

You know what a big tennis fan I am. So it was a happy coincidence that my husband and I arrived in Auckland on July 10th, the day before the Australian Open tennis tournament. As soon as we checked in at our hotel, I took a cab to the stadium, bought tickets for me and my wife, and hurried back to the hotel for dinner.

The tournament is held on two main courts. It's a good thing that they both have retractable roofs, so they can close them if there's rain or it gets too hot. It can be swelteringly hot during the tournament. That night, despite our long tiring journey, I was so excited about the tournament that I couldn't sleep.

## Puzzle 5

They call it the waiting room for a reason, you know. Waiting an hour or more to be seen by your doctor is most people's idea of fun. That's why I always bring lots of things to do. Usually, I fill a bag with stuff like knitting, magazines, candles and stationery to catch up on my letter writing. Sometimes, thankfully not too often, there are actually more people waiting than there are seats in the waiting room. When that happens, I walk to the library just a block away and browse the fiction section for the newest books from my favourite authors. The last time I was there, I took out two whodunits, the latest John Grisham legal thriller and a dieting book.

## Puzzle 6

Our neighbours recommended Mario's Italian restaurant, which has just opened on the other side of the town. They raved about it: 'Great food, great service, great prices – what more can you ask?' So we had to check it out for ourselves. It really was everything they said it was. We were greeted warmly by Mario himself the moment we walked in the door: 'Welcome back, Mr and Mrs Williams'. The menu was enormous, with five pages of main courses alone. We finally decided what to order. Michele had the veal Marsala, and I decided on the moussaka. The food was great, the portions were huge, and the bill was really reasonable. So we've added Luigi's to our own list of dining favourites.

*Answers on page 269*

# If ...then ...

Clear, careful thinking will help you to solve the logic problems here.

## If ... then 1

Bill's sock drawer has eight pairs of socks in it, each pair has a different pattern, and they're scattered about individually in the drawer. There's a power failure in his home one night, just as he opens the drawer to take out a pair of socks. He takes nine socks out of the drawer, but he can't see them, since the room is dark. Does he have at least one matching pair of socks among the nine?

Answer.............................

## If ... then 2

If in a yearly calendar of events National Egg Month comes before National Peanut Butter Month, National Strawberry Month comes after National Potato Month, and National Potato Month comes after National Egg Month, is National Egg Month before or after National Strawberry Month, or do we not have enough information to tell?

Answer.............................

## If ... then 3

If we know that Brazil has more people than Russia, Russia has more people than Mexico, and Mexico has fewer people than Pakistan, does Brazil or Pakistan have more people, or do we not have enough information to tell?

Answer.............................

## If ... then 4

If Amber's birthday is February 20, and her classmate Amanda was born 10 days later in the same year, do we know what Amanda's birthday is?

Answer.............................

*Answers on page 269*

## If ... then 5

If City B is due east of City A, City C is due north of city B, city D is due south of city B, and City E is due south of City A, what is the direction from City C to City D, or do we not have enough information to tell?

Answer.............................

## If ... then 6

A certain restaurant's lunch menu has three choices for sandwiches: tuna fish for £3, chicken salad for £4, and ham for £4.50. Three friends come into the restaurant for lunch, and each one orders a sandwich. If the total cost of the three sandwiches ordered is £10, do we know how many of each sandwich was ordered?

Answer.............................

## If ... then 7

If we know that a bushel of wheat weighs more than a bushel of oats, a bushel of barley weighs less than a bushel of sweetcorn, and a bushel of oats weighs more than a bushel of sweetcorn, what weighs more, a bushel of wheat or a bushel of sweetcorn, or do we not have enough information to tell?

Answer.............................

## If ... then 8

The fuel tank in Marie's car holds 90 litres (20 gallons). Her car gets 15 miles per gallon in city driving and 25 miles per gallon in motorway driving. If she drives 250 miles on a half-tank of fuel, do we know how many motorway miles and city miles she drove?

Answer.............................

*Answers on page 269*

# Seating plan ...

Kate and Larry are getting married.
It's your job to help them design a seating plan
for the table at which their relatives will sit – but there are
a few restrictions. See if you can figure out who should sit where.

## PEOPLE TO SEAT

Kate's Aunt Alice and Uncle Bob
(married couple)

Larry's Cousin Carl

Kate's Cousin Dave

Larry's Aunt Ella and Uncle Frank
(married couple)

Kate's Uncle George

Larry's Aunt Harriet

Kate's Cousin Ida

Larry's Uncle Jack

## SEATING RESTRICTIONS
## (in order of importance)

**1** All of Kate's relatives sit
together, and all of Larry's
relatives sit together

**2** Married couples must sit
together

**3** Cousin Dave plays in a rock
band and wants to sit as close to
the band as possible

**4** You're trying to get Cousin Carl
to date Cousin Ida, so seat them
together

**5** Uncle Frank isn't talking to
Uncle Jack, so they can't sit next
to each other

**6** Uncle George owes money to
Cousin Dave, so he wants to sit as
far from Dave as possible

**7** Uncle Bob hasn't seen Uncle
George for 20 years, and they
have a lot to catch up on

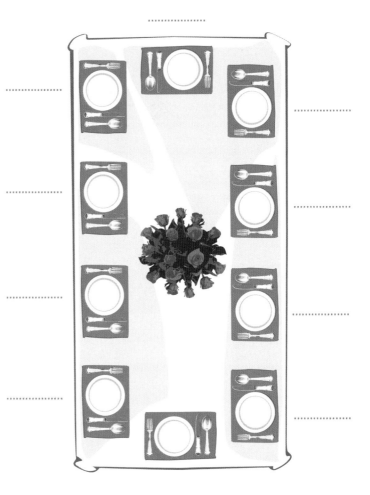

**ROCK BAND**

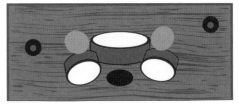

*Answers on page 269*

# Next in line ...

Study the sequence below and figure out which image should come next.

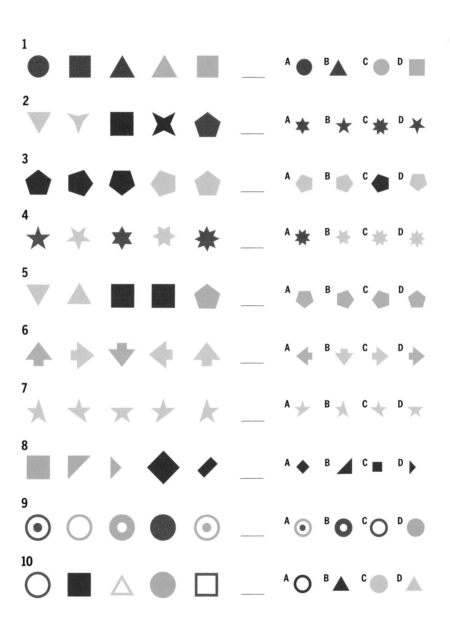

Answers on page 269

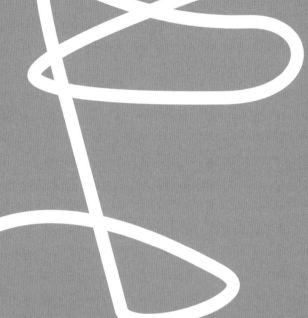

ANSWERS

## Name that shape 1

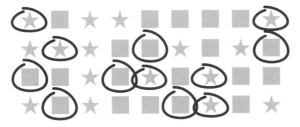

## Name that shape 2

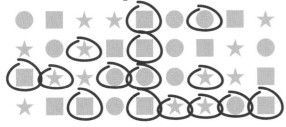

## Name that shape 3

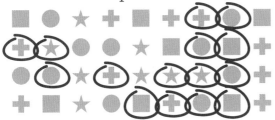

## Name that shape 4

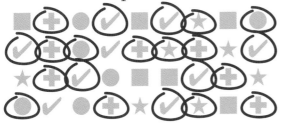

## Name that shape 5

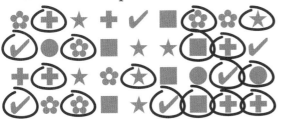

## Odd one out 1
second row, third item:

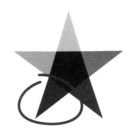

## Odd one out 2
second row, fourth item:

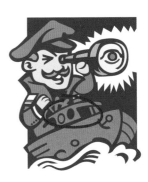

## Odd one out 3
first row, third item:

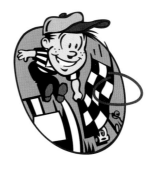

## Odd one out 4
first row, second item:

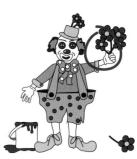

## Odd one out 5
second row, second item:

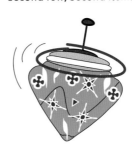

## Odd one out 6
first row, third item:

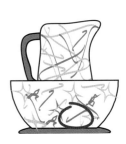

## Spot the difference 1

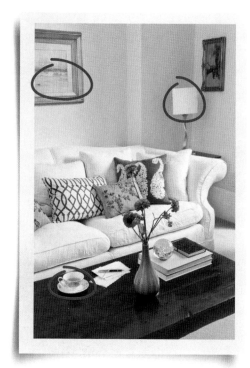

## Spot the difference 2

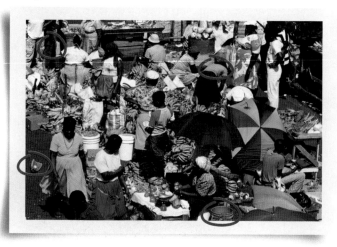

## Spot the difference 3

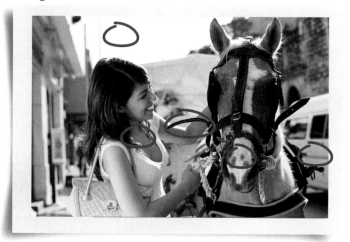

## Spot the difference 4

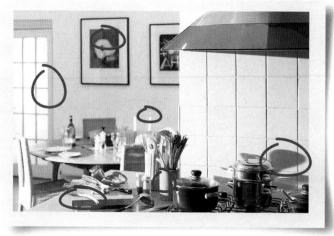

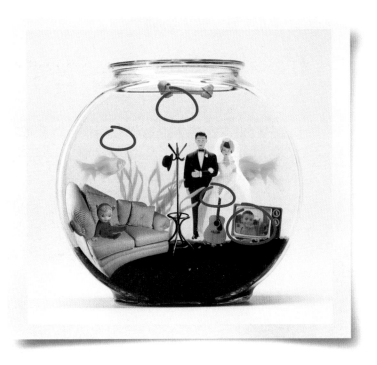

Picture recall 1

Picture recall 2

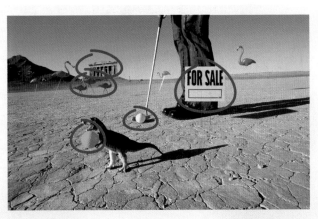

Picture recall 3

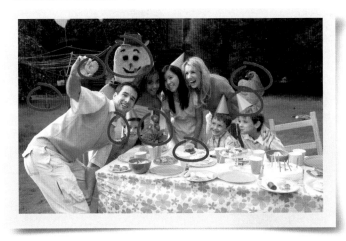

## Letter search 1
43 capitals, 33 lowercase, 6 red

## Letter search 2
28 capitals, 30 lowercase, 6 blue

## Letter search 3
10 capitals, 32 lowercase, 7 green

## Irregular words
**1** carrots (not green)
**2** brick (not spherical)
**3** ostrich (can't fly)
**4** rugby (oval ball, no net)
**5** inspire (not negative)
**6** zebras (don't have dots)
**7** camel (can't be a verb)
**8** watch (not four letters)
**9** money (the only word without the vowel 'a')
**10** radio (not something you watch)

## Link-up
**1** snow **2** year **3** atlas **4** racket **5** ruby **6** buzz
**7** colt **8** pothole **9** slither **10** rubber

## Circle-grams
**1** quality **2** realise **3** deserve **4** pianist **5** cheeses
**6** theatre **7** hopeful **8** ominous **9** abdomen

## Opposites attract 1
**1** e **2** j **3** f **4** i **5** a **6** c **7** b **8** d **9** h **10** g

## Opposites attract 2
**1** g **2** e **3** h **4** d **5** a **6** j **7** f **8** i **9** c **10** b

## Matching pairs 1
**1** b **2** h **3** j **4** i **5** g **6** d **7** e **8** a **9** f **10** c

## Matching pairs 2
**1** f **2** j **3** h **4** b **5** c **6** i **7** a **8** d **9** e **10** g

## Words & numbers 1
20 minutes

## Words & numbers 2
67p

## Words & numbers 3
Eight pennies, four 20p pieces, three 5p pieces

## Words & numbers 4
Jar of snacks, travel iron, gift for mother and laptop computer. Total weight: 11kg.

## Sums without symbols
**1** $8 \times 6 - 4 \div 11 = 4$
**2** $10 - 3 + 8 \times 2 = 30$
**3** $9 - 2 \times 8 + 4 - 10 = 50$
**4** $15 \div 5 + 11 + 6 \times 5 = 100$
**5** $5 \times 4 \times 2 - 4 \div 6 = 6$
**6** $12 \times 2 \div 8 \times 4 \div 3 - 4 = 0$

## Logical or not 1
The store closes early on weekends, but the dinner is on a Wednesday; Bill puts cash in his pocket but pays with a credit card; he walks to the store but puts the items in the car boot.

## Logical or not 2
St. Patrick's Day is annual, not semi-annual; it originated in Ireland, not Iceland; cellos are not marching band instruments; men in kilts would play bagpipes, not accordions.

## Logical or not 3
There are no stock-market listings on Mondays; the speaker is retired, so he would not go to the office.

## Logical or not 4

Auckland is in New Zealand, not Australia; the wife is speaking, yet she buys tickets for her and her wife; July is winter in Australia.

## Logical or not 5

'Is' should be 'isn't' most people's idea of fun; one can't use candles in a doctor's surgery; the diet book would not be found in the library's fiction section.

## Logical or not 6

The restaurant owner said 'welcome back' but the couple had never eaten there before; moussaka is a Greek, not Italian, dish; the restaurant name is Mario's, not Luigi's.

## If ... then 1

Yes

## If ... then 2

National Egg Month is before National Strawberry Month

## If ... then 3

Not enough information to tell

## If ... then 4

No.
It could be March 1 (if a leap year) or March 2 (if not)

## If ... then 5

City D is due south of City C

## If ... then 6

Yes.
Two tuna fish and one chicken salad.

## If ... then 7

A bushel of wheat

## If ... then 8

Yes.
250 motorway miles.

## Seating plan

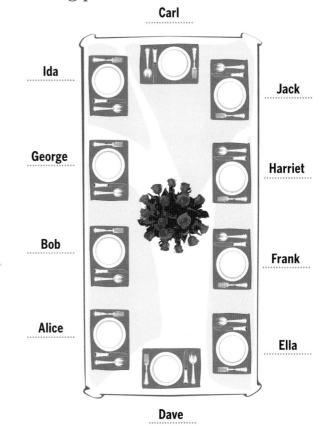

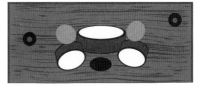

## Next in line

1 c  2 b  3 d  4 c  5 a  6 d  7 b  8 a  9 c  10 b

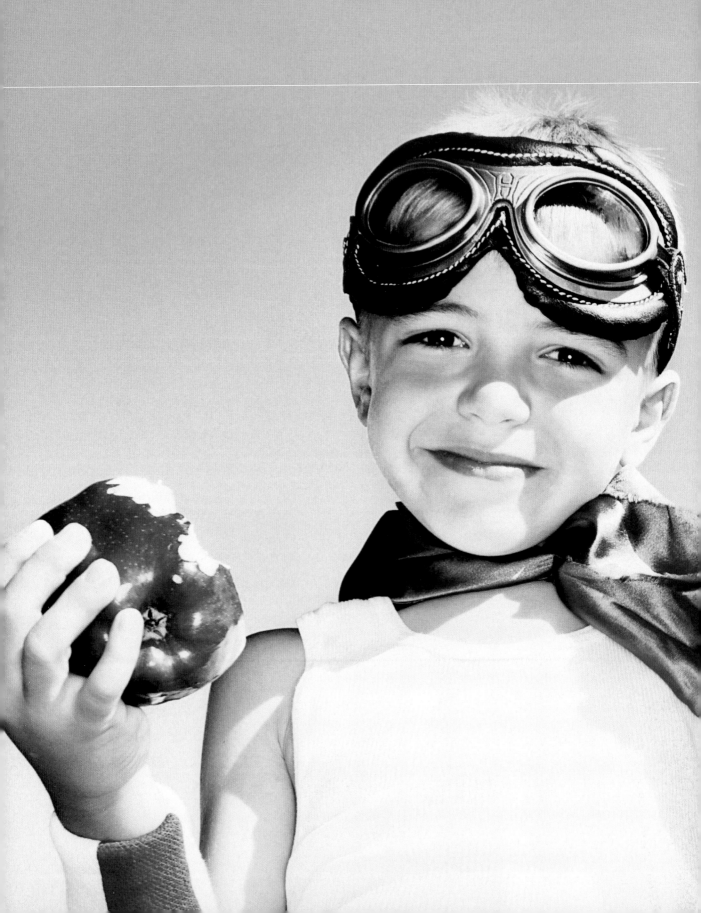

# RESOURCES

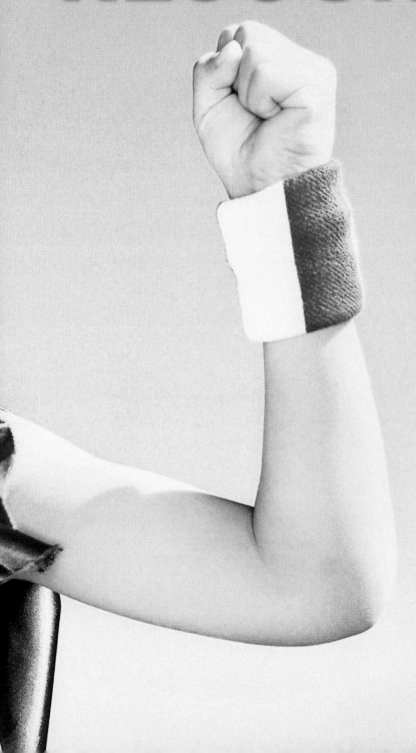

# The ten day
# JUMP-START PLAN

**By now, your brain may be whirling with all the new Sharp Brain ideas and tips you've picked up throughout this book.** Perhaps you've already tried a few of the brain-saving tactics. Every minute of every day presents a new opportunity to nourish, nurture and grow your grey matter. But what's the best way to ensure you use those opportunities, now and in the future? Here's a suggestion: start with *The ten-day jump-start plan*.

In the next few pages you'll find a calendar of possibilities to explore. You can do as many or as few as you like but they're all worth trying as each one will benefit your brain in some way. They're not onerous tasks. Scatter blueberries on your breakfast cereal. Make time for a phone call to a friend. Go ten-pin bowling on Saturday instead of watching TV. Guarding your brain against the forces that drain your memory and slow your thinking skills is that

simple. The key? Stepping outside your comfort zone just a little bit today … then choosing to do so over and over again in new and different ways. Protecting what goes on in your head also involves tasty brain-healthy foods, good-quality sleep – and plenty of it – fun with friends and family, and time in the great outdoors.

It's all well worth a try to help you get started on the path to an active, challenged brain.

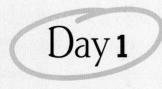

## Add zing to your cereal

Sprinkle a handful of blueberries and a tablespoon of chopped nuts onto your breakfast cereal. Voilà! You've just added a helping of brain-protecting antioxidants and good fats to your diet, in less than a minute. That's how easy it is to keep your brain sharp.

## Invest in some houseplants

Filling your home – and your outside space if you have one – with flowers and greenery helps to correct 'nature deficit disorder' and gives your brain the contact with nature it craves. It immediately puts you in touch with nature, which some studies suggest can foster sharper recall, quicker reactions and greater creativity.

## Prepare to walk

Find your walking shoes or trainers and put them where you'll see them first thing in the morning. You're going for a walk tomorrow.

*Recipe of the day*

Stir-fried beef with fine noodles, page 300

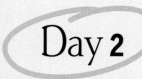

## Get out and about

Lace up your walking shoes and head out the door. A 10 to 15-minute walk is all it takes to boost the flow of oxygen-rich blood to brain cells. And morning sun exposure will help you to sleep better at night so that new memories can be locked into place.

## Plan a picnic

If it's summer, start arranging a healthy weekend picnic or barbecue. Plan to include dishes with as many different-coloured fruits and vegetables as you can for an added brain boost. If winter, meet friends for a weekend stroll and then a healthy lunch at a favourite pub.

## Get on the phone

Call up an old friend you haven't seen for a while. Have a chat – and before you hang up, make a date for lunch or coffee some time this month. Friendship is one of life's greatest joys ... social contact makes your heart sing and your brain thrive.

*Recipe of the day*

Fruity Bircher muesli, page 280

✳ *Sweet fruit, crunchy nuts, healthy oils and satisfying whole grains are part of the Mediterranean diet, which is known to help protect the brain.*

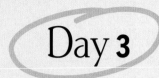

**Day 3**

## Choose brain-friendly oil

Drizzle olive oil on your salad at lunch. Not only does it taste delicious – it offers an important brain benefit. The healthy fats in olive oil can help to reduce inflammation. For an added boost make spinach one of your vegetables today.

## Swap tasks

Do a household chore that you always leave to your partner or which rarely gets done. Mow the lawn if you normally scrub the pots; weed the garden if you normally do the dusting. Cross-training your brain in this way builds new connections between brain cells – and your home's ripe with opportunities.

## And so to bed ...

Put on fresh, clean sheets and get your head down 15 minutes earlier than usual, then stick with your new bedtime all week. A good night's sleep is like a session at a spa for the mind, regenerating brain tissue, preserving memories and even boosting your IQ.

*Recipe of the day*

Millet with spinach and pine nuts page 302

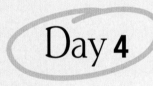

**Day 4**

## Start with a cuddle

Release the 'cuddle hormone' oxytocin by hugging someone you love (or stroking a beloved pet). As well as giving you a brain boost, it will strengthen your relationships, which helps to lower stress.

## Make space for fruit

Take your most attractive fruit bowl or plate and place it prominently on the kitchen table or counter. Fill it with all types of fruit, such as bananas, oranges and rinsed apples and pears. The more colour variety the better. This pretty-as-a-picture centrepiece will have you reaching for antioxidant-packed, brain-nourishing snacks.

## Me me me!

Indulge yourself. Soak in a bubble bath, ask your partner for a foot massage, have sex or savour a square or two of delicious dark chocolate (packed with antioxidants). Pleasure raises levels of dopamine, an attention-focusing brain chemical.

*Recipe of the day*

Quinoa with griddled aubergines page 300

**✳ Does walking benefit your brain? Yes! Exercise is like fertiliser for your mind – just a few minutes a day helps brain cell growth.**

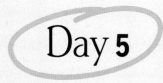

## Pack the good fats

Put a handful of walnuts into a resealable bag and slip it into your handbag or briefcase to have as your mid-morning snack. Walnuts are full of good fats that improve cell-to-cell communication in the brain.

## Say 'hello'

Make time to talk today: have a chat with colleagues, neighbours and friends in person instead of by email or phone. Smile and engage in conversation with shopkeepers. Even brief conversations boost brainpower.

## Major on the omega-3s

Serve fish, the ultimate brain food, for dinner. Go for salmon, trout, mackerel or even sardines. All are rich in omega-3 oils, critical for clear thinking, organisation, alertness, learning and reasoning.

*Recipe of the day*

Linguine with pan-fried salmon, page 294

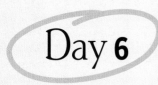

## Salute the day

Let the sun shine in. Throw open the curtains and pull up the blinds first thing this morning. A dose of early-morning sunlight resets your body clock, boosting mental alertness – which will improve your sleep tonight.

## Eat fresh

Shop at a farmers' market or at a nearby supermarket with the biggest fresh produce department. Stock up on a rainbow of brain-friendly and mouth-watering veggies and fruit – then reward yourself with a gourmet salad for lunch or dinner.

## Play some nutty games

Gather your family or close friends around the dining-room table for a games night. Brain-teasers such as Scrabble build extra neural connections that protect you from brain decline. Serve a fruity dessert or a platter of sliced fruit and nuts for even more brain benefits.

*Recipe of the day*

Cinnamon banana caramels, page 307

✳ **Your brain loves company. Fun with friends feels great – and people with active social lives tend to suffer less cognitive decline later in life.**

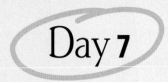

## Day 7

### Mix it up

Today is 'opposite' day, so step outside your usual routine. Brush your teeth with your non-dominant hand, take a different route to work, or stand when you normally sit. Shaking things up keeps your brain active – and takes it off autopilot.

### Soak up the details

Go to a park and pay close attention to everything you see (the shape and texture of the leaves), smell (freshly cut grass), feel (the wind on your face) and hear (birds chirping, children laughing). Flooding your brain with sensory data keeps your grey matter on its toes.

### Laugh or learn – or both

See a comedy or foreign film, or, even better, a foreign comedy. A funny film induces brain-healthy laughter, while watching it in a foreign language challenges your brain to keep track of the action and read the subtitles at the same time.

*Recipe of the day*

Cassoulet, page 294

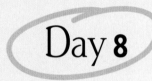

## Day 8

### Coffee time

Savour a hot cup of freshly brewed coffee. Studies show that coffee sharpens alertness and boosts processing speed. Not a coffee-drinker? Don't worry; tea also confers brain benefits.

### Go vegetarian

Make today a non-meat day. Choose porridge or cereal with dried fruits for breakfast, opt for veggie soup for lunch, then round off the day with some healthy grains such as bulghur wheat or quinoa, topped with beans, lentils or chickpeas in a spicy tomato sauce.

### Don't lose touch

Write out a 'call list' of friends, old and new. Starting tonight, catch up with one every day by phone or email. Widening your social circle significantly lowers your risk of cognitive impairment.

*Recipe of the day*

Spiced lentil dhal, page 298

**✳ Challenging your brain with new experiences keeps it young – the pleasure and surprise puts a sparkle in your eye and a spring in your step.**

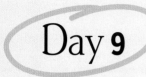

## Day 9

### Walk this way

Add 5 more minutes to your daily walk. From now on, plan to increase your walking time by an additional 5 minutes each week until you're on the go for 30 minutes. Vary your route and explore new places to increase the interest.

### Engage yourself

Turn off the TV and lose yourself instead in an absorbing new hobby or project (do a puzzle, read a new book or get out your knitting needles – anything that's different from the norm and gets you in a state of 'flow').

### Be thankful

Write down all the good things that happened today. Spending more of your mental energy on gratitude than on worry will help you reduce brain-sapping tension.

*Recipe of the day*

Chicken with apricots and cumin, page 292

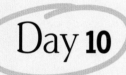

## Day 10

### Be breath aware

Sit in a comfortable chair in a quiet room for 10 minutes. Close your eyes, pay attention to your breath as it flows in and out, and let your muscles relax. You'll feel refreshed and reduce levels of stress hormones that are toxic to your brain.

### Have a massage

Arrange to have a massage – and book yourself in for one next week, and the week after that. If you can't afford it, get into the habit of taking turns with a partner or friend. It helps lower stress levels and reduces pain – good news for your brain.

### Treat yourself to more sleep

Turn back your bedtime another 15 minutes tonight, and keep it there. Your mind thrives on a good night's sleep

*Recipe of the day*

Borscht with crunchy mash, page 284

❋ Gentle stress-busters – hugging, laughter, relaxation – do more than shield your brain from tension's corrosive effects. They boost your happiness, right away.

**Do you want to boost your concentration and memory? Eating well is key. Science shows that poor nutrition damages our mental faculties** while good food protects against the effects of age, toxins and disease, and safeguards the neural networks that let you think, process, plan and dream.

# HEALTHY BRAIN

## recipes

Think of every meal as a chance not only to nourish your body but also your mind. The recipes that follow are designed to help you obtain important nutrients from their best sources – foods such as salmon and other oil-rich fish, olive oil, garlic, whole grains, nuts and flaxseeds, and antioxidant-rich vegetables and fruits and berries. Many of the recipes also feature anti-inflammatory spices, such as turmeric.

How much of a difference can your diet make? Plenty. Eating healthily and avoiding saturated fats and calorific fast foods can significantly improve your health which will in turn enhance your memory and thinking skills as well as lowering your risk of a brain-damaging stroke. Best of all, these recipes are as delicious as they are good for you. *Bon appétit!*

# RECIPE LIST

# BREAKFAST

## Fruity Bircher muesli

Serves 4
Preparation: 10 minutes, plus overnight soaking

115g rolled oats
115g sultanas
250ml semi-skimmed milk
1 crisp dessert apple, such as Cox's
2 tsp lemon juice
30g hazelnuts, roughly chopped
15g pumpkin seeds
1 tbsp sesame seeds
100g strawberries, chopped
4 tbsp plain low-fat bio yoghurt
4 tsp clear honey

Place the oats and sultanas in a large bowl and add the milk. Stir to mix evenly, then cover and place in the refrigerator. Leave to soak overnight.

The next day, just before eating, grate the apple, discarding the core. Toss the apple with the lemon juice to prevent browning.

Stir the hazelnuts, pumpkin seeds and sesame seeds into the oat mixture, then stir in the grated apple and strawberries.

To serve, divide the muesli among 4 cereal bowls and top each with a spoonful of yoghurt and honey.

Per serving: 366kcal, 11g protein, 12g total fat (2g saturated fat), 56g carbohydrate, 4g fibre

## Berry-flaxseed smoothie

Serves 2
Preparation: 5 minutes

2 tbsp whole flaxseeds
125ml orange juice
125g fat-free vanilla yoghurt
250g unsweetened frozen mixed berries or blueberries

Place the flaxseeds in a blender and blend until ground into a fine powder. Add the orange juice, yoghurt, mixed berries (or blueberries) and banana. Blend until smooth and creamy. Pour into two glasses and serve immediately.

Per serving: 200kcal, 9g protein, 6.5g total fat (0.7g saturated fat), 27g carbohydrate, 4g fibre

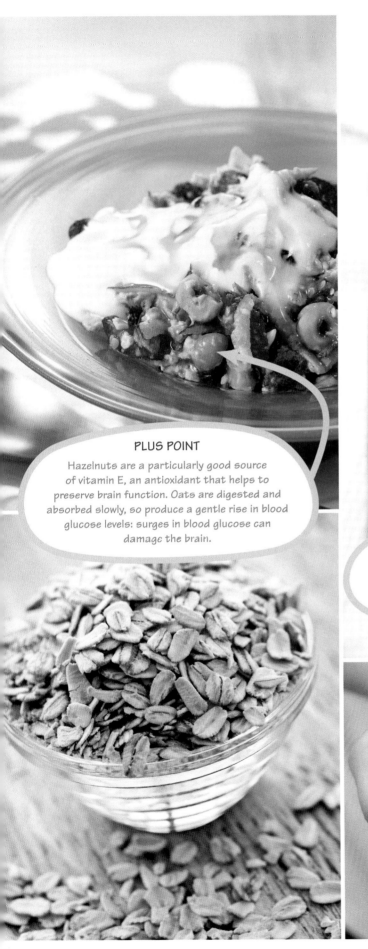

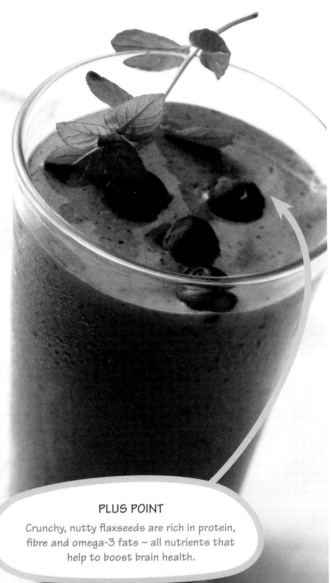

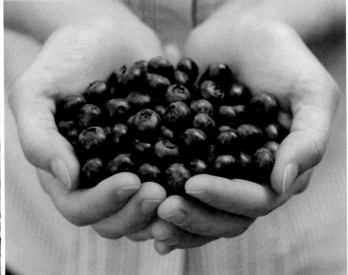

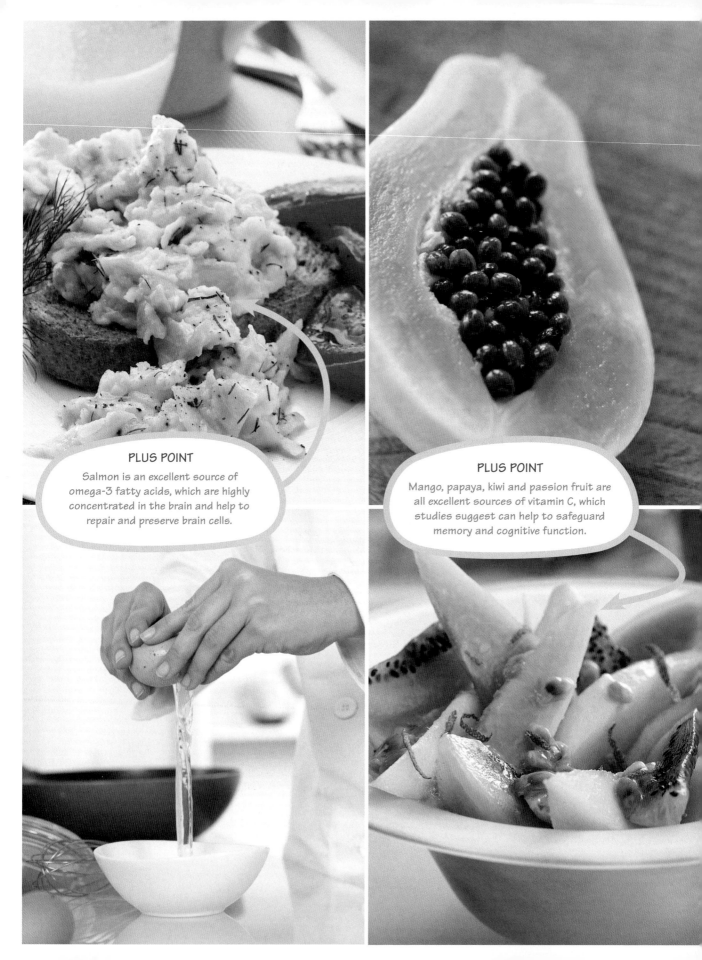

**PLUS POINT**

Salmon is an excellent source of omega-3 fatty acids, which are highly concentrated in the brain and help to repair and preserve brain cells.

**PLUS POINT**

Mango, papaya, kiwi and passion fruit are all excellent sources of vitamin C, which studies suggest can help to safeguard memory and cognitive function.

# Scrambled eggs with smoked salmon and dill

Serves 4
Preparation: 10 minutes  Cooking: 10 minutes

6 eggs
3 tbsp semi-skimmed milk
6 plum tomatoes, halved lengthways
4 thick slices wholemeal bread
3 tbsp crème fraîche
75g sliced smoked salmon, cut into thin strips
1 tsp lemon juice
1 tbsp chopped fresh dill
salt and pepper
sprigs of fresh dill to garnish

Lightly beat the eggs with the milk in a heatproof bowl or in the top of a double saucepan. Set over a saucepan containing barely simmering water – the base of the bowl or pan should just touch the water. Cook for 6–8 minutes or until the eggs begin to thicken, stirring frequently.

Preheat the grill to high. While the eggs are cooking, arrange the tomatoes cut side up on the rack of the grill pan, and sprinkle them with a little salt and pepper. Add the slices of bread to the rack. Grill for 4–5 minutes, turning the bread over halfway through, until the tomatoes are lightly browned and the bread is toasted on both sides.

Add the crème fraîche to the eggs, and season to taste with salt and pepper. Cook for a further 1 minute, stirring constantly, until the mixture is softly scrambled. Sprinkle the smoked salmon with the lemon juice, then add to the eggs together with the chopped dill. Immediately remove from the heat.

Place the toast on warmed serving plates and divide the smoked salmon scramble among them. Garnish each with a sprig of dill. Add 3 grilled tomato halves to each plate, and serve.

# Exotic fruit salad

Serves 4
Preparation: 15 minutes

1 large papaya
1 large mango
2 kiwi fruit
6 tbsp orange juice
2 tbsp lime juice
2 passion fruit

Peel and halve the papaya and scoop out the seeds. Slice the fruit crossways and arrange the slices in 2 rows on a serving platter, or cut into chunks and put into a large serving bowl.

Stone and peel the mango and cut lengthways into wedges. Arrange the wedges in a row between the papaya slices. Or cut into chunks and add to the serving bowl.

Peel the kiwi fruit and cut lengthways into wedges or chunks. Scatter them over the slices of mango and papaya.

Mix the orange juice with the lime juice. Halve the passion fruit and scoop out the seeds and pulp into the juice mixture. Spoon over the salad and serve immediately.

Per serving: 120kcal, 2g protein, 0.5g total fat (0g saturated fat), 27g carbohydrate, 5g fibre

Per serving: 363kcal, 22g protein, 21g total fat (9g saturated fat), 24g carbohydrate, 4g fibre

# SOUPS, SALADS & BITES

## Curried red lentil soup

Serves 8
Preparation: 15 minutes  Cooking: 25 minutes

2 tsp canola (rapeseed) oil
2 medium onions, chopped
4 garlic cloves, finely chopped
4–5 tsp mild curry powder
285g red lentils, rinsed and picked over
1.5 litres chicken or vegetable stock made without salt
180ml water
2 tbsp tomato purée
¼ tsp ground cinnamon
2 tbsp lemon juice
¼ tsp salt, or to taste
Freshly ground black pepper to taste
125g fat-free plain yoghurt
4 tbsp chopped spring onion greens

Heat the oil in a large saucepan over a medium heat. Add the onions and cook, stirring frequently, for 2–3 minutes or until softened. Add the garlic and curry powder, and cook, stirring, for 30 seconds.

Add the lentils and stir to coat. Add the stock, water, tomato purée and cinnamon. Bring to a simmer, then reduce the heat to low, cover and simmer for 20 minutes or until the lentils are very tender.

In batches, transfer the soup to a food processor or blender and process to a smooth purée. (Take care as the liquid will be very hot.) Return the purée to the pan and heat through.

Season with the lemon juice, salt and pepper. Ladle into bowls and garnish each serving with a dollop of yoghurt and a sprinkling of spring onion greens. The soup can be kept, covered, in the refrigerator for up to 2 days.

Per serving: 142kcal, 11g protein, 1g total fat (0.2g saturated fat), 23g carbohydrate, 2.3g fibre

## Borscht with crunchy mash

Serves 4
Preparation: 35 minutes  Cooking: 50 minutes

1 tbsp extra virgin olive oil
1 onion, chopped
1 large carrot
½ tsp lemon juice
1 bulb of fennel, quartered
500g raw beetroot, peeled and diced
1 litre vegetable stock
800g floury potatoes, peeled and cut into small cubes
120ml semi-skimmed milk
4 tbsp Greek-style yoghurt
2 spring onions, finely chopped

Place the oil in a large saucepan and add the onion. Set aside 55g of the carrot for the mash, then chop the rest and add it to the pan. Mix well, cover and cook over a moderate heat for 5 minutes to soften the onion.

Put the lemon juice in a small bowl. Finely grate a quarter of the fennel into the lemon juice and toss well. Add the reserved carrot, finely grated. Cover and set aside.

Chop the remaining fennel and add it to the saucepan with the beetroot. Pour in the stock and bring to the boil. Reduce the heat, cover the pan and simmer for about 30 minutes or until all the vegetables are tender.

Meanwhile, bring another pan of water to the boil. Add the potatoes and boil for 10 minutes or until very tender. Drain the potatoes well and return them to the pan. Toss over a low heat for about 1 minute to dry.

Purée the soup until smooth, then return it to the pan, if necessary, and reheat. Taste and adjust the seasoning. While the soup is reheating, set the pan of potatoes over a moderate heat and mash until smooth, gradually working in the milk. Stir in the yoghurt, grated fennel and carrot, spring onions and seasoning to taste.

Divide the mashed potato between 4 bowls, piling it up in the centre. Ladle the soup around the mash and sprinkle with chopped fennel or parsley. Serve at once.

Per serving: 300kcal, 11g protein, 4g total fat (1g saturated fat), 56g carbohydrate, 7g fibre

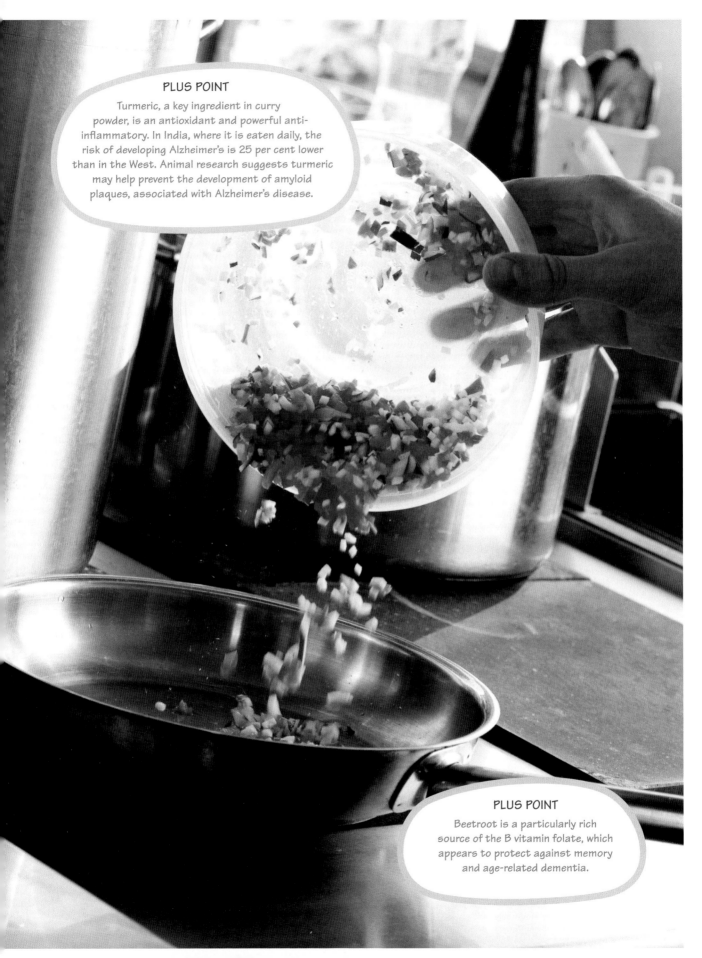

**PLUS POINT**

Turmeric, a key ingredient in curry powder, is an antioxidant and powerful anti-inflammatory. In India, where it is eaten daily, the risk of developing Alzheimer's is 25 per cent lower than in the West. Animal research suggests turmeric may help prevent the development of amyloid plaques, associated with Alzheimer's disease.

**PLUS POINT**

Beetroot is a particularly rich source of the B vitamin folate, which appears to protect against memory and age-related dementia.

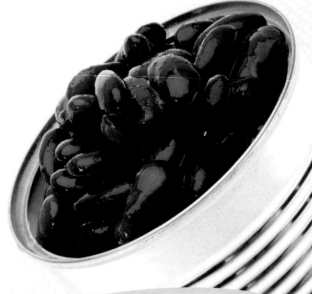

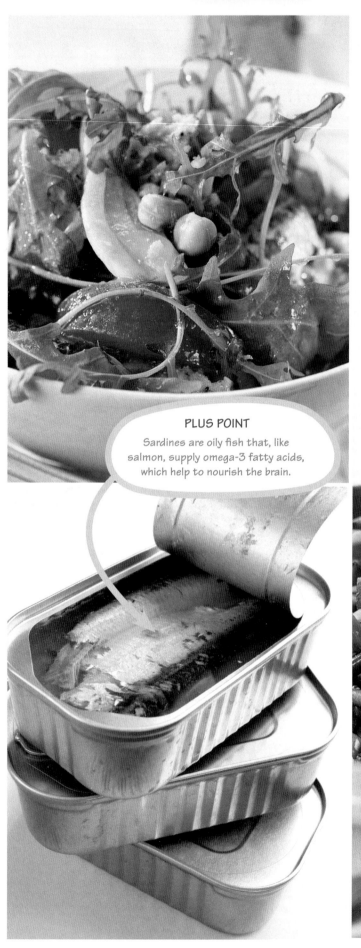

**PLUS POINT**

Sardines are oily fish that, like salmon, supply omega-3 fatty acids, which help to nourish the brain.

**PLUS POINT**

This salad supplies excellent amounts of both soluble and insoluble fibre, which help to prevent surges in blood glucose. Soluble fibre also helps to transport artery-clogging LDL cholesterol out of the body.

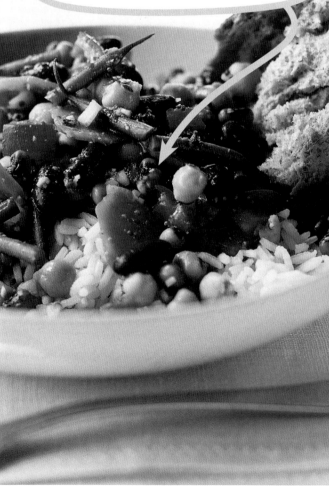

# Focaccia and fennel with sardines

Serves 4
Preparation: 30 minutes

170g frozen broad beans
2 cans sardines in oil, about 120g each, drained
3 tbsp extra virgin olive oil
2 tsp lemon juice
1 mild Spanish onion, halved and thinly sliced
2 tbsp drained capers
1 bulb of fennel
3 large or 4 medium-sized ripe beefsteak tomatoes, about 750g in total
1 herbed focaccia or ciabatta bread, about 280g, torn into 2.5cm pieces
100g rocket

Cook the broad beans in boiling water for 5–6 minutes. Meanwhile, split each sardine in half lengthways. Drain the broad beans and refresh under cold running water. Set aside.

Put the oil and lemon juice in a salad bowl and whisk together. Stir in the onion slices and capers.

Trim any feathery fronds from the fennel and finely chop them. Cut the fennel bulb in half lengthways, then cut into thin slices. Add the slices and chopped fronds to the salad bowl and toss to coat with the dressing.

Cut the tomatoes into quarters. Scoop out the seeds and put them in a sieve held over a large mixing bowl. Press with the back of a spoon to extract the juice – you should have about 150ml. Discard the seeds. Cut the tomato quarters into thin wedges.

Add the bread to the mixing bowl and toss to moisten with the tomato juice. Tip the bread into the salad bowl. Add the sardines and broad beans, the tomato wedges and rocket. Toss gently to coat everything with the dressing, taking care not to break up the sardines too much. Serve immediately.

Per serving: 449kcal, 25g protein, 20g total fat (3g saturated fat), 43g carbohydrate, 8g fibre

# Three beans and rice

Serves 4
Preparation: 50 minutes

250g long-grain rice
2 carrots, thinly sliced
125g thin green beans, cut into 2.5cm lengths
1 can red kidney beans, about 400g, drained and rinsed
1 can black-eyed beans, about 400g, drained and rinsed
1 can chickpeas, about 410g, drained and rinsed
1 large ripe tomato, coarsely chopped
1 small red pepper, seeded and chopped
1 small red onion, chopped
1 tbsp sunflower oil
1 tbsp mild wholegrain mustard
2 tsp caster sugar
3 tbsp red wine vinegar, or to taste
1 tbsp chopped fresh thyme
1 garlic clove, chopped
salt and pepper

Put the rice in a saucepan, cover with water and bring to the boil. Reduce the heat and simmer for about 15 minutes, or according to the packet instructions, until tender. Drain and leave to cool.

Meanwhile, drop the carrots into another pan of boiling water and cook for 3 minutes. Add the green beans and cook for a further 4 minutes or until the vegetables are tender. Drain and refresh under cold running water.

Place the carrots and green beans in a mixing bowl and add the kidney beans, black-eyed beans, chickpeas, tomato, red pepper and red onion.

Whisk together the oil, mustard, sugar, vinegar, thyme, garlic, and salt and pepper to taste in a small bowl. Drizzle this dressing over the bean salad and toss well to combine everything. Serve the bean salad over the rice, or gently fold the rice into the bean salad.

Per serving: 503kcal, 27g protein, 8g total fat (1g saturated fat), 85g carbohydrate, 18g fibre

# Chicken and sweet potatoes

Serves 4
Preparation: 40-45 minutes plus cooling

900g sweet potatoes, scrubbed and cut into 1cm slices
4 skinless boneless chicken breasts, about 140g each
pinch each of ground cinnamon and cumin
200g mixed salad leaves
¼ cucumber, thinly sliced
4 tomatoes, cut into thin wedges
2 tbsp chopped fresh coriander
2 tbsp toasted sunflower seeds
2 spring onions, finely shredded
**Pineapple salsa**
½ ripe pineapple, about 340g, peeled and chopped
½ small red onion, chopped
½ red pepper, seeded and finely diced
2 tbsp chopped fresh mint
¼ tsp mild chilli powder, or to taste
pinch each of ground cinnamon and cumin
juice of ½ lime
**Lime and soy dressing**
1 tsp caster sugar
juice of ½ lime
2 tbsp sunflower oil
dash of soy sauce, or to taste

Cook the sweet potato slices in a saucepan of boiling water for 6–8 minutes or until just tender. Drain and leave to cool.

Poach the chicken breasts in simmering water (use the water from the sweet potatoes, if liked) for 4–6 minutes or until cooked through. Drain and leave to cool, then cut into 1cm slices. Put the chicken and sweet potato slices in a bowl and sprinkle with the cinnamon and cumin.

To make the salsa, combine the pineapple, red onion, red pepper, mint, chilli powder, cinnamon, cumin and lime juice in a mixing bowl.

Whisk together the dressing ingredients in a large shallow salad bowl. Add the salad leaves and toss to coat with the dressing. Arrange the chicken and sweet potato slices, the cucumber slices and tomato wedges on top of the leaves, and scatter over the chopped coriander, sunflower seeds and spring onions. Serve with the pineapple salsa, to be added to taste.

Per serving: 459kcal, 25g protein, 13g total fat (2g saturated fat), 65g carbohydrate, 9g fibre

# Smoked trout wraps

Serves 8
Preparation: 15 minutes

8 large flour tortillas, about 340g in total
170g taramasalata
85g watercress
½ cucumber, thinly sliced
4 skinless smoked trout fillets, about 75g each, flaked

Preheat the oven to 180°C (350°F, gas mark 4). Wrap the stack of tortillas in foil and warm in the oven for 10 minutes or according to the packet instructions.

Spread a little taramasalata on the centre of each warm tortilla, then scatter over the watercress, cucumber slices and smoked trout pieces. Roll up tightly to enclose the filling. Cut each rolled tortilla in half diagonally and serve immediately.

Per serving: 275kcal, 12g protein, 14g total fat (1g saturated fat), 27g carbohydrate, 1g fibre

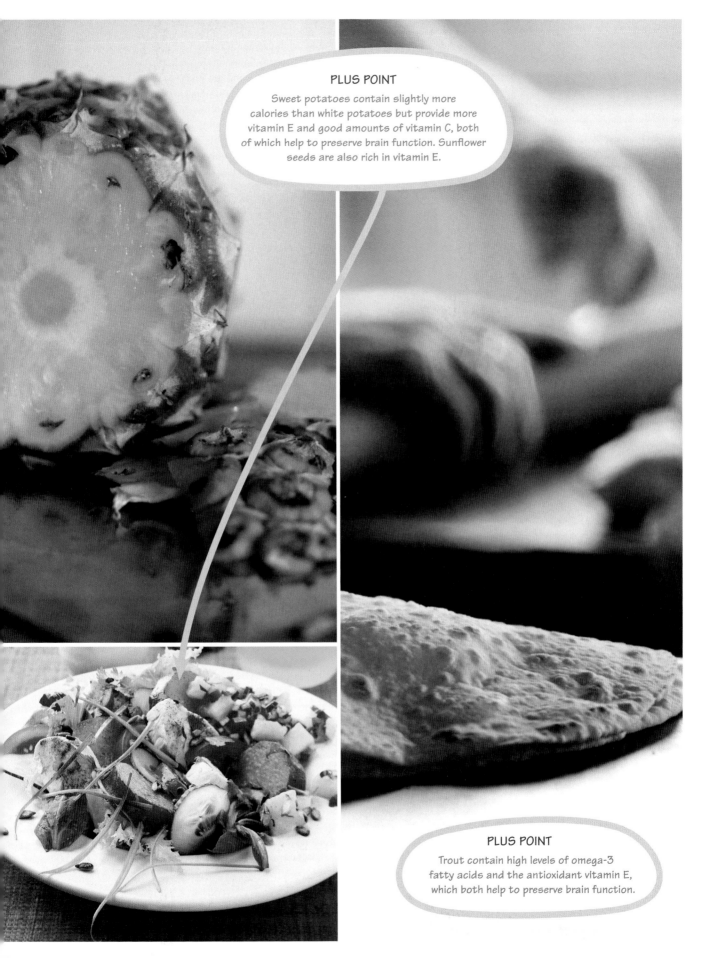

**PLUS POINT**
Sweet potatoes contain slightly more calories than white potatoes but provide more vitamin E and good amounts of vitamin C, both of which help to preserve brain function. Sunflower seeds are also rich in vitamin E.

**PLUS POINT**
Trout contain high levels of omega-3 fatty acids and the antioxidant vitamin E, which both help to preserve brain function.

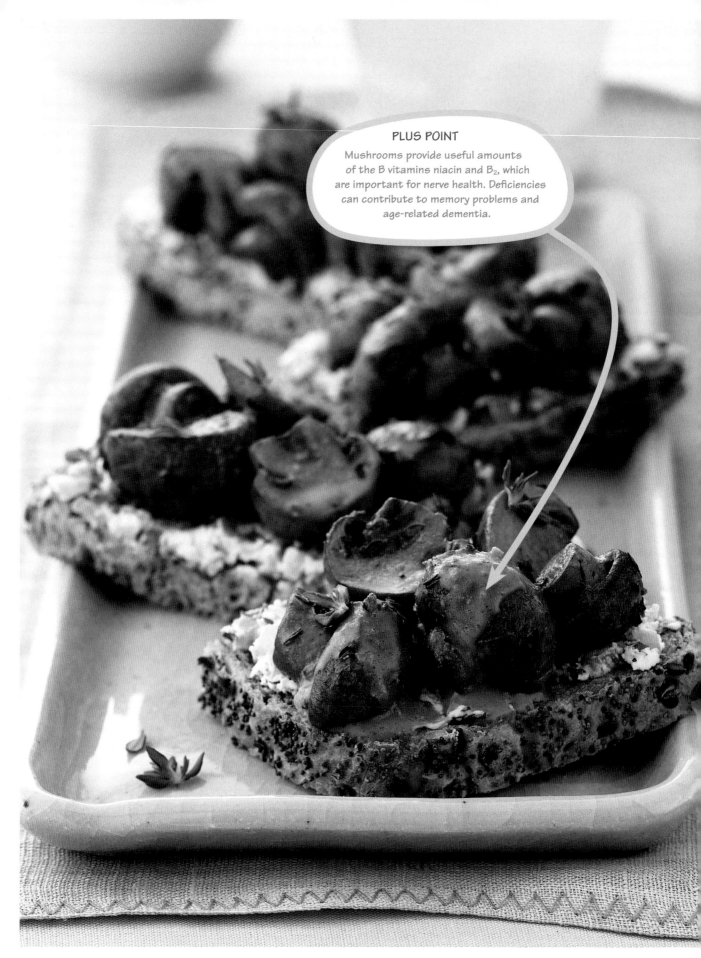

**PLUS POINT**

Mushrooms provide useful amounts of the B vitamins niacin and B$_2$, which are important for nerve health. Deficiencies can contribute to memory problems and age-related dementia.

# Mushroom and thyme toasts

Serves 4
Preparation: 25 minutes

125g ricotta cheese
2 celery sticks, finely chopped
3 tbsp finely chopped parsley
good pinch of cayenne pepper
500g chestnut mushrooms
1 garlic clove, crushed
2 tbsp chopped fresh thyme
2 tbsp crème fraîche
1 tsp lemon juice
8 thick slices cut from a small loaf of mixed seed bread, about 400g in total
salt and pepper

Put the ricotta, celery, parsley and cayenne pepper in a bowl and mix well together. Set aside in a cool place until needed. Preheat the grill to high.

Leave any small mushrooms whole and halve larger ones. Place them in a large, heavy frying pan, preferably non-stick, and add the garlic, thyme, crème fraîche and 1 tsp water. Cover and cook gently for 3–4 minutes or until the mushrooms are just tender and have given up their juices. Add the lemon juice and salt and pepper to taste.

While the mushrooms are cooking, toast the bread slices on both sides under the grill. While still warm, spread one side of each piece of toast with some of the ricotta mixture, then cut it in half.

Arrange the toasts on individual serving plates. Spoon the hot mushroom mixture over the toasts and serve immediately.

Per serving: 340kcal, 15g protein, 13g total fat (6g saturated fat), 44g carbohydrate, 5g fibre

# Leek and ham pizza muffins

Serves 4
Preparation: 15 minutes  Cooking: 4-5 minutes

1 tbsp extra virgin olive oil
2 leeks, about 250g in total, thinly sliced
4 wholemeal muffins, sliced in half
4 tbsp shredded fresh basil leaves
4 slices of Parma ham, about 50g in total, trimmed of fat and cut in half widthways
100g mozzarella cheese, cut into thin strips
4 tbsp coarsely shredded rocket
salt and pepper

Heat the oil in a saucepan, add the leeks and cook over a moderately high heat, stirring frequently, for about 5 minutes or until the leeks are tender and greatly reduced in volume. The juices they yield should have evaporated by this time – if not, increase the heat and cook for a few more seconds. Season with salt and pepper to taste.

Preheat the grill to high. Place the muffins, cut side down, in the grill pan without the rack. Grill to toast the bases, then turn the muffins over. Divide the leeks equally among the muffins, spreading evenly. Top with the basil, then lay a piece of Parma ham on each muffin half. Gently pinch the ham up into loose folds. Scatter the strips of mozzarella cheese over the ham.

Cook the muffin pizzas under the hot grill for 4–5 minutes or until the mozzarella cheese has melted and is bubbling. The ham and cheese should be lightly browned in places. Sprinkle with the shredded rocket and serve.

Per serving: 310kcal, 17g protein, 14g total fat (4g saturated fat), 32g carbohydrate, 3g fibre

### PLUS POINT
Leeks supply vitamin E, which has powerful antioxidant properties and helps to preserve brain function.

# DINNER

## Chicken with apricots and cumin

Serves 4
Preparation: 15 minutes  Cooking: 50 minutes

2 tbsp sunflower oil

8 chicken thighs, about 450g in total

1 onion, sliced

2 garlic cloves, chopped

2 tsp ground cumin

2 tsp ground coriander

300ml chicken stock

3 carrots, halved crossways, then each half cut into 6–8 thick fingers

1 bulb of fennel, halved lengthways, then cut crossways into slices

300g ripe but firm apricots, stoned and quartered

salt and pepper

Heat the oil in a large flameproof casserole and fry the chicken thighs for 5–10 minutes, turning occasionally, until golden brown all over. Remove from the pan. Add the onion and garlic to the casserole and fry for 5 minutes or until soft and golden.

Stir in all the spices and fry for 1 minute, then add the stock. Return the chicken to the casserole, together with the carrots and fennel. Bring to the boil. Stir well, then cover and simmer gently for 30 minutes or until the chicken is tender. Remove the lid. If there is too much liquid, boil to reduce it slightly.

Add the apricots to the casserole and stir gently to mix. Simmer over a low heat for a further 5 minutes.

Season to taste with salt and pepper. Sprinkle with the fennel leaves and serve with rice or potatoes, chopped fennel leaves from the bulb, or herb fennel, to garnish

Per serving: 370kcal, 26g protein, 24g total fat (6g saturated fat), 12g carbohydrate, 4g fibre

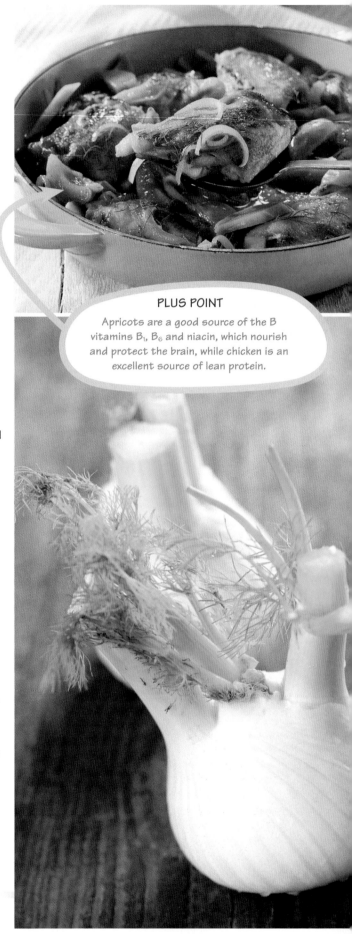

**PLUS POINT**

Apricots are a good source of the B vitamins $B_1$, $B_6$ and niacin, which nourish and protect the brain, while chicken is an excellent source of lean protein.

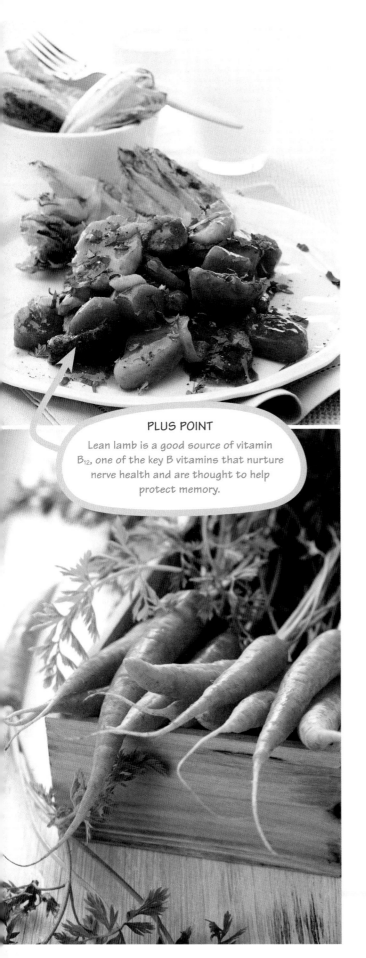

# Irish stew

Serves 4
Preparation: 20 minutes, plus optional marinating
Cooking: about 2 hours 20 minutes

4 boneless lean lamb leg steaks, about 500g in total, trimmed of fat and each steak cut into 4 pieces

1 kg floury potatoes, peeled and thickly sliced

1 large onion, sliced

500g carrots, thickly sliced

2 tbsp chopped parsley

1 tsp fresh thyme leaves

1 tbsp snipped fresh chives

450ml hot lamb or vegetable stock

salt and pepper

Preheat the oven to 160°C (325°F, gas mark 3). In a large casserole, make layers of the lamb, potatoes, onion and carrots, sprinkling each layer with parsley, thyme, chives, and salt and pepper to taste. Finish with a layer of potatoes, then pour over the stock.

Cover the casserole with a tight-fitting lid and place in the oven to cook for about 2 hours or until both the meat and vegetables feel tender when tested with a skewer.

Increase the oven temperature to 200°C (400°F, gas mark 6). Remove the casserole lid and cook for a further 20 minutes or until the potatoes on top are golden brown and crisp. Serve hot, sprinkled with more thyme and parsley.

Per serving: 508kcal, 32g protein, 19g total fat (8g saturated fat), 58g carbohydrate, 7g fibre

# Cassoulet

Serves 4
Preparation: 1½ hours, plus 8 hours soaking
Cooking: 1¾ hours

150g dried haricot beans, soaked for at least 8 hours
1 tbsp extra virgin olive oil
280g pork fillet (tenderloin), cut into 2.5cm dice
85g coarse-cut, dry-cured garlicky French sausage
1 onion, chopped
2 celery sticks, chopped
2 carrots, thickly sliced
1 turnip, chopped
1 can chopped tomatoes, about 400g
150ml dry white wine
400ml pork or chicken stock
1 tbsp tomato purée
2 bay leaves
4 sprigs of fresh thyme
**Breadcrumb crust**
1 tbsp extra virgin olive oil
85g fresh white breadcrumbs
15g parsley, chopped

Drain the soaked beans and rinse under cold running water. Put in a saucepan, cover with plenty of fresh water and bring to the boil. Boil rapidly for 10 minutes, then partly cover and simmer for 50–60 minutes or until tender. Drain and set aside.

Heat the oil in a large flameproof casserole, add the pork fillet and cook over a moderate heat for 5–6 minutes or until browned. Remove and set aside. Dice the sausage, add to the casserole and brown lightly. Remove and set aside with the pork. Add the onion, celery, carrots and turnip to the casserole and cook for 5 minutes, stirring occasionally, until softened and lightly browned.

Return the pork and sausage to the casserole. Add the beans, tomatoes with their juice, the wine, stock, tomato purée, bay leaves and thyme. Bring to the boil, then reduce the heat, cover and simmer for 1½ hours or until the meat and vegetables are very tender.

Next, prepare the breadcrumb crust. Heat the olive oil in a frying pan, add the breadcrumbs and parsley. Cook over a moderate heat, stirring constantly, for 3–4 minutes or until the crumbs are golden and quite dry. Season the cassoulet to taste, scatter the breadcrumb mixture evenly over the top and serve immediately.

# Linguine with pan-fried salmon

Serves 4
Preparation: 10 minutes, plus optional marinating
Cooking: 15 minutes

400g salmon fillet, skinned
grated zest and juice of 1 lemon
2 tbsp chopped fresh dill
340g linguine
225g carrots, cut into matchstick strips
225g courgettes, cut into matchstick strips
1 tsp sunflower oil
100g reduced-fat crème fraîche
salt and pepper

Cut the salmon into chunks and place in a dish. Add the lemon zest and juice, and the dill. Turn the chunks of salmon to coat them evenly. If time permits, cover and marinate in the fridge for at least 10 minutes.

Cook the linguine in boiling water for 10 minutes, or according to the packet instructions, until al dente. Add the carrots to the pasta after 8 minutes cooking, then add the courgettes 1 minute later.

Meanwhile, brush a non-stick or heavy-based frying pan with the oil and heat thoroughly. Drain the salmon, reserving the lemon juice marinade. Add the salmon to the hot pan and cook, turning the pieces occasionally, for 3–4 minutes, or until the fish is firm and just cooked.

Add the reserved marinade and the crème fraîche to the salmon, and cook for a few seconds. Remove from the heat and stir in seasoning to taste.

Drain the pasta and vegetables, and  transfer them to a serving dish or to individual plates. Add the salmon mixture, garnish with fresh dill, if liked, and serve with lemon wedges.

Per serving: 560kcal, 33g protein, 18g total fat (5g saturated fat), 70g carbohydrate, 4.5g fibre

Per serving: 434kcal, 31g protein, 14g total fat (3g saturated fat), 42g carbohydrate, 10g fibre

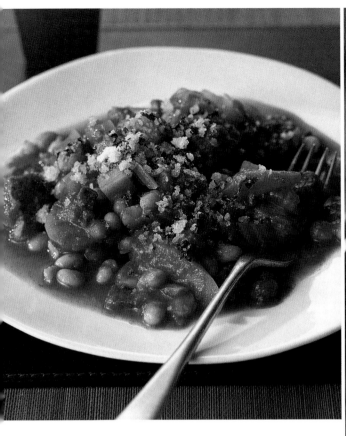

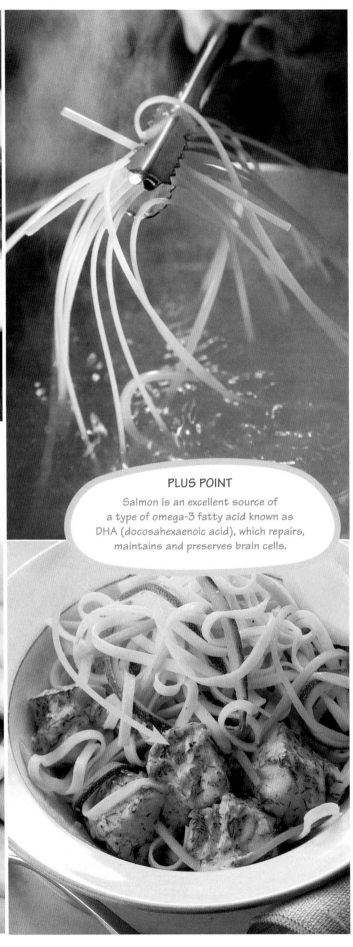

## PLUS POINT
Haricot beans provide both protein and B vitamins, especially brain-protective $B_6$, while lean pork is lower in fat than beef or lamb.

## PLUS POINT
Salmon is an excellent source of a type of omega-3 fatty acid known as DHA (docosahexaenoic acid), which repairs, maintains and preserves brain cells.

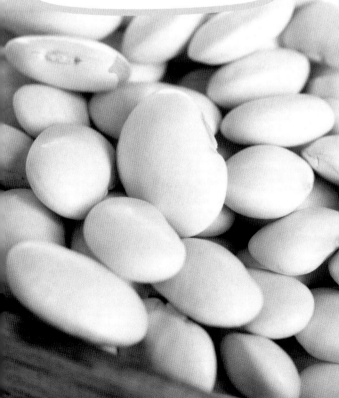

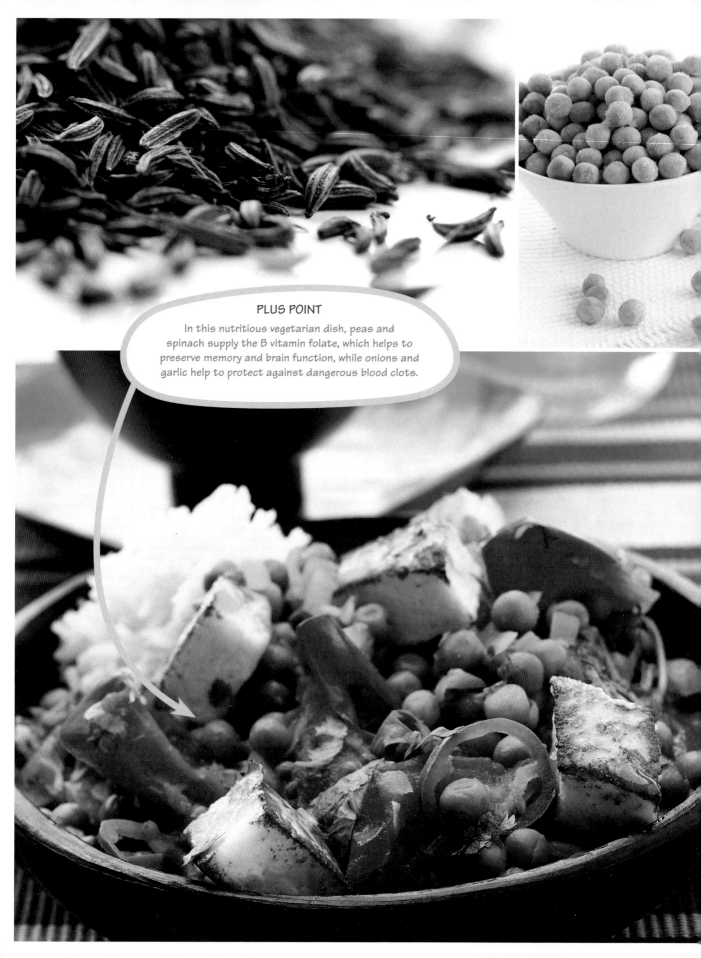

**PLUS POINT**

In this nutritious vegetarian dish, peas and spinach supply the B vitamin folate, which helps to preserve memory and brain function, while onions and garlic help to protect against dangerous blood clots.

# Pea curry with Indian paneer

Serves 4
Preparation: 15 minutes, plus about 45 minutes draining and 3 hours pressing
Cooking: about 20 minutes

**Paneer**

2.3 litres full-fat milk

6 tbsp lemon juice

**Pea and tomato curry**

3 tbsp sunflower oil

1 large onion, chopped

2 garlic cloves, finely chopped

5cm piece fresh root ginger, finely chopped

1 fresh green chilli, seeded and thinly sliced

1 tbsp coriander seeds, crushed

1 tbsp cumin seeds, crushed

1 tsp turmeric

1 tbsp garam masala

450g firm tomatoes, quartered

340g frozen peas

85g spinach leaves

15g fresh coriander, roughly chopped

salt

First make the paneer. Pour the milk into a large saucepan and bring to the boil. Immediately reduce the heat to low and add the lemon juice. Stir for 1–2 minutes or until the milk separates into curds and whey. Remove the pan from the heat.

Line a large sieve or colander with muslin, or a clean, tight-knit dishcloth, and set over a large bowl. Pour in the milk mixture. Leave to drain for about 15 minutes or until cool.

Bring together the corners of the muslin or cloth to make a bundle containing the drained curds. Squeeze them, then leave to drain for a further 30 minutes or until all the whey has dripped though the sieve into the bowl. Reserve 240ml of the whey.

Keeping the curds wrapped in the muslin or cloth, place on a board. Set another board on top and press down to flatten the ball shape into an oblong block. Place cans or weights on top and leave in a cool place for about 3 hours or until firm.

Carefully peel off the muslin and cut the cheese into squares about 2cm. Heat 1 tbsp of the oil in a large non-stick frying pan and cook the paneer for 1–2 minutes on each side or until golden. As the pieces are browned, remove from the pan with a draining spoon and set aside.

For the curry, heat the remaining 2 tbsp oil in the pan. Add the onion and cook gently for 5 minutes or until softened. Stir in the garlic and ginger, and cook gently for 1 minute, then stir in the chilli, coriander and cumin seeds, turmeric and garam masala. Cook for 1 more minute, stirring constantly.

Add the tomatoes, the reserved whey and a pinch of salt, and stir well to mix. Cover and cook gently for 5 minutes.

Add the peas and bring back to the boil, then reduce the heat, cover again and simmer for 5 minutes. Add the spinach, stirring it in gently so as not to break up the tomatoes too much. Simmer for 3–4 minutes or until the spinach has just wilted and the peas are hot and tender.

Stir in most of the chopped fresh coriander, then transfer the curry to a serving dish and scatter the paneer on top. Spoon the curry gently over the paneer to warm it, then sprinkle with the rest of the coriander and serve.

Per serving: 298 kcal, 20g protein, 15g total fat (5g saturated fat), 22g carbohydrate, 7g fibre

# Fragrant lamb with spinach

Serves 4
Preparation: 20-25 minutes
Cooking: 1 hour 20 minutes

2 tbsp sunflower oil
2 onions, finely chopped
4 garlic cloves, crushed
5cm piece fresh root ginger, peeled and chopped
1 red chilli, seeded and sliced
2 tsp paprika
2 tsp ground cumin
2 tsp ground coriander
1 tsp ground white pepper
½ tsp ground cinnamon
seeds from 8 green cardamom pods, crushed
2 bay leaves
½ tsp salt
200g Greek-style yoghurt
500g lean boneless lamb, cubed
2 large tomatoes, chopped
225g fresh baby spinach
4 tbsp chopped fresh coriander

Heat the oil in a large saucepan or flameproof casserole. Add the onions, garlic and ginger, and fry for about 15 minutes, stirring frequently, until the onions are golden.

Stir in the chilli, paprika, cumin, coriander, white pepper, cinnamon, crushed cardamom seeds, bay leaves and salt. Stir briefly over a moderate heat, then stir in the yoghurt and 150ml water. Add the lamb, mix well and cover the pan. Simmer gently for 1¼ hours or until the lamb is tender.

Add the tomatoes, spinach and chopped coriander. Cook for 2–3 minutes, stirring, until the tomatoes have softened slightly and the spinach has wilted. Taste for seasoning and remove the bay leaf. Serve garnished with fresh coriander.

Per serving: 350kcal, 32g protein, 22g total fat (8g saturated fat), 7g carbohydrate, 2g fibre

# Spiced lentil dhal

Serves 4
Preparation: 25 minutes  Cooking: about 55 minutes

2 tbsp sunflower oil
1 large onion, coarsely chopped
1–2 garlic cloves, crushed
2 tbsp finely chopped fresh root ginger
2 tbsp mild curry paste
170g red lentils
1 tsp ground cumin
1 tsp turmeric
1 tsp salt
400g small new potatoes, halved
1 small cauliflower, broken into florets
1 red pepper, seeded and coarsely chopped
4 tomatoes, skinned and quartered
225g baby spinach leaves
handful of fresh coriander leaves, coarsely chopped
**Carrot and coriander chutney**
3 carrots, coarsely grated
1 green chilli, seeded and finely chopped
juice of 1 lime
2 tbsp chopped fresh coriander
**Banana and almond raita**
2 firm bananas
280g plain low-fat yoghurt
55g flaked almonds, toasted

Heat the oil in a large saucepan. Add the onion, garlic and ginger, and cook for 5 minutes. Stir in the curry paste and stir for a further 2 minutes over a gentle heat.

Stir in the lentils, cumin, turmeric, salt and 1 litre water. Bring to the boil, then cover the pan and simmer gently for 10 minutes. Stir in the potatoes and cook for 10 minutes, then add the cauliflower and cook for another 10 minutes. Add the pepper and tomatoes, and simmer for 5 minutes.

Meanwhile, prepare the side dishes. Mix together the carrots, chilli, lime juice and coriander for the chutney. Transfer to a serving dish. For the raita, slice the bananas into a serving bowl. Stir in the yoghurt and sprinkle with the almonds.

Stir the spinach into the curry and cook for 2 minutes or until just wilted. Stir in the coriander and serve, with the chutney and raita.

Per serving: 550kcal, 26g protein, 17g total fat (3g saturated fat), 77g carbohydrate, 11g fibre

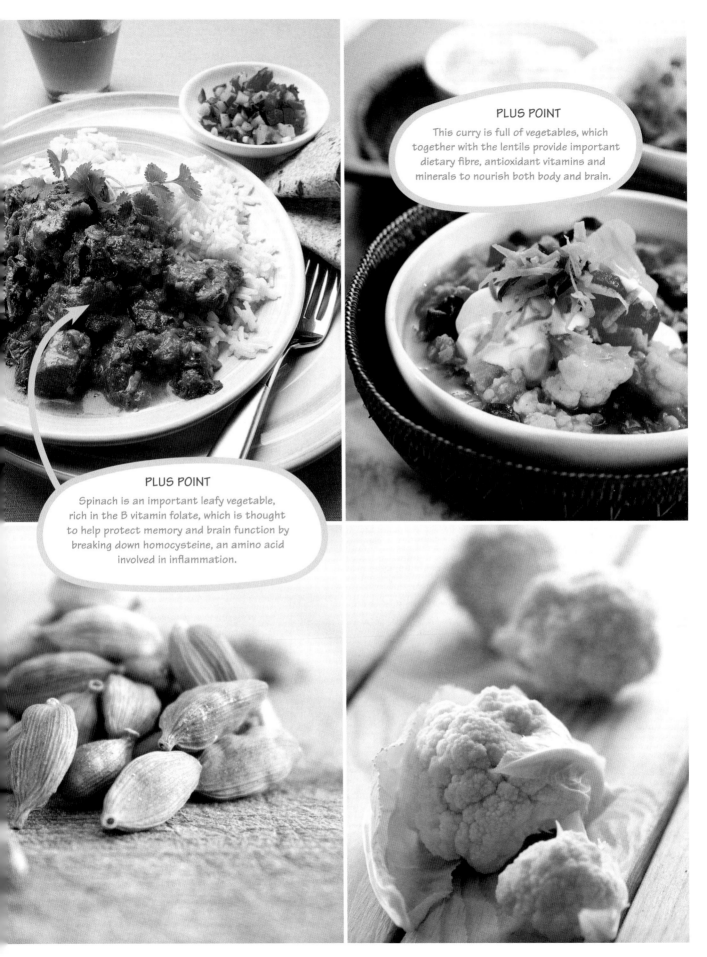

**PLUS POINT**

This curry is full of vegetables, which together with the lentils provide important dietary fibre, antioxidant vitamins and minerals to nourish both body and brain.

**PLUS POINT**

Spinach is an important leafy vegetable, rich in the B vitamin folate, which is thought to help protect memory and brain function by breaking down homocysteine, an amino acid involved in inflammation.

# Quinoa with griddled aubergines

Serves 4
Preparation: 35 minutes  Cooking: 35 minutes

300g quinoa
3–4 sprigs of fresh thyme
1.2 litres vegetable stock
250g baby aubergines, cut lengthways into quarters
1 red pepper, seeded and cut into chunks
1 red onion, cut into chunks
2 tbsp extra virgin olive oil
200g cherry tomatoes
2 garlic cloves, crushed
300ml tomato juice
200g goat's cheese log with herbs, cut into 8 slices
salt and pepper

Preheat the oven to 190°C (375°F, gas mark 5). Put the quinoa in a sieve and rinse thoroughly under cold running water. Place in a saucepan with the thyme sprigs and stock, and bring to the boil. Cover and simmer gently for 20 minutes or until all the stock has been absorbed and the quinoa is tender.

Meanwhile, heat a ridged cast-iron grill pan. Brush the aubergines, red pepper and onion with the olive oil, then cook them on the grill pan (in batches if necessary) for 4–5 minutes or until softened and lightly charred on both sides. Transfer to a plate.

Put the whole tomatoes on the grill pan and cook for about 2 minutes or until they are just beginning to burst their skins. Remove from the heat.

When the quinoa is cooked, tip it into an ovenproof dish. Add the griddled vegetables, garlic and tomato juice, and season with salt and pepper to taste. Fold together gently.

Arrange the slices of goat's cheese on top of the quinoa mixture. Cover with foil and bake for 35 minutes or until the vegetable are tender. Serve hot.

Per serving: 438kcal, 20g protein, 18g total fat (6.5g saturated fat), 53g carbohydrate, 3g fibre

# Stir-fried beef with fine noodles

Serves 2
Preparation: 20 minutes  Cooking: 10 minutes

1 tsp tamarind paste
3 tbsp boiling water
2 tbsp soy sauce
2 tsp toasted sesame oil
1 tbsp rice wine (sake or mirin) or sherry
100g fine rice noodles, such as vermicelli
1 tbsp sunflower oil
225g lean rump steak, cut into strips
85g onion, cut into wedges
2 tsp chopped lemongrass
1 fresh red chilli, seeded and chopped
2 large garlic cloves, crushed
85g mange-tout, halved diagonally
6 baby sweetcorn, sliced
100g fresh shiitake or chestnut mushrooms, sliced

In a small bowl, combine the tamarind paste and boiling water and leave to soak for 10 minutes, stirring frequently to break down the paste. Mix the resulting tamarind liquid with the soy sauce, sesame oil and rice wine or sherry.

While the tamarind is soaking, soak the rice noodles in boiling water for 4 minutes, or according to the packet instructions. Then drain, rinse under cold running water and set aside to drain thoroughly.

Heat the sunflower oil in a wok or very large frying pan and stir-fry the beef over a high heat for about 3 minutes or until cooked. Use a draining spoon to remove the beef from the wok and set it aside.

Add the onion, lemongrass, chilli and garlic to the wok and stir-fry over a high heat for 1 minute. Add the mange-tout, sweetcorn and mushrooms, and continue stir-frying for 2 minutes.

Return the beef to the wok. Add the tamarind liquid and the noodles and stir for about 1 minute to heat through. Serve immediately, offering soy sauce for extra seasoning as required.

Per serving: 460kcal, 30g protein, 15g total fat (3g saturated fat), 49g carbohydrate, 3g fibre

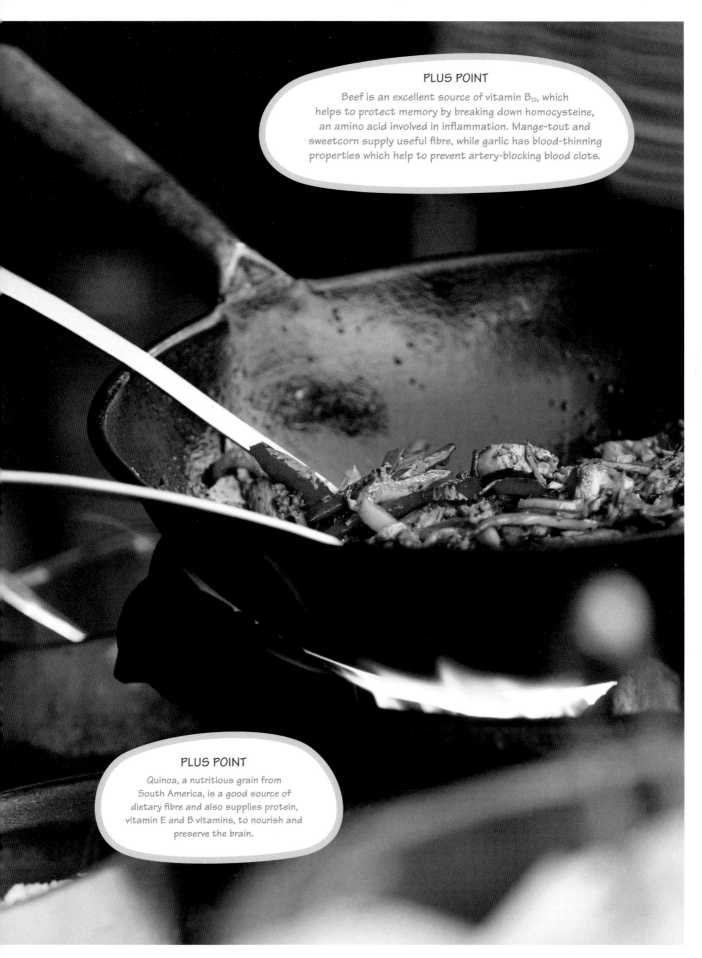

**PLUS POINT**

Beef is an excellent source of vitamin B$_{12}$, which help to protect memory by breaking down homocysteine, an amino acid involved in inflammation. Mange-tout and sweetcorn supply useful fibre, while garlic has blood-thinning properties which help to prevent artery-blocking blood clots.

**PLUS POINT**

Quinoa, a nutritious grain from South America, is a good source of dietary fibre and also supplies protein, vitamin E and B vitamins, to nourish and preserve the brain.

# SIDE DISHES

## Fragrant basmati rice

Serves 6
Preparation: 15 minutes, plus standing
Cooking: 15–20 minutes

1 tbsp sunflower oil

55g split blanched almonds, any tiny pieces discarded

250g basmati rice, rinsed

pinch of saffron strands

1 cinnamon stick

450ml boiling vegetable stock

1 ripe pomegranate

2.5cm piece of fresh root ginger, grated

1 tsp clear honey

1 tbsp chopped fresh mint

2 tbsp chopped fresh coriander

salt and pepper

Heat the oil in a large saucepan, add the almonds and cook gently for 2–3 minutes or until golden. Remove from the pan with a draining spoon and set aside.

Add the rice to the oil and cook, stirring, for 1 minute. Stir in the saffron and cinnamon stick, then add the stock and season with salt and pepper to taste. Bring to the boil. Stir, then cover and cook over a very low heat for 10–15 minutes or until the rice is tender and the stock has been absorbed.

Meanwhile, cut the pomegranate in half and remove all the seeds from the membranes. Reserve about one-third of the seeds for garnish. Put the rest of the seeds in a sieve placed over a mixing bowl and crush with a spoon to extract the juice.

Put the grated ginger into a garlic crusher, hold over the mixing bowl and squeeze out the ginger juice. Stir the honey into the juices.

When the rice is cooked, stir in the pomegranate juice mixture. Cover again and leave to stand for 2 minutes. Then remove the cinnamon stick, fork the mint and coriander through the rice, and transfer to a warmed serving dish. Scatter over the almonds and reserved pomegranate seeds, and serve.

## Millet with spinach and pine nuts

Serves 4
Preparation: 10 minutes  Cooking: 20–25 minutes

200g millet

50g ready-to eat dried apricots, roughly chopped

900ml vegetable stock

55g pine nuts

250g baby spinach leaves

juice of ½ lemon

salt and pepper

Put the millet and dried apricots into a large saucepan and stir in the stock. Bring to the boil, then lower the heat. Simmer for 15–20 minutes or until all the stock has been absorbed and the millet is tender.

Meanwhile, toast the pine nuts in a small frying pan until they are golden brown and fragrant. Set aside.

Add the spinach and lemon juice to the millet, with salt and pepper to taste. Cover the pan and leave over a very low heat for 4–5 minutes to wilt the spinach.

Stir the millet and spinach mixture gently, then spoon into a serving bowl. Scatter the toasted pine nuts on top and serve immediately.

Per serving: 307kcal, 7g protein, 11g total fat (1g saturated fat), 44g carbohydrate, 2g fibre

Per serving: 249kcal, 6g protein, 7g total fat (0.5g saturated fat), 40g carbohydrate, 2g fibre

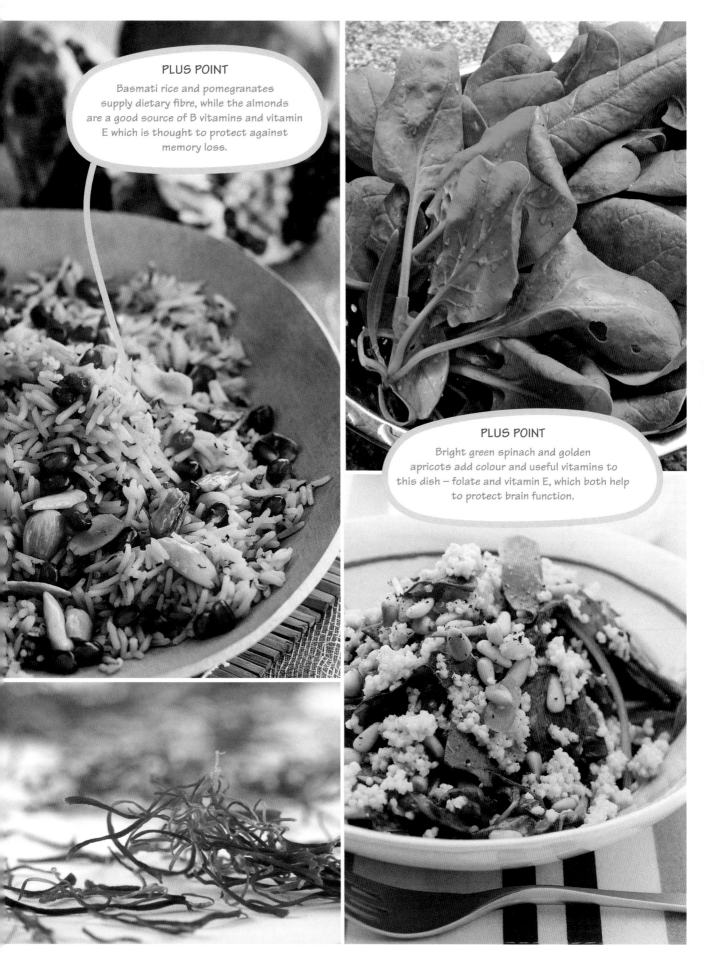

**PLUS POINT**

Basmati rice and pomegranates supply dietary fibre, while the almonds are a good source of B vitamins and vitamin E which is thought to protect against memory loss.

**PLUS POINT**

Bright green spinach and golden apricots add colour and useful vitamins to this dish – folate and vitamin E, which both help to protect brain function.

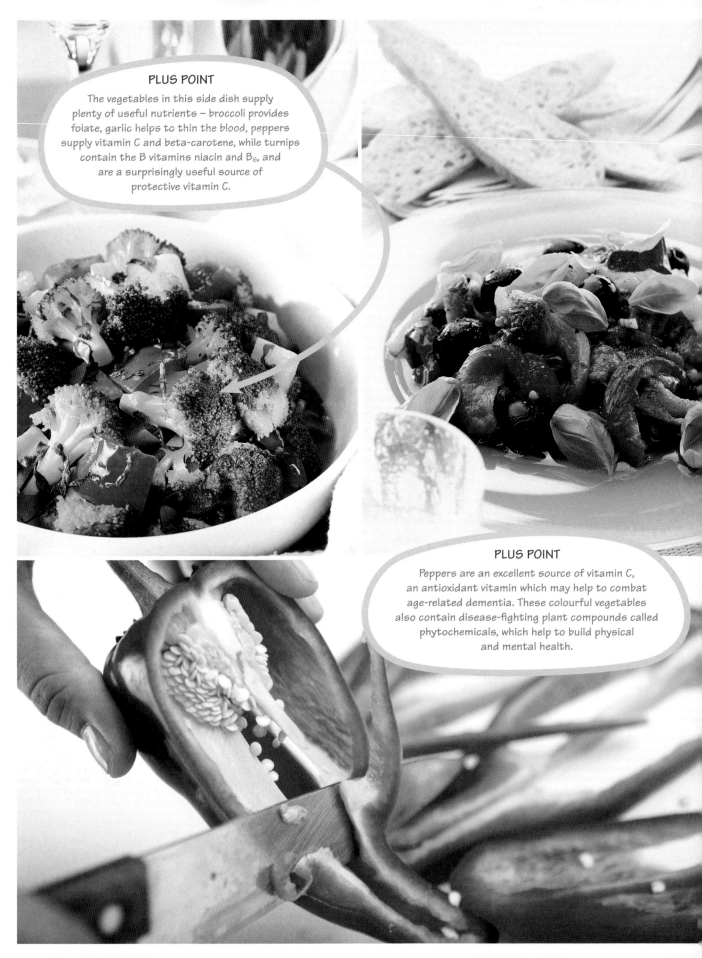

**PLUS POINT**

The vegetables in this side dish supply plenty of useful nutrients – broccoli provides folate, garlic helps to thin the blood, peppers supply vitamin C and beta-carotene, while turnips contain the B vitamins niacin and $B_6$, and are a surprisingly useful source of protective vitamin C.

**PLUS POINT**

Peppers are an excellent source of vitamin C, an antioxidant vitamin which may help to combat age-related dementia. These colourful vegetables also contain disease-fighting plant compounds called phytochemicals, which help to build physical and mental health.

# Basil-scented sautéed vegetables

Serves 4
Preparation: 10 minutes  Cooking: 7–8 minutes

500g broccoli
1 tbsp extra virgin olive oil
3–4 large garlic cloves, thinly sliced (optional)
1 large or 2 small red peppers, seeded and cut into chunks
1 turnip, about 150g, cut into bite-sized chunks
pinch of sugar
8 sprigs of fresh basil, stalks discarded, then finely shredded
salt

Cut the broccoli into small florets; trim and thinly slice the stalks. Heat the olive oil in a large non-stick frying pan or wok. Add the garlic, if using, the red pepper, turnip and slices of broccoli stalk. Sprinkle in the sugar and salt to taste. Cook for 2–3 minutes, turning frequently.

Add the broccoli florets and stir. Pour in 6 tbsp of water to provide a thin covering on the bottom of the pan. Cover and cook over a fairly high heat for 3–4 minutes. The broccoli should be just tender and bright green.

Stir in the basil, replace the lid and leave on the heat for a few more seconds. Serve immediately.

Per serving: 90kcal, 6g protein, 4g total fat
(1g saturated fat), 7g carbohydrate, 5g fibre

# Roasted pepper salad

Serves 6
Preparation: 45 minutes, plus cooling

2 large red peppers
2 large yellow or orange peppers
2 large green peppers
2½ tbsp extra virgin olive oil
2 tsp balsamic vinegar
1 small garlic clove, very finely chopped or crushed
**To garnish**
12 black olives, stoned
a handful of small fresh basil leaves

Preheat the oven to 200°C (400°F, gas mark 6). Brush the peppers with 1 tbsp of the olive oil and arrange them in a shallow roasting tin. Roast for about 35 minutes or until the pepper skins are evenly darkened, turning them 3 or 4 times. Place the peppers in a polythene bag and leave until they are cool enough to handle.

Working over a bowl to catch the juice, peel the peppers. Cut them in half and discard the cores and seeds (strain out any seeds that fall into the juice), then cut into thick slices.

Measure 1½ tbsp of the pepper juice into a small bowl (discard the remainder). Add the vinegar, garlic and salt and pepper to taste, and whisk in the remaining 1½ tbsp olive oil.

Arrange the peppers on a serving platter or on individual salad plates. Drizzle over the dressing and garnish with the olives and basil leaves.

Per serving: 97kcal, 2g protein, 6g total fat
(1g saturated fat), 10g carbohydrate, 3g fibre

# DESSERTS

## Rice pudding with apricots

Serves 4
Preparation: 15 minutes  Cooking: about 1¼ hours

850ml full-fat milk
45g caster sugar
finely grated zest of 1 orange
100g short-grain 'pudding' rice
55g sultanas
ground cinnamon to sprinkle
**Apricot compote**
300g fresh ripe apricots, halved and stoned
juice of 1 orange
1 cinnamon stick

Preheat the oven to 160°C (325°F, gas mark 3).
Pour the milk into a saucepan, and add the sugar
and orange zest. Heat gently, stirring, until the
sugar dissolves and the milk is almost boiling.

Put the rice and sultanas in a shallow 1.5 litre
ovenproof dish. Pour over the milk mixture and stir.

Bake the pudding for 30 minutes, then stir well.
Leave to bake for a further 45 minutes or until the
rice is tender and the pudding is creamy.

Meanwhile, to make the compote, combine the
apricots, orange juice and cinnamon stick in a
heavy-based saucepan. Cover and cook over a low
heat for 10 minutes. Remove the lid and cook for a
further 5 minutes or until the juice is reduced.

Remove the cinnamon stick from the compote.
Sprinkle the top of the rice pudding with a little
cinnamon, then serve hot, with the compote.

Per serving: 334kcal, 9g protein, 8g total fat
(5g saturated fat), 59g carbohydrate, 2g fibre

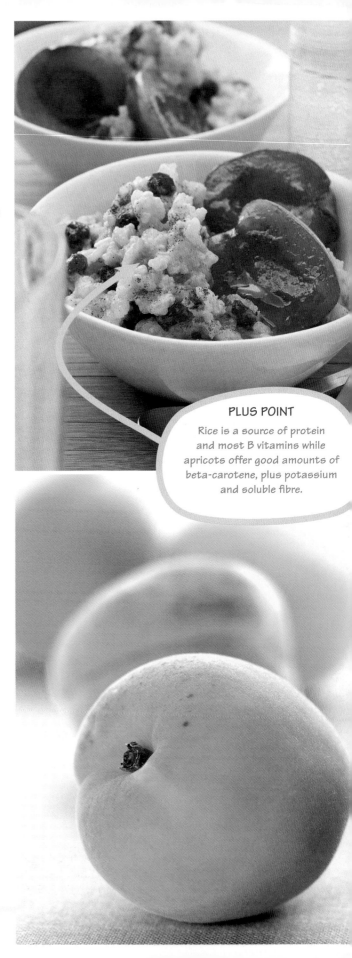

### PLUS POINT

Rice is a source of protein
and most B vitamins while
apricots offer good amounts of
beta-carotene, plus potassium
and soluble fibre.

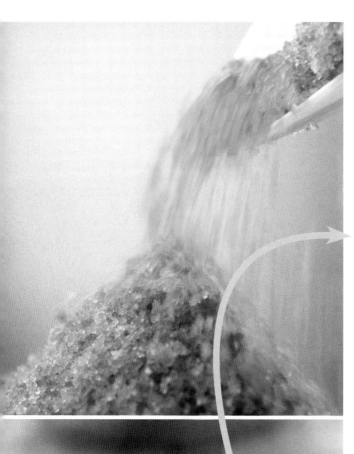

# Cinnamon banana caramels

Serves 4
Preparation: 8 minutes  Cooking: 1 minute

4 bananas
¼ tsp ground cinnamon
300g Greek-style yoghurt
4 tbsp demerara sugar

Preheat the grill. Peel and slice the bananas, cutting each one into about 16 slices. Divide the slices among four 250ml ramekin dishes and sprinkle with the ground cinnamon. Spoon the yoghurt over the banana slices to cover them completely. Sprinkle 1 tbsp of sugar evenly over each dessert.

Place the dishes on a baking sheet and put them under the grill. Cook for about 1 minute or until the sugar melts into the yoghurt – keep watch to make sure that it does not burn. Remove from the grill and leave to cool for a few minutes before serving.

Per serving: 240kcal, 6g protein, 7g total fat (4g saturated fat), 40g carbohydrate, 1g fibre

### PLUS POINT

Bananas are one of the best sources of potassium, a mineral which can help to regulate blood pressure. Yoghurt is a useful source of several minerals and calcium.

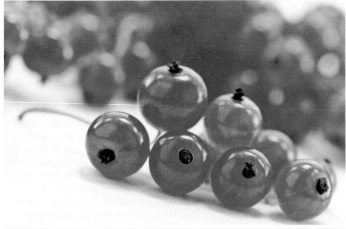

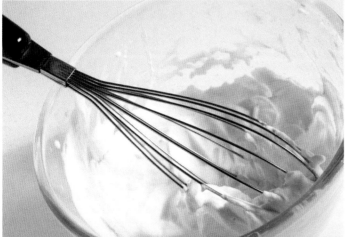

# Summer fruit fool

Serves 4
Preparation: 20 minutes, plus cooling and chilling

300g mixed soft fruit, such as raspberries, blackberries, blueberries or currants
55g caster sugar
150ml whipping cream
grated zest of ½ orange
150g plain low-fat bio yoghurt
finely shredded orange zest to decorate (optional)

Reserve about 55g of the mixed fruit for decoration. Put the remaining mixed fruit in a saucepan with 2 tbsp water. Bring just to the boil, then reduce the heat and cook gently for 5 minutes or until soft and very juicy. Stir in the sugar.

Remove from the heat and leave to cool slightly. Pour into a food processor or blender and purée. Press the purée through a sieve to remove all the pips. Alternatively, just press the fruit through a sieve to purée it. Set aside to cool completely.

Whip the cream with the grated orange zest until thick. Add the yoghurt and lightly whip into the cream, then mix in the cooled fruit purée.

Spoon into dessert dishes or goblets. Chill well before serving, decorated with the reserved berries and orange zest, if using.

Per serving: 230kcal, 3g protein, 15g total fat (9g saturated fat), 22g carbohydrate, 2g fibre

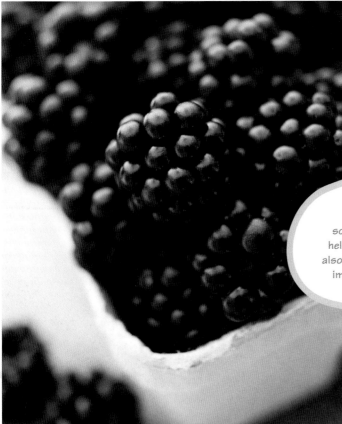

### PLUS POINT
The soft fruits are all excellent sources of vitamin C, an antioxidant which helps to protect brain function. The yoghurt also supplies B$_{12}$, a B vitamin that is especially important for maintaining a healthy brain.

# Fragrant gooseberry crumble

Serves 6
Preparation: 25 minutes  Cooking: 20–25 minutes

1kg gooseberries, topped and tailed
2 sprigs of fresh mint
2 tbsp elderflower cordial
50g caster sugar, or to taste
**Crumble topping**
55g plain white flour
30g plain wholemeal flour
55g cool unsalted butter, diced
55g light soft brown sugar
30g jumbo oats
30g hazelnuts, chopped
2 tbsp wheatgerm

Preheat the oven to 200°C (400°F, gas mark 6). Put the gooseberries in a saucepan with the mint sprigs and elderflower cordial. Cover and cook over a very low heat for 8–10 minutes or until the gooseberries start to soften and release their juices.

Stir in the caster sugar until it has dissolved, then transfer to a deep 1.7 litre baking dish, discarding the mint sprigs.

Sift the white and wholemeal flours into a mixing bowl, tipping in the bran left in the sieve. Rub the butter into the flour until the mixture resembles breadcrumbs. Stir in the sugar, oats, hazelnuts and wheatgerm. Sprinkle over 1 tbsp cold water and mix in to make a rough crumbly mixture. Spoon the topping evenly over the fruit.

Bake for 20–25 minutes or until the topping is golden brown and the fruit filling bubbling. Serve hot or warm, with custard, if liked.

Per serving: 275kcal, 5g protein, 12g total fat (5g saturated fat), 39g carbohydrate, 6g fibre

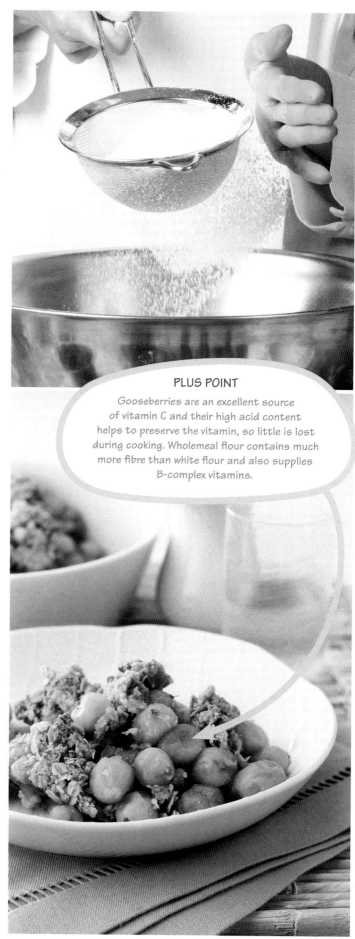

### PLUS POINT
Gooseberries are an excellent source of vitamin C and their high acid content helps to preserve the vitamin, so little is lost during cooking. Wholemeal flour contains much more fibre than white flour and also supplies B-complex vitamins.

# INDEX

and creativity 51
intuition 22
positive thinking 114
three beans and rice 287
TIAs (transient ischaemic attacks)
181
tilapia 68
tilefish 68
time, sense of 136
time management 99
tip-of-the-tongue phenomenon
242
tiredness 130–1, 166
toasts, mushroom and thyme 291
tomatoes
cassoulet 294
focaccia and fennel with sardines
287
pea curry with Indian paneer 297
quinoa with griddled aubergines
300
tortillas
smoked trout wraps 289
total recall 13, 53
trainers 94
trans fats 65, 72–3
transcendance 104
triglycerides 159
trout 67, 68, 289
smoked trout wraps 289
tryptophan 129
tuna 67–8
turmeric 77, 285
turnips 304
basil-scented sautéed vegetables
305

## U,V

university 119
useful information, remembering
35
vascular dementia
abdominal fat and 158
alcohol and 190
blood sugar levels and 182
cardiovascular disease and 186,
187, 189
gender differences 186
smoking and 189–90
vegan diet 79
vegetable oils 65
vegetables 74–80
and blood pressure 177
and dementia prevention 195

fibre content 162
Mediterranean diet 64
phytochemicals 75–8, 80
ventilation 170–2
verbal memory 55
verbal skills 242–7
video games 13, 235, 236
violence, on television 129
visceral fat *see* abdominal fat
vision 23
vision loss 186
visual memory 55, 56
visual reminders 218
vitamins
and blood pressure 177
vitamin B complex 79
vitamin C 78–9
vitamin D 91–2
vitamin E 78–9
volunteering 107, 114

## W

waist-to-hip ratio 157–8
waistline measurements 159–60
walking 89
benefits of 13, 92–5, 166
and cholesterol 180
and dementia risk 191
and depression 154
pedometers 94
reducing abdominal fat 161
shoes 94
stress reduction 144
sunshine and 173
with friends 118
walnut oil 68–70
walnuts 67, 68
wasabi 77
water
dehydration 172
drinking 83
weight loss
and blood pressure 177
and cholesterol 178–80
exercise and 161
and forgetfulness 29
for sleep apnoea 131
weight training 89
white matter 21, 235
white noise 127–8, 170
whole grains 80–2, 162,
177, 195
wholemeal flour 309
widows 104

windows
double glazing 170
opening 172
wine 64, 83, 178
wisdom 15, 42–9
quiz 46–7
Women's Institute 117
words
remembering 243
verbal skills 242–7
work
after retirement 112–14
lunch breaks 141–2
reducing stress 152
workaholism 142
working memory *see* short-term
memory
'worry' jotters 138–9
worst-case scenarios 136–8
wraps, smoked trout 289
writing 112, 130, 205

## Y

yoga 92, 145
yoghurt 308
banana and almond raita 298
berry-flaxseed smoothie 280
cinnamon banana caramels 307
fragrant lamb with spinach 298
summer fruit fool 308

## A Sharp Brain for Life

Published in 2011 in the United Kingdom by Vivat Direct Limited (t/a Reader's Digest), 157 Edgware Road, London W2 2HR.

*A Sharp Brain for Life* is owned and under licence from The Reader's Digest Association, Inc. All rights reserved.

Adapted from *No More Brain Drain* published by The Reader's Digest Association, Inc. in 2009.

We are committed both to the quality of our products and the service we provide to our customers. We value your comments, so please do contact us on **0871 351 1000** or visit our website at **www.readersdigest.co.uk**

If you have any comments or suggestions about the content of our books, email us at **gbeditorial@readersdigest.co.uk**

**For Vivat Direct**
**Project editor** Rachel Warren Chadd
**Art editor** Simon Webb
**Senior editor** Ali Moore
**Senior designer** Jane McKenna

**Editorial director** Julian Browne
**Art director** Anne-Marie Bulat
**Managing editor** Nina Hathway
**Picture resource manager** Sarah Stewart-Richardson
**Pre-press technical manager** Dean Russell
**Product production manager** Claudette Bramble
**Senior production controller** Jan Bucil

Colour origination by FMG
Printing and binding by Neografia

ISBN: 978-1-78020-014-9
Concept code: US6069/IC–UK
Book code: 400-506 UP0000-1